ESSENTIALS OF
Oral Histology
and Embryology
A CLINICAL APPROACH

6th EDITION

ESSENTIALS OF

Oral Histology and Embryology

A CLINICAL APPROACH

Daniel J. Chiego, Jr., M.S., Ph.D.
Associate Professor, School of Dentistry
Department of Cariology, Restorative Sciences and Endodontics
University of Michigan
Ann Arbor, Michigan

ELSEVIER

Elsevier
3251 Riverport Lane
St. Louis, Missouri 63043

Essentials of Oral Histology and Embryology, SIXTH EDITION

ISBN: 978-0-323-87664-3

Notice

Practitioners and researchers must always rely on their own experience and knowledge in evaluating and using any information, methods, compounds or experiments described herein. Because of rapid advances in the medical sciences, in particular, independent verification of diagnoses and drug dosages should be made. To the fullest extent of the law, no responsibility is assumed by Elsevier, authors, editors or contributors for any injury and/or damage to persons or property as a matter of products liability, negligence or otherwise, or from any use or operation of any methods, products, instructions, or ideas contained in the material herein.

Previous editions copyrighted 2019, 2014, 2006, 2000, and 1992.

Content Strategist: Kelly Skelton
Content Development Specialist: Rishabh Gupta
Publishing Services Manager: Ranjana Sharma
Project Manager: Sindhuraj Thulasingam
Design Direction: Margaret Reid

Printed in India

Last digit is the print number: 9 8 7 6 5 4 3 2 1

Working together
to grow libraries in
developing countries

www.elsevier.com • www.bookaid.org

PREFACE

It seems that the last time I looked, Jim Avery and I were working on editing the third edition of *Essentials of Oral Histology and Embryology: A Clinical Approach*, and now I am completing the sixth edition. It's truly amazing that time seems to travel at the speed of light the more you have to accomplish.

The sixth edition has many changes from previous editions. One of the major additions is a section on viruses of the oral cavity. The stimulus for this section was the COVID-19 pandemic the world is/was experiencing. Viruses of the oral cavity have been playing an increasingly more common role in the various pathologies of the mouth. Before COVID, herpes simplex 1 was diagnosed with increasing frequency. Then came human papillomavirus and finally, COVID.

Of course, this is a simplistic timeline, but the world was changed. Today, we live with the new guidelines for prevention of and protection from a virus that didn't exist in its present form until recently. In a very short amount of time, a vaccine was developed and administered to the world. We are all grateful to the many different professions and healthcare providers who worked together to develop and administer the vaccine. There was some turmoil and trepidation in between, but the outcome was as good as or better than predicted.

Throughout the sixth edition, there have been many editorial changes that clarify and enhance the subject matter of each chapter, including new references. I sincerely hope that the reader—whether that be a student, instructor, or interested lifelong learner—finds this edition easy to read and informative.

Daniel J. Chiego, Jr., M.S., Ph.D.

ACKNOWLEDGMENTS

Even though it is my name that appears on the cover of the sixth edition of *Essentials of Oral Histology and Embryology: A Clinical Approach*, it was definitely a team that brought this book to fruition. Kelly Skelton, senior content strategist, contacted me about a year and a half ago, suggesting that I think about new edition of this textbook. Kelly gave me plenty of time to think about the idea, and we finalized the timeline about a year later. I was very slow at the beginning, since I had to move many items already on the agenda forward. Kelly would call, ask how I was proceeding, and give me many helpful suggestions to get past any stumbling blocks I was encountering. Kelly was always supportive and understanding, and I thank her for her helpfulness during every step of the process.

Rishabh Gupta has helped me over many hurdles along the way. As the senior content development specialist, his vast understanding of how this edition should look was comforting when I was in some sort of quandary or other. Rishabh always had a solution.

I also thank Sindhuraj Thulasingam, project manager, for all his work during the production process of this book. I am sure there are many others in the development team and within Elsevier who I do not know but are working hard behind the scenes to get this sixth edition published on time and as "perfect" as possible. I thank you for your dedication, perseverance, and work ethic.

I would like to thank my colleagues, friends, and family for their support and encouragement during the writing of the sixth edition. It is very gratifying to hear positive feedback from friends and fellow academics from around the world about something you had a major role in.

And finally, I would like to thank my family and my adult children, Daniel III and Nadia, for making my life enjoyable and for teaching me the ways of the "young." And, as always, I would like to thank my parents, Daniel Sr. and Josephine, for making all things possible—especially my mother, who always stressed the strength of education.

Daniel J. Chiego, Jr., M.S., Ph.D.

CONTENTS

Development and Structure of Cells and Tissues

LEARNING OBJECTIVES

- Describe the cell and how it divides.
- Discuss how cells change from a stem cell to a terminally differentiated state.
- Discuss the origin of tissue and the ovarian cycle and the development of the embryonic disk.

- Describe the various tissues of the human body and some of the adverse factors, such as environmental stress, heredity, and diet, that may affect development of these tissues.

OVERVIEW

The smallest unit of structure in the human body is the cell, composed of a nucleus and cytoplasm. The nucleus contains **deoxyribonucleic acid (DNA)** and **ribonucleic acid (RNA)**, the fundamental structures of life. The cytoplasm functions in absorption and cell duplication, in which organelles perform specific actions. The cell cycle is the time required for the DNA to duplicate before mitosis. This chapter discusses the four stages of mitosis: prophase, metaphase, anaphase, and telophase. Also described are the three periods of prenatal development: proliferative, embryonic, and fetal. The fertilization of the ovum in the distal one-third of uterine tube, zygote migration, and the zygote's implantation in the uterine wall are discussed. In addition, the origin of human tissues—ectoderm, mesoderm, and endoderm—is presented, followed by the differentiation of tissue types, such as those of ectodermal origin, epithelium and skin with its derivatives, and the central and peripheral nervous systems. This chapter also delineates development of the mesodermal components involving connective tissues of the body, such as fibrous tissue, three types of cartilage, two types of bone, three kinds of muscles, and the cardiovascular system. The reader will better comprehend the origin, development, organization, and structure of the various cells and tissues of the human body.

CELL STRUCTURE AND FUNCTION

The human body is composed of cells, intercellular substance (the products of these cells), and fluid that bathes these tissues. Cells are the smallest living units capable of independent existence. They carry out the vital processes of **absorption, assimilation, respiration, irritability, conductivity, growth, reproduction**, and **excretion**. Cells vary in size, shape, structure, and function, which are determined by the cytoskeletal elements. Regardless of function, each cell has a number of characteristics in common with other cells, such as **cytoplasm** and a **nucleus**, which contains a **nucleolus**. However, some cell characteristics are related to function. A cell on the surface of the skin, for example, serves best as a thin, flattened disk, whereas a respiratory cell functions best as a cuboidal or columnar cell to facilitate adsorption with mobile cilia to move fluid from the lung to the oropharynx. Surrounding each cell is the **intercellular material** that provides the cell with nutrition, takes up waste products, and provides the body with form. It may be as soft as loose connective tissue or as hard as bone, cartilage, or teeth. **Fluid**, the third component of the body, is the blood and lymph that travel throughout the body in vessels or the tissue fluid that bathes each cell and fiber of the body.

Cell Nucleus

A nucleus is found in almost all cells except mature red blood cells and blood platelets. The nucleus is usually round to ovoid, depending on the cell's shape. Ordinarily, a cell has a single nucleus; however, it may be binucleate, as are cardiac muscle cells or parenchymal liver cells, or multinucleate, as are osteoclasts and skeletal muscle cells. The nucleus is important in the production of DNA and RNA. DNA contains the genetic information in the cell, and RNA carries information from the DNA to sites of actual protein synthesis, which are located in the cell cytoplasm. The nucleus is bound by a membrane, the **nuclear envelope**, which has openings at the **nuclear pores**. This envelope is composed of two phospholipid layers similar to the plasma membrane of the cell. The pores are associated with the **endoplasmic reticulum (ER)** that forms at the end of each cell division. The nucleus contains from one to four nucleoli, which are round, dense bodies constituting the RNA contained in the nucleus. Nucleoli have no limiting membrane (Fig. 1.1).

Cell Cytoplasm

Cytoplasm contains structures necessary for adsorption and for creation of cell products. The **cytosol** is the part of the cytoplasm

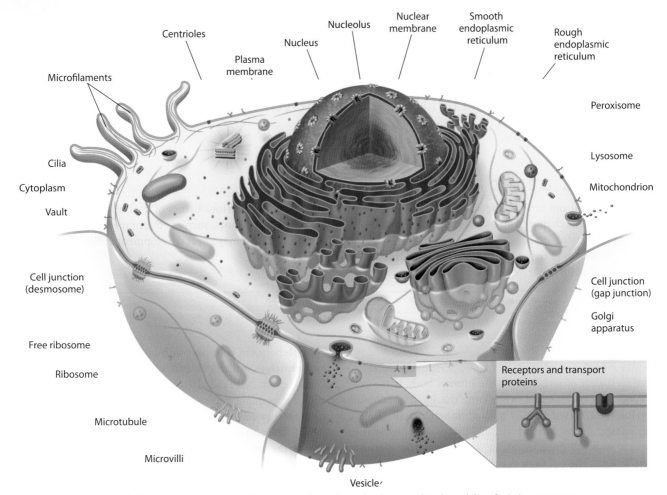

Fig. 1.1 Nucleus, rough surface endoplasmic reticulum, mitochondria, Golgi apparatus, centrioles, and gap junctions as viewed by electron microscopy (artist's rendition). Cells communicate with each other to regulate organization, growth, and development.

that contains the organelles and solutes. The cytosol uses the raw materials brought into the cell to produce energy. It also functions in the excretion of waste products. These functions are carried out by the ER-parallel, membrane-bound cavities in the cytoplasm that contain newly acquired and synthesized protein. Two types of ER—smooth surfaced and granular or rough surfaced—can be found in the same cell. Rough-surfaced ER is caused by ribosomes on the surface of the reticulum and is the site at which protein production is initiated. Proteins are vital to the cell's metabolic processes, and each type of protein is composed of a number of different amino acids linked in a specific sequence. Amino acids form protein-containing groups, which, in turn, form acids or bases.

Ribosomes are particles that translate genetic codes for proteins and activate mechanisms for their production. They can be found as separate particles in the cytoplasm, clustered as polyribosomes, or attached to the ER membranes. Ribosomes are nonspecific as to what type of protein they synthesize. The type is dependent on the **messenger RNA (mRNA)**, which carries the message directly from the DNA of the nucleus to the RNA in the ER. This molecule attaches to the ribosomes and gives orders about the formation of the amino acids. **Transfer RNA**

(tRNA) is another type of RNA that acts at the level of the ribosome by carrying amino acids for the synthesis of proteins.

The ER transports substances in the cytoplasm. The ER is connected to the Golgi apparatus via small vesicles. The **Golgi apparatus** or **complex** is critical for posttranslational modifications that help sort, condense, package, and deliver proteins arriving from the ER. The Golgi apparatus is composed of cisternae (flat plates) or saccules, small vesicles, and large vacuoles. From here, the secretory vesicles move or flow to the cell surface, where they fuse with the cell membrane and the plasmalemma and release their contents by exocytosis.

Lysosomes are small, membrane-bound organelles that contain a variety of acid hydrolases, hydrogen peroxide, and digestive enzymes to help break down substances both inside and outside the cell. They are in all cells except red blood cells but are prominent in macrophages and leukocytes. Peroxisomes, another intracellular organelle, are also important for breaking down fatty acids.

Mitochondria are membrane-bound organelles that lie free in the cytoplasm and are present in all cells. They are important in generating energy, are a major source of adenosine triphosphate (ATP), and therefore are the site of many metabolic reactions. These organelles appear as spheres or rods, or ovoid or threadlike bodies. Usually, the inner layer of their trilaminar bounding membrane inflects to form transverse-appearing plates, the cristae (see Fig. 1.1). Mitochondria lie adjacent to areas that require their energy production. They also have the ability to store ionic calcium and to release it when needed by the cell for various reactions, including signal transduction. They are self-replicating and contain maternal DNA.

Cytoskeletal Elements

Intermediate filaments are a family of proteins that function as cytoskeletal elements and are categorized as VI types, including acid and basic keratins, desmin, glial fibrillary acidic protein, vimentin, neurofilaments, laminins, and nestin.

Microtubules are small tubular structures in the cytoplasm that are composed of the protein tubulin. These structures may appear as singles, doublets, or triplets. They function as structural and force-generating elements and relate to cilia (motile cell processes) and to **centrioles** in relation to mitosis. They have cytoskeletal functions in maintaining cell shape. Centrioles are short cylinders appearing near the nucleus. Their walls are composed of nine triplets of microtubules. Centrioles are microtubule-generating centers and are important in mitosis, self-replicating before mitosis begins.

CLINICAL COMMENT

Drugs that can adversely affect microtubule formation by binding tubulin, a major component of microtubules, include colchicine, vinblastine, and vincristine. Inhibiting microtubule formation prevents cells from being able to undergo mitosis. Vinblastine and vincristine are antimitotic drugs commonly used in the treatment of cancer. They are not specific for cancer cells, but since certain kinds of cancer cells divide more often than normal cells, the cancer cells are affected more.

Surrounding the cell is the **plasma membrane** or plasmalemma, which envelops the cell and provides a selective barrier that regulates transport of substances into and out of the cell. All membranes are composed mainly of lipids and proteins, with a small amount of carbohydrates. The plasma membrane receives signals from hormones, growth factors, and neurotransmitters by having them bind to receptors located on the surface and within the plasma membrane, eventually activating a second messenger (e.g., cyclic adenosine monophosphate) that signals intracellular organelles or the nucleus/nucleolus to modify cell activity, such as increasing the production of a protein. Also included in the plasma membrane are many kinds of ion channels that can activate many different cell functions. In addition, cells contain proteins, lipids, or fatty substances that provide energy in the cell and are important components of cell membranes and permeability. Carbohydrates are also important in cells as the most available energy component in the body. These carbohydrates may exist as polysaccharide-protein complexes, glycoprotein complexes, glycoproteins, and glycolipids. Carbohydrate compounds are important in cell function and for development of cell products, such as supportive tissues and body lubricants.

Genetic mechanisms help a cell to develop and maintain a high degree of order. This ability is dependent on the genetic

information that is expressed within the cell. The basic genetic processes in the cell are RNA and protein synthesis, DNA repair, and replication and genetic recombination. These processes produce the proteins and nucleic acids of a cell. These genetic events are relatively simple compared with other cell processes.

CELL DIVISION

Cell Cycle

Cell division is a continuous series of discrete steps by which the cell component divides. This function is related to the need for growth or replacement of tissues and is partly dependent on the length of the cell's life. Continually renewing cells line the gastrointestinal tract and compose the epidermis and the bone marrow. A second type of cell is part of an expanding population—the cells of the kidney, liver, and some glands. The third type of cell does not undergo cell division or DNA synthesis. An example is the neurons of the adult nervous system. For a somatic cell to undergo cell division, it must pass through a **cell cycle**, which ensures time for DNA genetic material in the daughter cells to duplicate that of the parent cell. However, in a sex cell—an ovum or spermatozoon—the process of meiosis occurs, in which a reduction division of chromosomes in the daughter cell takes place. The result is that half as many chromosomes are in the daughter cell as are in the parent cell. Through meiosis, after fertilization of the ovum by the male sperm, the original (diploid) number of chromosomes is regained. The duration of the cell cycle in somatic cells is now known (Fig. 1.2). After mitosis, the cells enter the reduplication or **G1 phase** of the interphase, the initial resting stage. This is followed by the **S phase**, in which DNA synthesis is completed. Next, the cell enters the **G2 phase** or quiescent phase of the post-DNA

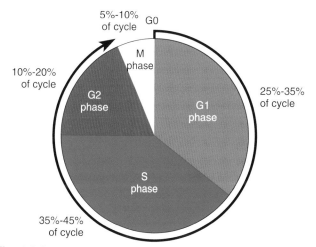

Fig. 1.2 Periods of cell cycle indicate relative time needed for each phase. G1 is the reduplication phase, or resting phase, which takes about 6 to 8 hours. In the S phase, DNA duplication takes place in 8 to 10 hours. The G2 phase is the postduplication phase, which takes about 4 to 6 hours. In the M phase, mitosis takes about 35 to 40 minutes. These figures are for cultured mammalian cells. The total is 18 to 24 hours for these four stages of cytokinesis. Other types of cells can have a longer or shorter cell cycle.

duplication and proceeds into the mitotic stages of prophase, metaphase, anaphase, and telophase (Fig. 1.3). The cell then reenters and remains in the interphase stage until duplication resumes the mitotic process of developing two daughter cells identical to the parent cells.

Mitosis

Before mitosis, the cell exists in the interphase, as seen in Fig. 1.3A. The first step of mitosis is **prophase**, in which four structural changes occur (see Fig. 1.3B). The chromatin thread of the nucleus thickens into rodlike structures called **chromosomes**. Each chromosome then splits, forming two **chromatids**. These chromatids line up along the central area of the cell, called the **equatorial plate**. Each chromatid pair is attached to a spherical body called a **centromere**. The centriole pair duplicates, and the chromatids accompany the centrioles' migration to the opposite ends of the cell. Those fibers not formed between the migrating centrioles are **spindle fibers**, and those that form around the centrioles are **astral rays** or **asters** (see Fig. 1.3C). At this time,

the nucleolus disappears, and its components become attached to the chromatids. Finally, the nuclear envelope breaks down and changes into granular elements, such as the ER (see Fig. 1.3D).

Chromatids have moved to the cell center by the **metaphase** stage. They are arranged along an equatorial plate at right angles to the long axis of the spindle (see Fig. 1.3E). The two chromatids of each chromosome become attached centrally at the equatorial plate to a centromere. These chromatids then split at the centromere into two sets of chromosomes.

In **anaphase**, the daughter chromosomes move to the opposite poles of the cell with the full complement of 46 at each end (see Fig. 1.3F and G). This is thought to occur by movement

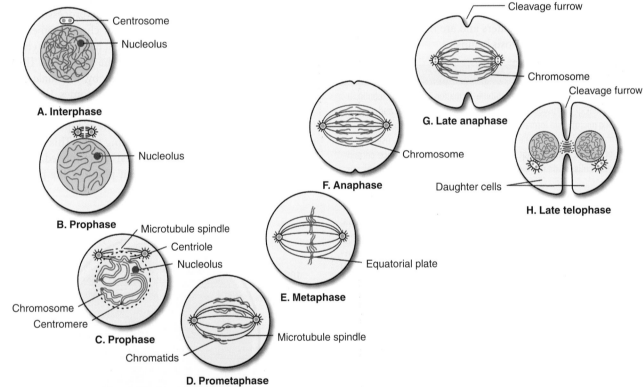

Fig. 1.3 Mitosis of somatic cell. The continuous process of cell division is shown. Mitosis is replication of parent chromosomes and distribution of two sets of chromosomes into two separate and equal nuclei. Stages are as follows: **A**, Interphase, resting cell. **B** and **C**, During prophase, chromatin thread shortens and thickens and becomes chromosomes, which then split into pairs of chromatids. Nuclear membrane disappears, and centrioles appear and begin migration to opposite poles of cell. **D**, In prometaphase, or early metaphase, chromatid pairs attach to centromere and line up in equatorial plate of cell. **E**, Metaphase occurs when centromeres and chromatids line up in middle of cell. Centrioles are at opposite ends of cell and attach to chromosomes by mitotic spindles. **F**, Anaphase is a division and movement of completed identical sets of chromatids (chromosomes) to opposite ends of cells. **G**, In late anaphase, identical sets of chromosomes have reached opposite ends of the cells as cleavage begins. **H**, In telophase, a nuclear membrane reappears, nucleoli appear, and chromosomes lengthen and form chromatin thread. Mitotic spindles disappear, and centrioles duplicate so that each cell has completely identical properties.

of the chromosomal microtubules that attract the chromatids toward the poles. A constriction begins to appear around the midbody of the cell (see Fig. 1.3G).

In **telophase**, the chromosomes detach from the chromosomal microtubules, and the microtubules disintegrate. The chromosomes next elongate and disperse, losing their identity and regaining the chromatin thread appearance. Both the nucleoli within the nucleus and the nuclear envelope then reappear. As each nucleus matures, the cleavage furrow deepens in the midcell until the two daughter cells separate (see Fig. 1.3H).

Meiosis

Meiosis is the process of reduction of the number of chromosomes to half the normal number in the germ cells to allow fusion of the male and female germ cells. There are two cell divisions in meiosis (Fig. 1.4). In the first meiotic division, the chromosomes divide equally with pairing of the homologous chromosomes and the appropriate synthesis of DNA. In the second meiotic division, the DNA is not synthesized, and three of the daughter cells divide into polar bodies that become inactive; the one remaining germ cell containing half the amount of DNA pairs with the germ cell of the opposite sex. This pairing of the XY chromosomes of the male and female germ cells provides the needed mature somatic cell and results in a zygote.

Apoptosis

Apoptosis, or programmed cell death, is the fragmentation of a cell into membrane-bound particles, which are then eliminated by phagocytosis by specialized cells. Cell death is the usual accompaniment of embryonic growth and differentiation. It is a means of eliminating transient and obsolete tissues. Thus cell death, as well as histogenesis and morphogenetic movement, accomplishes the final form of the structure. Cell death typically occurs at sites during folding or invagination of tissues. Cell death is a useful way of eliminating tissues or organs that provided a function during early embryonic life (e.g., the tadpole's tail and gills) and during development of the central nervous system.

Adult stem cells (Fig. 1.5) are found in hematopoietic cells in bone marrow as well as in many other tissues, and they have the multipotent capacity to form a number of cell types. Early embryonic stem cells from the morula stage are totipotent and can divide and produce all the differentiated cells in an organism. However, as they divide and go through a developmental lineage to the blastocyst stage, they become pluripotent during gastrulation, which then limits further differentiation to any of the three germ layers. Stem cells have been found in the dental pulp as well as in the brain, hair, muscle, adipose tissue, skin, intestinal tract, and blood vessels. It is the hope of the future that these cells will be able to replace damaged, dead, or malfunctioning tissue. It has recently been reported that damaged corneal cells of the eye can be replaced with bits of oral epithelium using the patient's own stem cells to aid in the healing process and in restoring vision.

CLINICAL COMMENT

All cells have a limited lifetime. For example, the life span of a white blood cell is only a few hours to a few days. Red blood cells live approximately 120 days before they are ingested by macrophages. Surface-covering cells—such as those of the skin, hair, or nails—renew as they are replaced, as do cells lining the respiratory, urinary, and gastrointestinal tracts. Other cells in the body—such as those of the liver, kidneys, and thyroid gland—do not normally renew after maturity unless they are injured.

ORIGIN OF HUMAN TISSUE

Epithelial-Mesenchymal Interaction

The following definitions are important to understanding the basic processes of early development.

Induction

Induction is the process in which an undifferentiated cell is instructed by specific organizers to produce a morphogenic effect.

Cell Differentiation

The **organizer** is the part of an embryo that influences another part to direct histologic and morphologic differentiation. Chemical substances called **growth factors** and **morphogens** induce cells to initiate specific cellular processes, including DNA synthesis, in a specific temporal and spatial manner.

Periods of Prenatal Development

Implantation and enlargement of the blastocyst, which contains the embryonic tissue, occur rapidly in the **proliferative period**, which lasts for 2 weeks. During this time, fertilization, implantation, and formation of the embryonic disk take place.

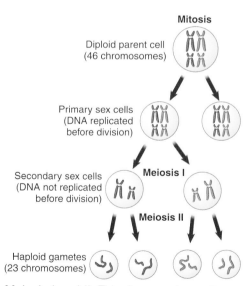

Fig. 1.4 Meiosis I and II. This diagram shows the process of meiosis, in which the diploid complement of chromosomes (46) is reduced to haploid (23) in the gamete (sperm or ovum). Meiosis occurs as meiosis I and II and results in half the complement of chromosomes from each parent that has been recombined representing various genetic combinations from each parent. (Patton KT, Thibodeau GA. *Human body in health and disease*, 7th ed. St. Louis: Elsevier; 2018.)

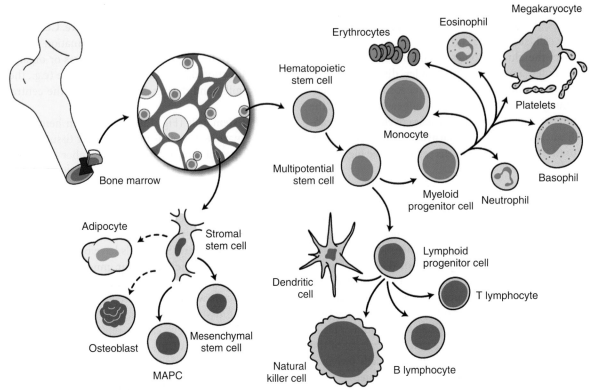

Fig. 1.5 Stem cells in the bone marrow (hematopoietic) have been studied extensively. These cells can differentiate into blood and immune cell lines. Other stem cells in the bone marrow are stromal stem cells, which have been reported to be able to differentiate into fat and bone cell precursors. Other stem cells have been discovered in the brain, eyes, skin, muscle, dental pulp, blood vessels, and gastrointestinal tract.

After the second week, this mass of cells begins to take the form of an embryo, so the period of 2 to 8 weeks is termed the **embryonic period**. During this period, the different types of tissue develop and organize to form organ systems. The heart forms and begins to beat by the fourth week, and the face and oral structures develop during weeks 4 to 7. The embryo takes on a more human appearance in the eighth week and moves into the **fetal period**, which extends until birth (Fig. 1.6). During this period, the tissues that developed in the embryonic stage enlarge, differentiate, and become capable of function.

> **CONSIDER THE PATIENT**
>
> An expectant mother has reason for concern about the health of her baby. She asks whether tests are available to find out if her baby is healthy. She wants to know what the tests would reveal and if any risks are involved. (See discussion at end of chapter.)

Ovarian Cycle, Fertilization, Implantation, and Development of the Embryonic Disk

The origin of tissue begins with fertilization of the egg, or ovum, which occurs when sperm contact the egg in the distal part of the uterine tube (Fig. 1.7). The fertilized egg then grows and is termed the **zygote**. The cell mass produces a ball of cells (the **morula**) in the uterine tube. The morula grows and begins migration medially to the uterus, which it reaches at the end of the first week. The uterine cavity, meanwhile, prepares for the arrival of the fertilized ovum. The uterine lining (**endometrium**) thickens, and capillaries and glands develop to nourish the ovum. Estrogen and progesterone control this cyclical event (Fig. 1.8). The morula increases in size and is termed a **blastocyst**. As the blastocyst swells, it becomes hollow and develops a small inner cell mass. When this blastocyst or zygote reaches the uterine cavity, it attaches to the sticky wall of the uterus and becomes embedded in its surface. The cells of the zygote enzymatically digest the uterine endometrium, permitting deeper penetration. This process is known as **implantation**. If no fertilized ovum reaches the uterine cavity, the development of capillaries and glands is terminated by menstruation (Fig. 1.9).

Two small cavities develop on either side of the inner cell mass. They reach each other in the center, where a small disk (the **embryonic disk**) is formed (Fig. 1.10). The embryonic disk becomes the embryo, composed of the common walls of the two adjacent sacs. One sac is lined with **ectodermal** cells, which will form the outer body covering (**epithelium**). The other sac is lined with **endodermal** cells. On the dorsal surface of the embryonic disk, the ectoderm forms the **neural plate**, whose lateral boundaries elevate to form a **neural tube** that will become the brain and spinal cord (Fig. 1.11). The endodermal cells also form a tube, which will become the **gastrointestinal**

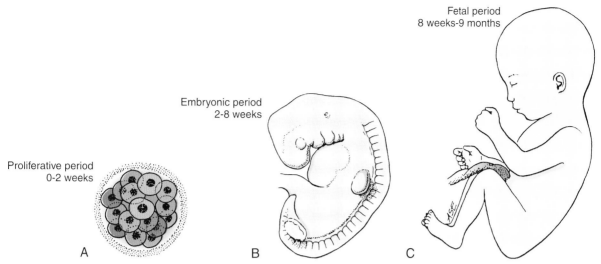

Fig. 1.6 The developing human passes through three periods of growth. **A**, Proliferative period: the first 2 weeks when cell division is prevalent. **B**, Embryonic period: from the second to the eighth weeks. **C**, Fetal period: from the eighth week to birth.

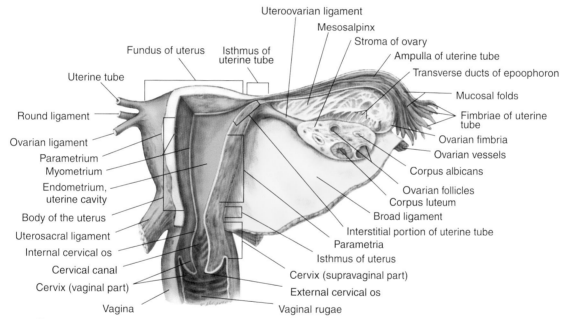

Fig. 1.7 Schematic diagram of the uterus and uterine tubes reveals the path of sperm to the distal tube, in which fertilization of the newly appearing ovum from the adjacent ovary occurs. The resultant zygote travels to uterus while undergoing cleavage, and implantation occurs on seventh day after conception. (Lentz GM, Lobo RA, Gershenson GM, et al. *Comprehensive gynecology*. 7th ed. St. Louis: Mosby; 2017.)

tract. As this tube elongates, it anteriorly develops outpouchings that form the pharyngeal pouches, lung buds, liver, gallbladder, pancreas, and urinary bladder (Fig. 1.12).

Next, cells develop between the ectodermal and endodermal layers in the embryonic disk. This area becomes the **mesodermal** layer. These cells will develop into the muscles, skeleton, and blood cells of the embryo (Fig. 1.13). Mesodermal cells also accompany the elongating digestive tube and support its walls with muscle growth. This enables function and assists in the formation of organs arising from the developing gastrointestinal tube. From these three layers—ectoderm, mesoderm, and endoderm—develop all tissues of the body, as well as the complex organs (see Fig. 1.12).

CLINICAL COMMENT

Environmental teratogens may affect the development of normal cells, tissues, organs, or organ systems. A defect in the development of a group of cells is considerably less damaging than a defect in an organ or organ system. The smaller and less complex the development, the less extensive the problem created. Development is also related to timing. **Tissues are most susceptible to defective development when they begin to differentiate in the embryonic period (2 to 8 weeks)**.

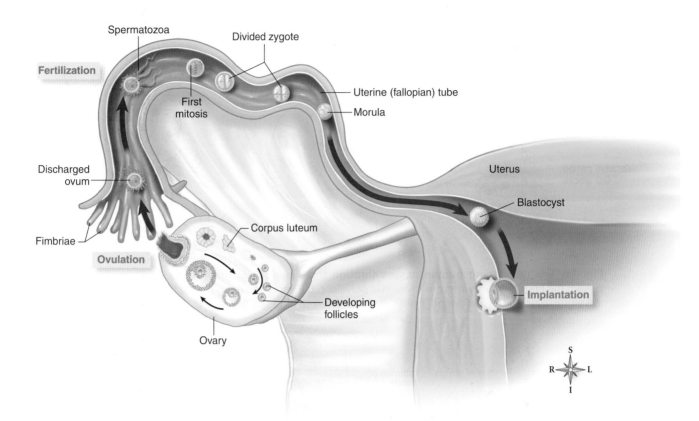

Fig. 1.8 Implantation of a fertilized ovum (zygote) in the wall of the uterus. Outer cells of trophoblast digest uterine cells to implant. An embryoblast develops within cell mass. As the mass expands, a surrounding cavity is formed. (Patton K, Thibodeau G. *Human body in health and disease.* 7th ed. St. Louis: Elsevier; 2018.)

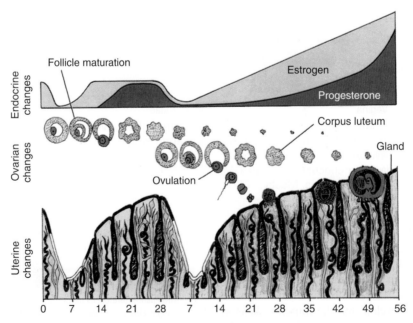

Fig. 1.9 Cyclical events of ovulatory cycle. *Top*, Endocrine changes: ovulation is controlled by estrogen and progesterone. *Center*, Ovarian changes: the ovum matures, is expelled from ovary on fourteenth day, and if fertilized, becomes implanted in uterine wall 7 days later. *Bottom*, Uterine changes: uterine wall thickens and prepares for implantation each month. If implantation does not occur, uterine wall erodes with loss of blood vessels and gland ducts (menstruation).

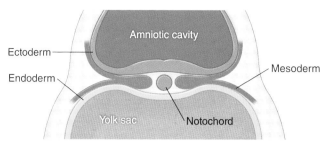

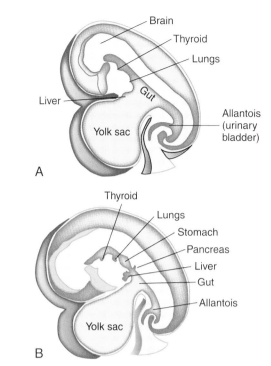

A

Fig. 1.10 Second small cavity lined with ectoderm develops (amniotic cavity). The other cavity (yolk sac) is lined with endoderm. The two cell layers contact in the center to form an area of ectoderm and endoderm for embryonic disk.

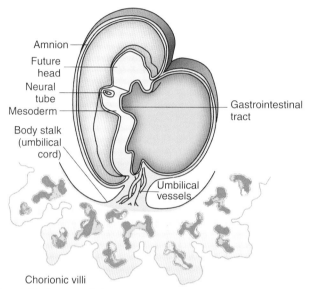

Fig. 1.11 A 3-week human embryo. The embryo is viewed from the ventral-lateral aspect, illustrating an elongating gastrointestinal tube and a dorsally located neural tube.

B

Fig. 1.12 Further development of the gastrointestinal tract. **A**, At 4½ weeks, and **B**, at 5 weeks. Outpouchings of the intestinal tube form gastrointestinal organs.

DEVELOPMENT OF HUMAN TISSUES

Epithelial Tissue

The skin is a dual organ that has an **epidermis**, a surface cell layer that develops from the surface of ectodermal cells, and a **dermis**, which arises from the underlying mesoderm. The dermis originates in the **somites**, the masses of mesoderm that lie on either side of the neural tube. From this mesoderm come both the dermis of the epithelium and the visceral mesoderm that covers the yolk sac and later becomes the gastrointestinal tract (Fig. 1.14). Therefore all the muscles functioning in intestinal peristalsis (the wavelike movements of the gastrointestinal tract) arise from this mesoderm.

Initially, the embryo is covered with a single layer of ectodermal cells (Fig. 1.15A). By 11 to 12 weeks, this ectodermal layer of epithelium thickens into four layers. From the basal layer of cells come the more superficial cells of the epithelium (see Fig. 1.15B). Later, **melanocytes** invade and pigment the skin. At birth, the skin may show varying degrees of keratinization. Hair, teeth, and nails, and mammary, sebaceous, and salivary glands all develop from a combination of epidermal and dermal cells (epithelial-mesenchymal

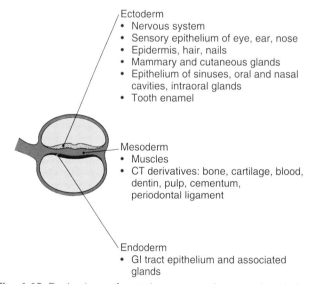

Fig. 1.13 Derivatives of ectoderm, mesoderm, and endoderm germ layers.

interactions). This development occurs when epithelial cells proliferate, invade the underlying dermis, and finally differentiate into glands or teeth, with both the epidermis and dermis contributing to each of these structures.

Epithelial-mesenchymal interactions are the necessary interactions of an epithelium and underlying mesenchyme that determine the terminally differentiated tissue. There are many examples of this process, including tooth and salivary gland induction and differentiation during normal development and during cancer metastasis.

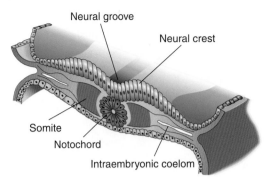

Fig. 1.14 Neural folds and somites in transverse section at approximately 20 days after conception. Medial somite (mesoderm) forms the axial skeleton that surrounds neural tube. Intermediate mesoderm forms striated muscle of body, and lateral mesoderm forms dermis of the epithelium of the body wall (somatic) and gastrointestinal tract (splanchnic). (Moore KL, Persaud TVN, Torchia MG. *Before we are born: essentials of embryology and birth defects*. 9th ed. St. Louis: Saunders; 2016.)

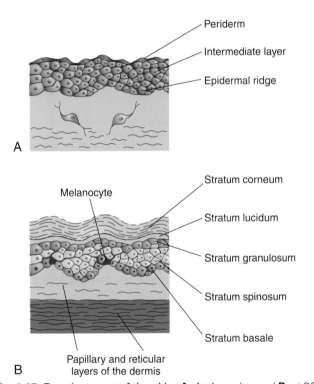

Fig. 1.15 Development of the skin. A, At 4 weeks, and **B,** at 36 weeks. Initial layer of epithelial cells thickens into multiple layers, and underlying connective tissue becomes dermis. Dermis and epithelium combine to become skin. (Moore KL, Persaud TVN, Torchia MG. *The developing human: clinically oriented embryology*. 10th ed. St. Louis: Saunders; 2016.)

Nervous System

Brain and Spinal Cord

The neural folds appear during the third prenatal week. The lateral edges of the neural plate begin to elevate as folds arising dorsally (see Fig. 1.10). These folds represent the first change in shape of the embryo's body from the flat sheet of cells (see Fig. 1.9).

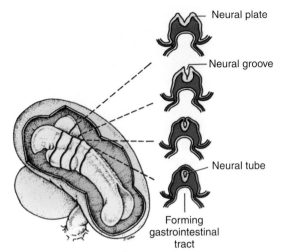

Fig. 1.16 *Left,* Dorsal view of closing neural tube of 3-week human embryo. Closure occurs initially in the dorsal area, then anteriorly and posteriorly. *Right,* Transverse sections of neural folds appear anteriorly, and those of closed neural tube are in the midbrain region.

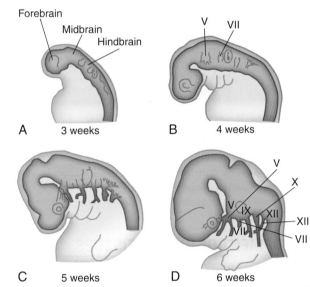

Fig. 1.17 Development of cranial nerves. A, 3 weeks; **B,** 4 weeks; **C,** 5 weeks; **D,** 6 weeks. At 3 weeks, the forebrain has enlarged, and sensory vesicles are laterally located. At 4 and 5 weeks, the forebrain has bent forward, and cranial nerves have grown into tissues they innervate. At 6 weeks, the anterior brain has enlarged and bent back on the posteriorly located cerebellum.

These folds reach the midline, first in the cervical region, and then the neural tube closes both anteriorly and posteriorly (Fig. 1.16). When the anterior tube closes, it shows three dilations that form the primary brain vesicles, the **forebrain, midbrain**, and **hindbrain** (Fig. 1.17A). The neural tube bends forward just behind the midbrain and backward behind the hindbrain (see Fig. 1.17C and D). The **cerebral hemispheres** develop from the forebrain vesicles. The midbrain is a pathway from the cerebral cortex to centers in the **pons** and **cerebellum** of the hindbrain. The fifth cranial nerve develops in the

Neural crest cells

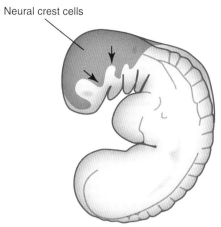

Fig. 1.18 Migration pathway of neural crest cells from neural folds to the developing face.

midbrain (see Fig. 1.17B–D) and grows peripherally to innervate structures derived from the first pharyngeal arch. The cerebral hemispheres of the forebrain develop into the **frontal, temporal**, and **occipital lobes**.

Cranial Nerves

The ventricles of the brain are continuous and connect posteriorly with the spinal cord. The walls of the neural tube are lined with neuroepithelium. As these cells proliferate, they differentiate into **neuroblasts** and become the white and gray matter of the spinal cord. Neuroblasts are primitive nerve cells that develop into adult nerve cells called the **neurons**. These cells do not divide further. Along the surface of the developing brain and spinal cord, neural crest cells form the sensory system of the dorsal root ganglia of the cranial and spinal nerves (Fig. 1.18) Table 1.1. The neural crest cells also contribute to tissues of the face, such as cartilage, muscles, teeth, and ligaments (Box 1.1).

BOX 1.1 Neural Crest Derivatives
Neural and Other Than Neural

Structures Arising From the Cranial Neural Crest
Skeletal and Connective Tissue
- Bones and cartilage of the head and face
  - Upper and lower jaw
  - Dental papilla (odontoblasts)
  - Palate
  - Cranial vault floor
- Connective tissues
  - Corneal stromal fibroblasts
  - Contributions to dermis and subcutaneous adipose tissue of face, jaw, and upper neck
  - Lining of forebrain (meninges)
- Muscles
  - Ciliary muscles (striated)
  - Smooth muscle of cranial blood vessels and dermis
Endocrine and Exocrine Tissues
  - Mesenchyme of pituitary, thyroid, parathyroid thymus, and salivary glands

Structures Derived From Both Cranial and Trunk Neural Crest
Neural Derivatives
- Sensory neurons of cranial and spinal ganglia
- Symptomatic neurons of pre- and paravertebral ganglia (noradrenergic)
- Parasympathetic neurons of visceral ganglia and plexuses (cholinergic, serotonergic)
- Neurosecretory cells
  - Calcitonin-producing (c) cells of the thyroid
  - Adrenal medullary cells (adrenergic)
  - Possible contribution to neuroactive peptide-secreting cells of pituitary
Supportive cells of the peripheral nervous system
- Glia
- Schwann sheath cells
- Satellite cells of ganglionic neurons
Pigment (melanin or other pigment granule-containing)
- Cells of skin, hair (feathers), and iris

TABLE 1.1 Cranial Nerves: Functions and Test

Cranial Nerve	Function	Test
I. Olfactory	Smell	Odorous substance
II. Optic	Vision	Vision chart
III. Oculomotor	Eyelid and some eyeball	Coordinated following of an object
IV. Trochlear	Superior oblique muscle: eyeball	Look down at nose
V. Trigeminal	Mastication, sensory for face and mouth	Bite down, touch face and gingiva
VI. Abducens	Lateral rectus muscle: eyeball	Gaze to the side
VII. Facial	Muscles of facial expression, controls secretion of tears and saliva; taste (anterior two-thirds of tongue)	Smile, frown, raise eyebrows, use a sweet or salty substance on anterior two-thirds of tongue
VIII. Vestibulocochlear	Hearing and equilibrium	Tuning fork; equilibrium
IX. Glossopharyngeal	Taste (posterior one-third of tongue), salivary secretion, carotid blood pressure, and sensory posterior one-third of tongue, stylopharyngeus muscle	Gag reflex, use a sweet or salty substance on posterior one-third of tongue
X. Vagus	Motor to muscles of pharynx and larynx; parasympathetic to neck, thorax, and abdomen; sensory from pharynx, larynx, and gut; external ear; taste	Hoarseness, muscles' responses after saying, "Ah"
XI. Spinal accessory	Motor to trapezius and sternocleidomastoid muscles	Raise shoulders; turn head
XII. Hypoglossal	Motor to tongue muscles except palatoglossal	Protrude tongue

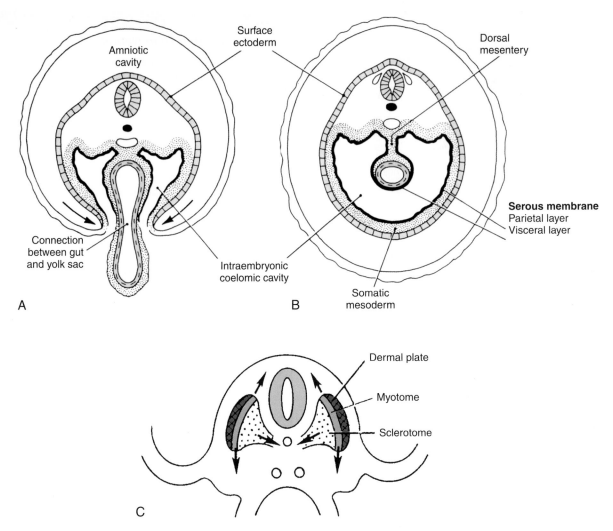

Fig. 1.19 Cross sections of embryo. A and **B** illustrate the yolk sac's role in development of the gastrointestinal tube. The developing body wall is growing ventrally, closing the ventral opening. **C**, Contributions of somite to skin, muscles, and cartilage. Cartilage forms a support for the spinal column (sclerotome), which surrounds neural tube. Contribution of somatic mesoderm (dermal plate) to the body wall seen in B. Muscles arise from intermediate mesoderm (myotome).

Connective Tissue

Connective Tissue Proper

Connective tissue develops from the somites as fibroblasts migrating from either side of the neural tube (see Fig. 1.14). Early in formation, the ventromedial part of the somite differentiates into the **sclerotome**, the dorsolateral part becomes the **dermatome**, and a third division becomes the intermediate mesoderm, or **myotome**. The medial sclerotome differentiates into **mesenchymal cells**, which become **osteoblasts, chondroblasts,** and **fibroblasts**. A large part of the embryonic skeleton develops from these cells. Dermatome cells form the dermis, the subcutaneous tissue, and the **visceral mesoderm**, which supports the endoderm of the gastrointestinal tract, as well as a system of mesenteries that stabilize and support the gastrointestinal tract (Fig. 1.19). Also, connective tissue arises from the somites, providing supporting connective tissues, bones, cartilage, tendons, and ligaments. The tendons connect the muscles to the skeleton as they develop. Connective tissue also functions as capsules of glands and the supporting tissues within them.

Blood and Lymphatic Tissues

Blood is a specialized connective tissue that is composed of 7 liters of fluid and cells in the body. The blood contains formed elements that are the red blood cells or **erythrocytes**, white blood cells or **leukocytes**, and blood platelets suspended in a liquid termed **plasma**. The red blood cells are most numerous (5×10^3 per mm^3), and they carry oxygen from the lungs by means of a substance termed **hemoglobin** and also carry carbon dioxide from the cells of the tissue to the lungs by both the hemoglobin of the red blood cell and the plasma of the blood. Thus blood is a pathway for conducting blood cells throughout the body. The white blood cells or leukocytes are few compared with the red (6500 to 10,000 mL) and function in defending the body against bacteria and other invasive organisms and foreign substances. The leukocytes only travel in the blood vessels from their site of origin to the area of infection, where they leave the blood vessel, migrating between the endothelial cells by a process known as *diapedesis*, to travel in tissue spaces to the site of infection. Three types of **granulocytes** exist: **neutrophils, eosinophils**, and **basophils**, and two types of **agranulocytes: lymphocytes** and **monocytes**. The neutrophils (polymorphonuclear leukocytes) are the most numerous of the white blood cells, representing 60% to 70%, and function in destroying bacteria that invade the tissue spaces. The platelets are small, disk-shaped cell fragments carried in the blood and originate from megakaryocytes in the bone marrow spaces. There are 300,000 to 350,000 platelets in 1 mm^3 of blood; they function to limit hemorrhage to the endothelium of the vessel.

The **lymphatic system** is composed of the lymph nodes, thymus, and spleen, as well as the vessels that carry the lymph throughout the body and back to the venous system at the right brachiocephalic vein and the left subclavian vein. The lymphatic system is a protective mechanism in the immunologic defense of the body. The lymphoid system destroys bacteria, viruses, and invasive microorganisms. The lymphatics are made up of the innate and the adaptive immune systems. The cells that constitute the innate and adaptive immune systems are the B cells, the T cells, the natural killer cells, and macrophages, all of which are formed in the bone marrow. The T cells migrate to the thymus to become immunocompetent. The thymus consists of a cortex and medulla, and is composed of epithelia and reticular cells and macrophages. The medulla consists primarily of thymocytes that are immunocompetent T cells. Throughout the lymphatic vascular system are lymph nodes that act as filters for all bacteria or substances foreign to the body. The lymph nodes are composed of a cortex and a medulla, the cortex is composed of lymph nodules, and the medulla is composed of lymph sinuses interposed with cords of lymph cells. The spleen is the other lymphatic organ and is composed of a cortex and the hilum, where the blood vessels enter and exit. The spleen functions in T- and B-cell formation and also in blood formation if the need arises.

Cartilage and Bone

The initial skeletal component in the embryo is **cartilage**. Cartilage cells arise from the sclerotome and migrate to surround the notochord and spinal cord, which form the spinal column (see Fig. 1.19C). The skeleton develops in the same segmental pattern as the muscles do (Figs. 1.20 and 1.21). Chondroblasts also form cartilage in the appendages, the cranium, and the face, which first appear in the fifth prenatal week. Cartilage cells undergo both **appositional** (exogenous) and **interstitial** (endogenous) growth (see Fig. 1.20B).

Apposition of new layers of cartilage occurs on the surface of cartilage, and interstitial growth involves the proliferation and expansion of the cells within the matrix (see Fig. 1.20B). A supportive cartilage skeleton is produced rapidly to support the soft tissues of the growing embryo. Later, most of this same cartilage skeleton is replaced by bone, which offers more rigidity and strength as muscles attach to it, making movement possible (see Fig. 1.20C). Most cartilage appears clear and glasslike and is called **hyaline cartilage**. Cartilage may also contain elastic fibers and be termed **elastic** or **fibrous cartilage**. The intervertebral disks, for example, are fibrous cartilage, but the external ear contains elastic cartilage. Cartilage combines the properties of elasticity and strength.

Bone replaces cartilage by a process termed **endochondral bone development** (Fig. 1.22). In this case, a small blood vessel enters the cartilage shaft (diaphysis), the cartilage calcifies and disintegrates in the center, and a marrow space is formed (see Fig. 1.22B). New bone develops on the surface of cartilage spicules that border the marrow space (see Fig. 1.22C). Small blood vessels enter the head of the long bones, and secondary ossification centers appear, repeating the process that took place in the shaft of the long bone (see Fig. 1.22D). During the growth period, a developing cartilage disk remains in the neck of each long bone, and bone forms on either side. This disk is known as the **epiphyseal line** (plate) and will remain as long as the bone is forming. The wider part of the diaphysis adjacent to

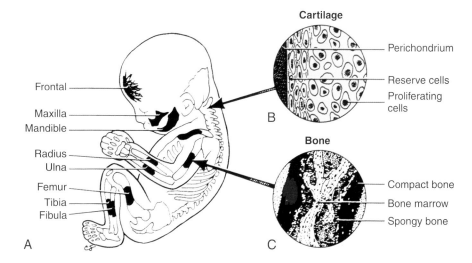

Fig. 1.20 Embryo's skeleton. **A,** Development of cartilage and bones. **B,** Cartilage development by both surface apposition and internal interstitial growth. **C,** Endochondral bone development in the shaft of a long bone.

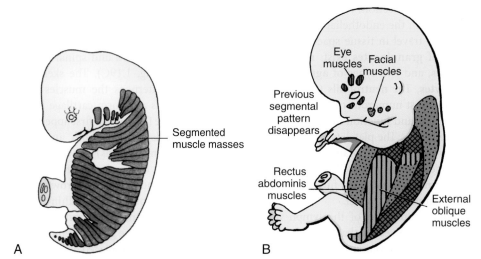

Fig. 1.21 A, Primitive myotome in skeletal muscle formation in an embryo. **B**, Differentiation of skeletal muscle by enlargement of fibers and attachment to bony skeleton to become functional units. The previous segmental pattern disappears.

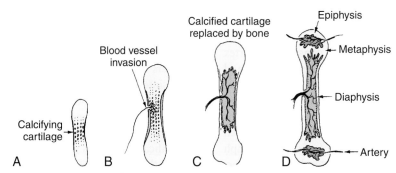

Fig. 1.22 Schematic diagram of endochondral ossification as seen in developing long bones of the body. A, Original hyaline cartilage is calcified in the center of the diaphysis. **B**, A blood vessel invades the center of the shaft. **C**, Marrow space appears in the center of the shaft, and bone forms around the diaphysis. **D**, Bone formation continues in the shaft, and secondary ossification sites appear in the heads (epiphysis) of the bones. A disk of cartilage remains between bone forming in the head and the shaft (epiphyseal line).

the epiphyseal line is known as the **metaphysis** (see Fig. 1.22D). Cartilage develops and expands by **interstitial growth**, which is growth within the cartilage matrix by each cartilage cell enlarging and forming matrix around each cell. New bone forms along the cartilage margins of the epiphyseal line. After bone replaces the epiphysis, cartilage is limited to covering the heads of long bones, the nasal septum, the ears, the temporomandibular joint, and a few other sites.

Direct transformation of connective tissue into bone may also take place. In this case, collagen fibers of connective tissue organize into closely knit meshwork, and this matrix gradually calcifies into bone by a process termed **intramembranous bone formation** or *membranous bone formation* (Fig. 1.23). It is much simpler for bone cells to organize in this manner and to form spicules of bone through coalescence with neighboring spicules until a bony plate is formed. The majority of the flat bones of the face and cranium develop in this manner.

Muscle

By the tenth prenatal week, muscle cells (myoblasts) have begun migrating from the myotome, following a segmental pattern similar to that of the bony skeleton (see Figs. 1.20 and 1.21). They gradually differentiate into elongated, multinucleated muscle fibers, which are specialized cells with the property of contractility. In this manner, muscle is able to provide motion on the basis of structural and functional characteristics.

Muscle is divided into three types: skeletal, smooth, and cardiac. Later, these skeletal muscles lose their segmental pattern of development as they acquire insertion on skeletal elements. These muscle fibers become the **striated voluntary muscles**, which divide into groups that supply the dorsal and ventral parts of the limbs and provide both the deep and superficial muscle fibers (see Fig. 1.21B). These muscles are called *striated* because they have lines across them that are the contraction sites that allow the muscles to function.

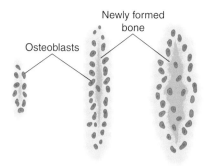

Fig. 1.23 Membranous bone formation that takes place in connective tissue. Initial membranous sites grow by apposition of new bone on their surfaces.

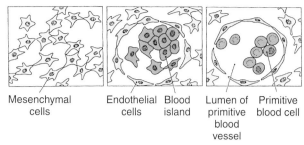

Fig. 1.25 Appearance of blood islands from mesenchymal cells in the location noted in Fig. 1.24. The more peripheral cells form capillary walls, and the inner cells form red blood cells. The tubes or capillaries then lengthen.

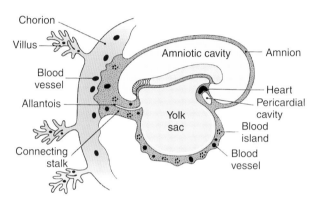

Fig. 1.24 Origin of blood cells and blood vessels in walls of yolk sac, placenta, and body stalk in a 2½-week-old embryo.

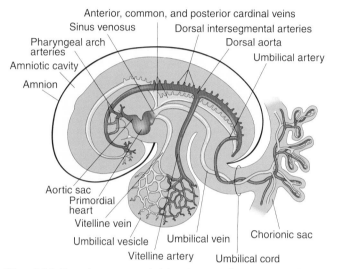

Fig. 1.26 Development of blood vascular system in an embryo. *1*, In the yolk sac, vitelline circulation develops, persisting for only a few weeks until this nutritional source is exhausted. *2*, The umbilical system develops in the umbilical cord, supplying the embryo and fetus with oxygen and nutrients until birth. (Moore KL, Persaud TVN. *The developing human: clinically oriented embryology.* 10th ed. Philadelphia: Saunders; 2016.)

Muscle cells also migrate to the gastrointestinal tract and support the trachea, bronchi, urogenital tract, and larger blood vessels. These muscle cells develop and become oriented in the direction in which their contractility will be exerted. They are termed **smooth muscle cells** and are under the control of the autonomic nervous system, not under conscious control, as are skeletal muscles. The blood vessels that develop in the head region, limbs, and body wall gain their muscular coat from local mesenchyme.

Cardiovascular System

The cardiovascular system originates from cells termed **angioblasts**, which arise from **angiogenic clusters** from the visceral mesoderm located in the walls of the yolk sac during the third week of prenatal life (Fig. 1.24). As these cells separate into clusters, the outer cells organize into a series of elongating tubes and the inner cells become blood cells (Fig. 1.25). For the first few weeks, nutrition moves from the yolk sac to the embryo through the developing **vitelline vascular system** (Fig. 1.26). The entire blood vascular system within the embryo is created in the same manner, with longitudinal growth of vessels and the appearance of blood cells within them. As vessels begin to develop in the embryo, they in turn form a vascular network connected to the placenta. Because it traverses the umbilical cord, this network is termed the **umbilical system** (see Fig. 1.26). Through this umbilical system, nutrition and oxygen are conducted to the embryo

and carbon dioxide and wastes to the placenta. By the fourth week, the heart begins to beat. This vascular system takes over the functions as the vitelline system expires because the yolk sac has nothing more to contribute (see Fig. 1.26).

Other mesenchyme cells migrate into the pericardial area to function in the development of heart tubes, and these cells later differentiate into cardiac muscle. Two angiogenic cell clusters initially form the straight bilateral endocardial heart tubes, which fuse during the third week. They then enlarge and bend back on themselves (Fig. 1.27). As the great vessels that bring blood to the heart enlarge and become more extensive, the heart grows and internal partitioning begins. An opening persists between the right and left atria (**foramen ovale**) until birth. As the heart tube enlarges and twists during development, strands of muscle take on the arrangement of parallel fibers. Like striated muscle, cardiac muscle fibers are also striated and have an array of specialized gap junctional complexes between adjacent cells, forming

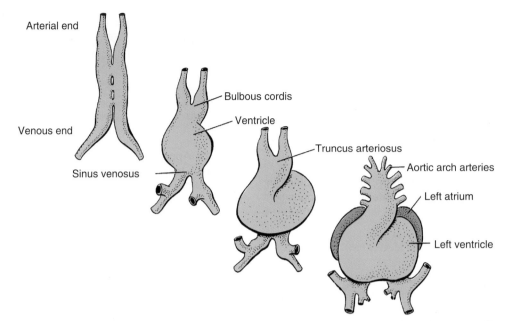

Fig. 1.27 Development of the four-chamber heart from fusion of two bilateral endocardiac heart tubes. Tubes fold laterally into a single tube, which is next divided by internal septa into a four-chamber heart.

intercalated disks. The myofibrils on either side of these disks exert contraction through the interaction of these many cells. Cardiac muscle is thus not under conscious control and begins to beat during the fourth week. Umbilical circulation then becomes active in transporting oxygen and nutrition from the placenta.

CLINICAL COMMENT

The human placenta is often considered in terms of its function in exchanging fetal oxygen and carbon dioxide. It also exchanges nutrients and electrolytes such as proteins and carbohydrates. The placenta produces hormones such as human chorionic gonadotropin, placental growth factor, human placental lactogen, and progesterone and estrogen, which can help maintain pregnancy. It also produces a lactogenic hormone that gives the fetus first priority on circulating maternal blood glucose.

Developmental Abnormalities

Developmental defects may be environmental or hereditary. Most developmental defects are usually an interaction between environmental and hereditary factors. Not much can be done to reduce hereditary factors in humans. However, a great deal has been learned about dietary and stress factors and when they may affect development. For example, it is known that the developing human is least susceptible to teratogens during the proliferative period, which is the first 2 weeks after conception. Because of multiple cell mitosis, compensation may occur. However, the third through the eighth weeks are the most critical time in development, because this is the period of differentiation. During this time, the embryo tissues and organs are developing into specific structures. Serious malformations may arise during this period. The fetal period from 8 weeks until

birth is a declining period of susceptibility. Only minor defects may occur during this period.

Hereditary causes of abnormalities may result from either genetic or chromosomal abnormalities. Many chromosomal abnormalities may result from an increase or a decrease in number from the normal number of chromosomes (46) in humans. DNA transcription is an example of **gene expression**. Transcription generates mRNA that carries information for protein synthesis, as well as transferring ribosomal and other RNA molecules that have structural and catalytic functions. RNA molecules synthesize RNA polymerase enzymes, which make an RNA copy of a DNA sequence.

Genetic abnormalities can perpetuate from one generation to the next. Abnormal development may be caused by expression of defective genes, which may be dominant or recessive. A dominant gene expresses itself whether it is on one member of the pair of homologous chromosomes or both pairs. A recessive gene expresses itself only when it is present on both members of the homozygous chromosomes. An example of a dominant genetic abnormality is dentinogenesis imperfecta, which results in defective dentin formation. Some examples of autosomal recessive genetic disorders include sickle cell disease and cystic fibrosis. There are also sex-recessive (X-linked) defects, including hemophilia and Duchenne muscular dystrophy.

Nerves develop in conjunction with the developing muscle fibers. By the end of the seventh week, the fibers of the fifth nerve have entered the mandibular muscle mass, as has the seventh nerve in the facial muscle mass in the second arch (see Fig. 3.12). As these muscle masses develop, the nerves are present and follow or lead them as they migrate to their position of differentiation, maturation, and function. The seventh nerve supplies the stylohyoid and stapedius muscles and the posterior belly of the digastric muscle. The ninth (glossopharyngeal)

TABLE 1.2 Summary of Structures That Develop From Pharyngeal Arches, Pharyngeal Grooves, and Pharyngeal Pouches

Branchial Grooves	Branchial Arch Structures					Pharyngeal Pouches
Adult derivative	Arch number	Cranial nerve	Branchiomeric muscles	Skeletal derivative	Aortic arch	Adult derivative
External auditory meatus	I Mandibular	V Trigeminal	Muscles of mastication, anterior belly of digastric, mylohyoid, tensor tympani, tensor palatini	Malleus, incus, sphenomandibular ligament, sphenomalleolar ligament (Meckel cartilage)	I	
	1					1. Middle ear Eustachian tube
	II Hyoid	VII Facial	Muscles of facial expression, stapedius, stylohyoid, posterior belly of digastric	Stapes, styloid process, stylohyoid ligament, lesser cornu of hyoid, upper part of body of hyoid	II	
	2					
Cervical fistula	III	IX Glossopharyngeal	Stylopharyngeus	Greater cornu of hyoid, lower part of body of hyoid	III	2. Palatine tonsil
	3					3. Thymus, inferior parathyroid
	IV	X Vagus	Laryngeal musculature, pharyngeal constrictors	Laryngeal cartilages	IV	
	4					4. Superior parathyroid
	V	XI Spinal accessory	Sternocleidomastoid Trapezius		VI	5. Ultimobranchial body

nerve enters the third arch and supplies the stylopharyngeal and upper pharyngeal constrictor muscles. The tenth (vagus) nerve innervates muscles of the fourth arch, which are the inferior constrictors and laryngeal muscles. The tongue, which is primarily muscle, is innervated by branches of the ninth nerve (IX), which carries the sensory modality of taste from the taste buds located in the posterior one-third of the tongue and by the seventh nerve (VII), specifically the chorda tympani nerve, which carries the modality of taste from the taste buds on the anterior two-thirds of the tongue. Motor (efferent) innervation to the intrinsic muscles of the tongue is from the hypoglossal nerve (XII). The fifth nerve is the sensory nerve to the same area of the anterior tongue (see Fig. 3.12). The tongue is a good example of muscle cell migration because it originates in the occipital myotome and migrates anteriorly into the floor of the mouth. During migration, the nerves mentioned enter the muscle mass and later carry out their functions (see Fig. 3.12). Functions and tests for cranial nerves are discussed in Table 1.1. Structures derived from Pharyngeal Arches, Grooves and Pouches are discussed in Table 1.2.

SELF-EVALUATION QUESTIONS

1. What is the smallest unit of structure, and what are its eight functions in the body?
2. Name the structures found in cell cytoplasm and describe their functions.
3. Discuss the mitochondrion relative to where it is found, its function, and some unique characteristics.
4. Name the cells that do not undergo division.
5. Describe apoptosis and discuss why it is critical during development.
6. Describe changes in the embryonic disk during the third and fourth prenatal weeks.
7. Define the cell cycle and describe the activities that occur in the G1, S, and G2 phases.
8. What is the significance of the angiogenic clusters found in the vitelline and umbilical vascular systems?
9. What develops from the gastrointestinal tract?
10. Describe the characteristics of the three prenatal periods.
11. Name three types of cartilage and describe where they are in the human body.
12. Name and describe three types of muscle fibers.

CONSIDER THE PATIENT

Discussion: Two diagnostic tests are available. Amniocentesis is the withdrawal of a small amount of amniotic fluid; it reveals genetic disorders and the age of the fetus. Fetal ultrasound reflects body tissues to the video monitor; it reveals abnormal or normal development, vitality, sex, and fetal age. Neither test causes tissue damage. Ultrasound would be the choice in this case.

QUANDARIES IN SCIENCE

The ability to regenerate new organs is predicated on the principle that regeneration will recapitulate embryologic development. Embryologic development is a complex series of events that includes many steps that are highly regulated by a multitude of chemical signals including genes, transcription factors, and growth factors. Many scientists are actively engaged in research to better understand the role of specific molecules in the orchestration of the zygote's transformation from a single cell to an independent functional organism. Although scientists have made many advances into understanding the processes involved in development, including sequencing of the human genome, many aspects are still unknown and are under active investigation. What will happen and what will be the consequences when scientists can actually "make" a human and regenerate body parts?

CLINICAL CASE

A young nulliparous woman recently went on a honeymoon to the Caribbean. While she was surfing, she noticed a mosquito bite on her forearm. She was concerned because she and her partner were planning on having a family and were not using birth control. During the next week she noticed eye redness, a slight fever, intermittent headaches, muscle and joint pain, and a skin rash, all suggestive of having contracted a Zika virus infection. On return, the patient visits her primary care physician to test her blood or urine for evidence of Zika virus infection.

What are the potential consequences of a Zika infection on the developing child?

The Zika arbovirus is known to cause microcephaly and other neurologic deficits in a developing child. Microcephaly is due to failure of the brain to develop normally and can also be caused by other infectious agents such as rubella, toxoplasmosis, or cytomegalovirus. At present, there is no treatment or preventative measures against the Zika virus. Blood and urine tests for Zika are the most common ways to determine a positive diagnosis for Zika, although the virus is also present in seminal and vaginal fluids as well as saliva. There are guidelines issued by the World Health Organization (WHO) that discuss when to resume trying to become pregnant.

SUGGESTED READING

Abel E. Paternal contribution to fetal alcohol syndrome. *Addict Biol.* 2004;9(2):127–133. [discussion: 135–136].

Avery JK, ed. *Oral development and histology.* 3rd ed. Stuttgart: Thieme Medical; 2002.

Carlson BM. *Human embryology and developmental biology.* 5th ed. St. Louis: Mosby; 2014.

Garcia E, Yactayo S, Nishino K, et al. Zika virus infection: global update on epidemiology and potentially associated clinical manifestations. *Weekly Epidemiol Rec.* 2016;91:73–81.

Gourinat AC, O'Connor O, Calvez E, et al. Detection of Zika virus in urine. *Emerg Infect Dis.* 2015;21(1):84–86.

Hart TC, Marazita ML, Wright JT. The impact of molecular genetics on oral health paradigms. *Crit Rev Oral Biol Med.* 2000;11:26–56.

Hill SL, Russell K, Hennessey M, et al. Transmission of Zika virus through sexual contact with travelers to areas of ongoing transmission: continental United States, 2016. *MMWR Morb Mortal Wkly Rep.* 2016;65(8):215–216.

Jurisicova A, Acton BM. Deadly decisions: the role of genes regulating programmed cell death in human preimplantation embryo development. *Reproduction.* 2004;128:281–291.

Moore KL. *The developing human.* 10th ed. Philadelphia: WB Saunders; 2016.

Nishida K, Yamato M, Hayashida Y, et al. Corneal reconstruction with tissue-engineered cell sheets composed of autologous oral mucosal epithelium. *N Engl J Med.* 2004;351:1187–1196.

Sadler TW, ed. *Langman's medical embryology.* 9th ed. Baltimore: Lippincott Williams & Wilkins; 2004.

Sperber GH. *Craniofacial development.* Hamilton, Canada: BC Decker; 2001.

Tortora GJ. *Principles of human anatomy.* 7th ed. New York: Harper Collins; 1995.

Trasler JM, Doerksen T. Teratogen update: paternal exposures-reproductive risks. *Teratology.* 1999;60(3):161–172.

Structure and Function of Cells, Tissues, and Organs

LEARNING OBJECTIVES

- Discuss how the various tissues of the body build on one another.
- Describe the components of specific organ systems such as the skin and its accessories, the digestive system, the

respiratory system, the vascular system, the lymphatic system, the endocrine system, the urinary system, the reproductive system, and the special senses.
- List general functions of each of these organ systems.

OVERVIEW

This chapter describes the structure and function of the body's four primary tissues: epithelial, neural, connective, and muscle. This chapter continues with a description of the tissues and how they function in making up organs and organ systems. This chapter initially describes cells and tissue types and their structure, location, and function in the body. For example, simple squamous epithelium lines the blood vascular and respiratory systems, the kidney, most glands, and the intestine. Stratified squamous epithelium, on the other hand, covers the body and is the lining of the mouth, the pharynx, larynx, vagina, anus, and part of the urinary bladder.

Neural tissue is the first tissue type considered. Both the **central nervous system (CNS)**, which is composed of the brain and spinal cord, and the nerves and their ganglia, which comprise the peripheral nervous system, are described. The basic structural unit of the nervous system is the neuron. Along with the supporting neuroglial cells, this tissue forms a communication network. The two properties of a neuron are its excitability and conductivity, both of which enable neurons to react and respond to stimuli. The third tissue type discussed is connective tissue, characterized by its abundant extracellular matrix and composed of fibers and amorphous substance. This tissue is classified according to associated cells, fibers, location, and function. Connective tissue proper consists of loose and dense connective tissue and loose connective tissue with special properties. Two other specialized types of connective tissue are cartilage and bone. Three types of cartilage are described—hyaline, elastic, and fibrous—followed by both cancellous (spongy) and compact (dense) bone. A fourth type of connective tissue is blood and lymph, which function to carry oxygen and nutrients to the body tissues and to carry carbon dioxide to the lungs, where it is eliminated.

The three types of muscle—striated, smooth, and cardiac—are described according to cell shape, matrix, and their functions in the body. Organ systems are then described to illustrate how tissues combine to carry out specialized functions in the human body. These organ systems are integumentary, digestive, respiratory, vascular, lymphatic, endocrine, urinary, reproductive, and special senses. Correlative tables help explain this information. These descriptions are meant only as an introduction to tissues of the human body; for more complete information, refer to a comprehensive textbook of histology.

CELLS AND TISSUES

Epithelial Tissue

Epithelial tissue consists of different layers. One is a superficial layer of closely packed sheets of cells covering the external surface of the body, known as the epidermis. Another, the **dermis**, is the connective tissue layer of the skin underlying the epithelial tissue. A much thinner layer of epithelial tissue also lines the internal cavities of the body and the tubes that drain glands and carry blood throughout the body. Most epithelium has the capability of cell renewal by mitosis of the basal cell layer, and the rate of renewal is dependent on the location of the epithelium in the body. For example, human buccal mucosa (Fig. 2.1) renews in 10 to 14 days, whereas the junctional epithelium of the gingiva renews in 4 to 6 days.

The dermis is closely associated and adherent to the **epidermis** and has an interdigitating relationship with it in some areas. Because epithelium does not contain blood vessels, the skin depends on blood vessels located in the connective tissue of the dermis. The vessels are in close proximity, nourishing the skin and playing an important part in its function of thermal regulation. Nerves also exist in the dermis, and some penetrate the epithelial layer to function as receptors. Sweat glands, hair follicles and their associated sebaceous glands, and erector pili muscles are located in the dermis and subcutaneous tissues. Ectoderm is the source of the epithelial lining of some internal organs but not of all epithelial-lined surfaces. For example, the epithelial lining of the peritoneal cavity and endothelial lining of blood vessels are from mesoderm. Epithelium is described according to cell shape and cell arrangement in one or more layers. Some cells form a single layer known as **simple epithelium**. Epithelium with all cells in contact with the basal lamina but not with the surface is known as **pseudostratified**. The type consisting of several cell layers, with only the basal cell layer in contact with the basal lamina, is known as **stratified epithelium** (Fig. 2.2). Further modifications are based on cell shape. For example, the surface cells may be flattened, as in keratinized stratified squamous epithelium of the palm of the hand (see Fig. 2.2).

Epithelial membranes function in one or more of the absorptive processes: contractility, digestion, secretion, excretion, protection, and sensation. Table 2.1 illustrates the classification of epithelia by cell type, cell shape, cell modifications, characteristics, and location.

Neural Tissue

Neural tissue is a second type of tissue. Nerve tissue arises from neuroepithelial cells, which are highly organized areas for reception and correlation. The nervous system carries out numerous functions with only two principal types of cells, which are the **neurons** and the **neuroglia**. Neurons are the nerve cells that receive and conduct impulses and regulate muscle and gland activity. Neuroglial cells are the supporting cells of the nervous system. Each neuron consists of three parts. The first part is the **cell body** or **perikaryon**, which contains the nucleus and the **cytoplasm**. The cytoplasm contains a chromatophilic substance or rough endoplasmic reticulum (RER). The function of the RER, as in other cells, is protein synthesis. Sensory ganglia are accumulations of cell bodies outside the enlargements associated with, for example, each of the spinal nerves containing unipolar or pseudounipolar ganglion cells held together with a connective tissue capsule. These ganglia are called *dorsal root ganglia of the spinal cord* (Fig. 2.3). Some ganglia associated with the cranial nerves include the trigeminal, facial, glossopharyngeal, and hypoglossal cranial nerves (Fig. 2.4).

Proteins travel from the perikaryon by **axoplasmic transport** into the second part of the neuron, the **axon**, which is a long, thin, singular process that varies in length from a few millimeters to several feet or more. Anterograde axoplasmic transport is responsible for moving substances and organelles in the direction of the synapse, and retrograde axoplasmic transport moves substances and organelles in the opposite direction of the synapse. The axon conducts nerve impulses away from the nerve cell body. It terminates by branching into **axon terminals**, or synaptic terminals. Most axons outside the CNS are protected and insulated by a myelin sheath, which is a multilayer of phospholipid produced by the neurilemma

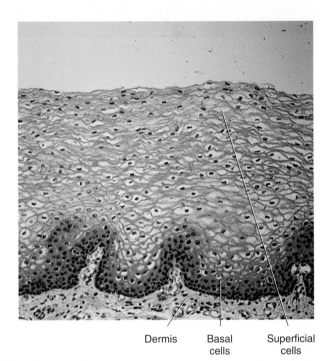

Fig. 2.1 Stratified squamous nonkeratinized epithelium from the oral cavity. Darker stained cells are basal cells. These are dividing to form more superficial layers. As the cells develop in the basal layer, they gradually migrate to the surface and are then lost by attrition.

Dermis   Basal cells   Superficial cells

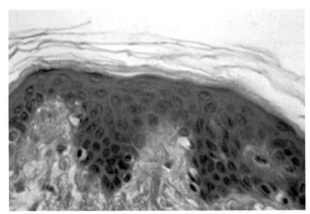

Fig. 2.2 Stratified squamous keratinized epithelium. This epithelium is distinctive in that its surface layers are dead and nonnucleated, and cell contents are filled with keratin. This skin is located on the palms of the hands and soles of the feet.

(Schwann cells) (Fig. 2.5). The third component of the neuron is the **dendrite;** usually there are multiple dendrites, which receive impulses and conduct these impulses to the cell body (Fig. 2.6).

Neuroglial cells carry out the functions of support. These are 5 to 50 times more numerous than neurons. Neuroglial cells protect and support nerve cells, and some are even **phagocytic**, meaning that they ingest bacteria.

TABLE 2.1 Classification of Epithelia

Cell Type	Cell Shape	Cell Modifications	Characteristics	Location
Simple				
1. Squamous				
a. Endothelial	Spindle			Lines heart, blood, lymph vessels
b. Mesothelial	Oval to polygonal			Lines pleural, pericardial, peritoneal cavities
2. Cuboidal	Cube		Cilia may appear	Kidney, glands, respiratory passages
3. Columnar	Rodlike		Cilia, stereocilia	Most glands, small intestines, respiratory passages
4. Pseudostratified	Rodlike with thin section		Microvilli, cilia may appear	Respiratory passages, male reproductive organs
Stratified				
1. Squamous	Polyhedral		Intercellular bridges	Covering of the body, mouth, pharynx, vagina
2. Columnar	Columnar cells on cuboidal or columnar on columnar			Oropharynx, larynx
3. Transitional	Cube to pear		Distension causes cell flattening	Urinary passages, bladder

Images from Gartner LP, Hiatt JL. *Color textbook of histology*. 3rd ed. St. Louis: Saunders; 2007.

CLINICAL COMMENT

Oral infections can cause pain, tenderness, swelling, and enlarged lymph nodes. Pain is the result of the response of a nerve receptor and its transmission to the brain, with corresponding efferent response to both autonomic and somatic systems, and includes a psychological component in humans. Physiologic pain is known as **nociception** and does not include the psychological component. This results in a change in vascular tone and permeability, causing swelling. Lymph nodes enlarge as defense cells proliferate and become active, filtering and destroying the bacteria and their products in the local lymph nodes.

CONNECTIVE TISSUE

Connective tissue varies in its proportion of cells, fibers, and intercellular substance and its location in the body. **Connective tissue proper** is classified as **loose** (Fig. 2.7), **dense** (Fig. 2.8), or **loose connective tissue with special properties**. It functions in tissue support and in protection of the body parts in areas of fluid exchange and storage of adipose (fat) tissue. The ligaments that attach bones and the tendons that attach muscles to bones are forms of dense connective tissue.

Cartilage

The three types of cartilage are **hyaline** (Fig. 2.9), **elastic** (Fig. 2.10), and **fibrous** (Fig. 2.11). These are known as specialized connective tissues. Hyaline cartilage is the most common type of cartilage and is present in the nose, the tracheal rings, the larynx, the articular rings and bronchi, the ventral ends of the ribs, and the articulating surfaces of the long bones. Elastic cartilage has abundant elastic fibers in its matrix and functions in the epiglottis, in the cuneiform cartilage of the larynx, and in the auditory canal and tube. Fibrous cartilage contains bundles of collagen fibers associated with either hyaline cartilage or dense regular connective tissue. It is located in the vertebral disks and intervertebral areas, the insertion of some tendons, and the pubic symphysis.

Bone

Bone is calcified connective tissue. Although it is one of the harder connective tissues that resists deformation, it is responsive to stress and strain. An example of this is during tooth movement, when fibers embedded in the bone are compressed

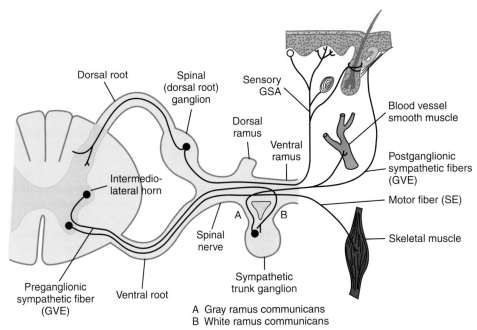

Fig. 2.3 Cross section of a spinal nerve. This figure is representative of a typical cross section of a spinal nerve. There are 31 pairs of spinal nerves in the human body: 8 cervical, 12 thoracic, 5 lumbar, 5 sacral, and 1 coccygeal. They emerge through the intervertebral foramen between the vertebrae. The dorsal roots have afferent nerve fibers (sensory-general sensory afferent *[GSA]*), while the ventral roots contain two types of efferent fibers (sympathetic-general visceral efferent *[GVE]* and somatic efferent *[SE]*). The sensory fibers of the dorsal root have cell bodies located in the dorsal root ganglia and terminate in a variety of receptors (e.g., Pacinian corpuscles). The ventral root contains SE nerves that innervate various skeletal muscles of the trunk. The preganglionic sympathetic GVE nerves synapse in the sympathetic trunk ganglion with the postganglionic fibers, innervating blood vessel smooth muscle as well as other structures containing smooth muscle (e.g., piloerector muscles).

on one side of the tooth, resulting in bone resorption and tension on the other, with subsequent bone remodeling. Bone is classified as **compact** (dense) or **cancellous** (spongy) (Figs. 2.12 and 2.13). Endochondral and intramembranous (membranous) are terms describing their origin, and are discussed in other chapters.

Blood

Blood conducts oxygen to the cells, returns carbon dioxide from the cells to the lungs, clots to prevent blood loss, and regulates pH through a buffer system (Fig. 2.14). It also regulates body temperature and provides protection from bacteria through its phagocytic and antigenic properties. Plasma is the fluid part of the blood in which the cells and particulate substances are suspended. Men have about 5 L of blood, and women have about 4.5 L, which is about 7% of body weight. The erythrocytes (red blood cells) are not true cells, because they have no nucleus or other organelles. However, these cells do have the ability to take oxygen from the lungs, transport it to the tissues, and return carbon dioxide from these tissues to the lungs. Leukocytes (white blood cells) are of two types, granular and nongranular. Leukocyte cell types and functions are shown in Table 2.2.

Details of cellular and other elements of blood are also noted in Table 2.2. Each type of connective tissue has specific associated cells and fibers with special functions and locations in the body (Table 2.3).

Lymphocytes

Lymphocytes arise and become functional in the bone marrow. They are responsible for the humorally activated (innate) immune system. Lymphocytes include natural killer cells, which are associated with cell-mediated, cytotoxic innate immunity; T cells associated with cell-mediated, cytotoxic adaptive immunity; and B cells associated with humoral, antibody-adaptive immunity. They are the main type of cell found in lymph.

Lymphocytes circulate in the lymphatic vessels and in the bloodstream, functioning wherever they are called on by antigen actions. T cells have several different surface molecules that have the function of calling the T cells into action. B memory cells also function as well as plasma cells to produce antibodies in response to various types of foreign substances.

Muscle Tissue

The reaction to stimulus is motion, and the basis of motion in a muscle cell is the change from chemical to mechanical energy by enzymatic cleavage of adenosine triphosphate (ATP). This is a result of the action of two proteins, **actin** and

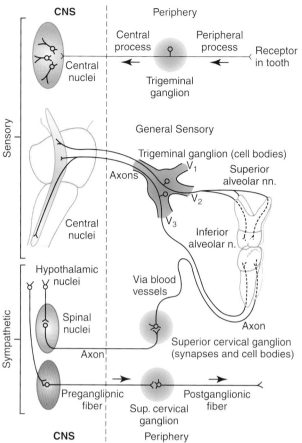

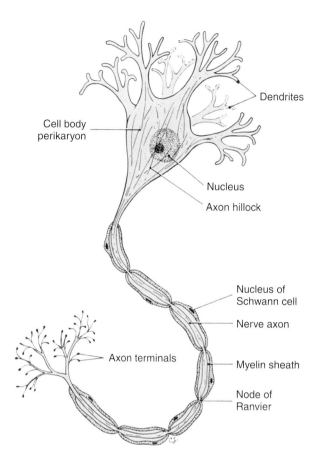

Fig. 2.4 Sympathetic-sensory/CNS-periphery. Using the sensory and sympathetic innervation to the head, this figure demonstrates the differences in the two systems and the nomenclature associated with each one. The peripheral nerves and ganglia are located to the right of the *dotted line*, and the nuclei in the central nervous system *(CNS)* are located to the left of the *dotted line*. (Beachey W. *Respiratory care anatomy and physiology: foundations for clinical practice.* 2nd ed. St. Louis: Mosby; 2007.)

Fig. 2.6 Diagram of a nerve cell and its processes. Myelin insulates the axon and is produced by Schwann cells. Impulses received by the dendrites travel to the cell body and then to the axon terminals, where they may contact the dendrites of an adjacent nerve cell.

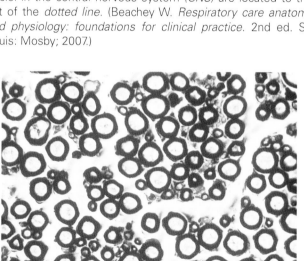

Fig. 2.5 A nerve fiber surrounded by a myelin sheath and a Schwann cell. Myelin insulates the nerve axon and is produced by Schwann cells. The axon is a single, thin process capable of transmitting impulses to other neurons. Impulses are received by the dendrites and travel to the cell body and then the axon terminals, where they may contact dendrites of an adjacent nerve cell.

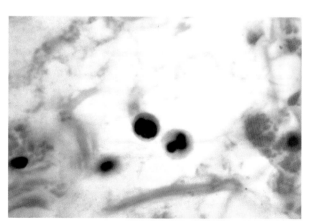

Fig. 2.7 Appearance of loose areolar connective tissue. Observe the collagen and elastin fibers and numerous fibroblasts seen in loose connective tissue.

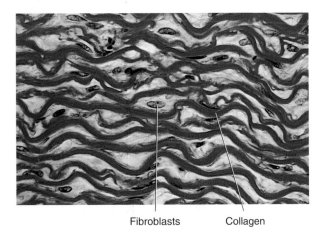

Fibroblasts Collagen
fibers

Fig. 2.8 Appearance of dense regular connective tissue. Large bundles of collagen fibers appear in longitudinal section, with a few pale-stained fibroblasts interspersed between them. The faint banding of these collagen fibers cannot be seen at this magnification.

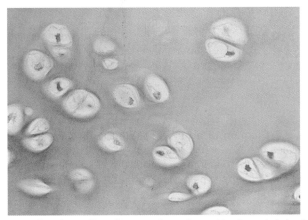

Fig. 2.9 Section of hyaline cartilage found in the adult in the thyroid or tracheal cartilages. The large cells (chondrocytes) are surrounded by a homogenous-appearing cartilage matrix. Only dark-stained nucleoli can be seen in the nucleus. Cells exist in lacunae, which are open spaces in the matrix. Some cells have divided, and two cells appear in the same lacunae.

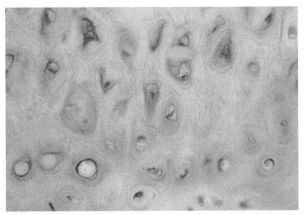

Fig. 2.10 Elastic cartilage present in ear, epiglottis, auditory tube, and auditory canal. Elastic fibers are present in the matrix, as well as type II collagen fibers, and a perichondrium is present.

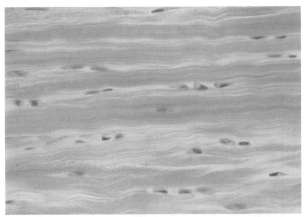

Fig. 2.11 Fibrous cartilage with bundles of collagen fibers in the matrix. This cartilage is present in the vertebral and articular disks and contains type I collagen. The chondrocytes are arranged in parallel rows between collagen bundles.

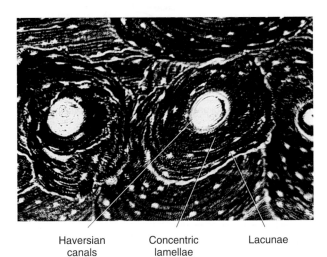

Haversian Concentric Lacunae
canals lamellae

Fig. 2.12 Cross section of compact bone. Tubular haversian canals are surrounded by concentric lamellae and lacunae appearing along the lamellae. This pattern indicates the deposition pattern of the bone. Between the haversian systems are some interstitial lamellae. In living bone, osteocytes would appear as live cells within the lacunae.

myosin, which are arranged in the direction of contraction. Muscle is located throughout the body and consists of three types: **skeletal** or **voluntary** (Fig. 2.15), **smooth** or **involuntary** (Fig. 2.16), and **cardiac** (Fig. 2.17). Skeletal muscle allows movement under voluntary control. Involuntary muscle (smooth muscle) is found in the walls of larger blood vessels and in the gastrointestinal tract and within glands, and it assists with digestion and movement of food through the alimentary tract. The cardiac muscle of the heart (involuntary) pumps blood through some 50,000 miles of blood vessels. Therefore the three muscle types in the body have specific characteristics permitting individualized functions. However, some features of muscle are common to all types. For example, each entire muscle is covered with a **perimysium**, each muscle fascicle (a group of muscle fibers) is covered with an **epimysium**, and each muscle fiber is covered

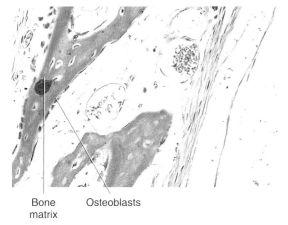

Bone   Osteoblasts
matrix

Fig. 2.13 Appearance of cancellous bone. Trabeculae of bone are seen with osteoblasts and osteoclasts appearing on their surface. In newly forming intramembranous bone, many osteoblasts would be on the surface of the trabeculae. A few elongated and flattened osteoblasts can be seen on the bone surface. Several thin-walled veins, which contain red blood cells, and scattered connective tissue cells can be seen in the field.

with an **endomysium**. Each muscle type contains actin and myosin, which enable the contractions so vital to muscle function. Table 2.4 shows the muscles' locations and the cells that function within each.

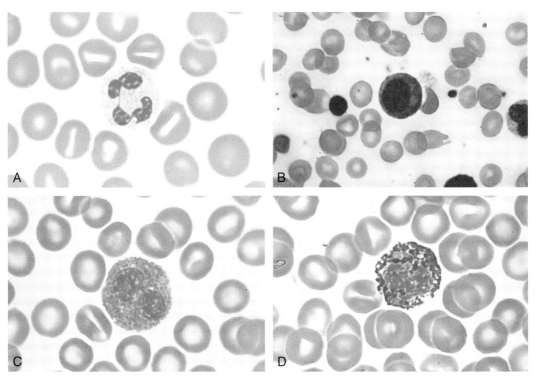

Fig. 2.14 A, Polymorphonuclear leucocytes are the most abundant of the white blood cells. Neutrophils can squeeze through the capillary walls and into infected tissue, where they kill invaders (e.g., bacteria) and engulf the remnants by phagocytosis. **B,** Monocytes leave the blood and become macrophages. A single macrophage surrounded by several lymphocytes and red blood cells can be seen. Macrophages are large phagocytic cells that engulf foreign material (antigens) that enter the body. They are also responsible for phagocytosing dead or dying cells. **C,** Eosinophils are a type of white blood cell that contains granules and takes up the red dye eosin. They accumulate wherever allergic reactions (e.g., asthma) take place. Their natural role is in the defense of parasites and other microorganisms. Allergies such as asthma are probably a malfunction of the body's protective mechanisms and are partially due to eosinophilic reactions. **D,** Basophils are a type of white blood cell that is filled with blue staining granules of chemicals including histamine, serotonin, bradykinin, heparin, and cytokines such as prostaglandins and leukotrienes. Basophils can also digest microorganisms and are responsible for allergy symptoms.

TABLE 2.2   Formed Elements of the Blood

Element		Number	Function
Erythrocytes		Male: 5.4 million/mL^3 Female: 4.8 million/mL^3	Oxygen and carbon dioxide pickup and transport
Leukocytes		5000–9000/mL^3	
Granular	Neutrophils	55%–65%	Phagocytic to infectious agents
	Eosinophils	1%–3%	Helminthic parasitic diseases
	Basophils	0%–0.7%	Histamine, serotonin, heparin
Nongranular	Lymphocytes	20%–35%	Immunologic response, B, T, and natural killer (NK) cells
	Monocytes	3%–7%	Phagocytic, contribute osteoclasts
Platelets		5000–9000/mL^3	Function in clot formation, stimulate cell division

TABLE 2.3   Classification of Connective Tissue

Tissue Type	Associated Cells	Fibers		Location and Function
I. Connective Tissue Proper A. Loose connective tissue	Fibroblasts, macrophages, mast cells	Yellow elastic White collagen		Fascia, superficial and deep; organ framework support
B. Dense connective tissue				
1. Dense regular	Fibroblasts, macrophages	White fibrous		Tendons, ligaments; muscle to bone attachment
2. Dense irregular	Fibroblasts, macrophages	Mostly white fibrous, elastic, and reticular fibers		Sheets, dermis, some sternum, capsules; support of organs
C. Loose connective tissue with special properties				
1. Mucous connective tissue	Stellate fibroblasts	Collagenous		Umbilical and vocal cords; support
2. Elastic tissue	Fibroblasts	Yellow elastic		Ligamenta nuchae, vocal cords; support
3. Reticular tissue	Reticular cells	Fine reticular		Framework of lymph node and spleen
4. Adipose tissue	Fat cells	None		Scattered in all loose connective tissue and in deposits
5. Pigment tissue	Melanoblasts	None		Corium of dark skin, choroid and iris of eye
II. Cartilage A. Hyaline cartilage	Chondrocytes	Fine collagenous		Articular and nasal cartilages, trachea, bronchi; support

TABLE 2.3   Classification of Connective Tissue—cont'd

Tissue Type	Associated Cells	Fibers		Location and Function
B. Elastic cartilage	Chondrocytes	Elastic, collagenous		External; ear, Eustachian tube, epiglottis; support
C. Fibrous cartilage	Chondrocytes	Collagenous (dense)		Intervertebral disks; support
III. Bone				
A. Spongy or cancellous	Osteocytes, osteoblasts, osteoclasts	Collagenous		Center of long bones
B. Compact or dense	Osteocytes, osteoblasts, osteoclasts	Collagenous		Outer shaft of bones
IV. Blood and Lymph				
	Erythrocytes, leukocytes			Blood, vascular, and lymphatic systems

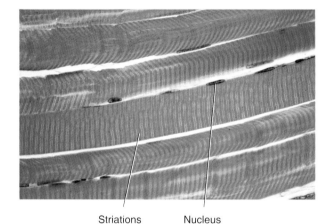

Striations   Nucleus

Fig. 2.15 Skeletal muscle fibers in longitudinal section. Cross striations are seen as alternating light and dark bands, indicating fiber contraction sites. Each large fiber contains a number of nuclei on the periphery. These are muscle fibers of the arms, legs, and body wall. They provide for body posture, locomotion, and arm movement, and are controlled voluntarily.

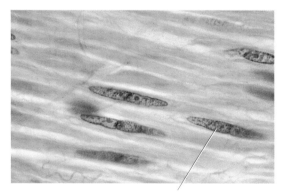

Nucleus of smooth
muscle cell

Fig. 2.16 Smooth muscle fibers in longitudinal section. These can be compared with skeletal muscle shown in Fig. 2.15. Smooth muscle fibers are spindle shaped, with a large, longitudinal nucleus in the center of the fiber. Small amounts of connective tissue surround the fibers. This muscle surrounds the gastrointestinal tract and muscular blood vessels. It is controlled involuntarily.

QUANDARIES IN SCIENCE

Understanding cells and cell signaling, tissues, and organs is vital to understanding how the body can respond to the variety of stimuli that is required for the body to maintain health and respond to injury. These are highly complex processes that are initiated by the stimulus of a particle binding to a receptor on the cell surface, which then is internalized and, eventually, after activating specific intracellular pathways, causes a response that is transmitted from the cellular layer into the tissues and organs. Many of these processes are beginning to be understood, resulting in great strides in the development of applications and treatments; however, much more needs to be accomplished before strategies for personalizing treatments can truly be designed. Since everyone is unique, how will personalized medical and dental treatments become cost effective enough to be available to everyone?

Organs and Organ Systems

Organ systems comprise the tissues in the body that are functionally integrated and specifically designed to perform designated functions. Cells, the basic structural and functional units of the body, may aggregate and form tissues or groups of tissues that are organized together to form organs. These organs consist of all four types of basic tissues, and they form for a specific function, which relates to other organs to form organ systems.

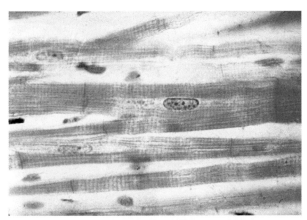

Fig. 2.17 Section of cardiac muscle found in the heart wall. Muscle fibers appear striated and are similar to skeletal muscle fibers, except that some of the fibers branch. The nuclei of these fibers are located centrally, as seen in smooth muscle, and the areas at the ends of the nuclei are pale staining.

Fig. 2.18 shows most of the body's organ systems, which are described in the following sections.

Integumentary or Skin System

The largest organ in the body is the skin, which has numerous functions (Fig. 2.19). One is the excretion of waste products, such as carbon dioxide, water, small amounts of salts, and urea. The skin also eliminates heat and serves as a protection against invasion of foreign materials. The nerves of the skin receive stimuli from outside the body to monitor temperature, pressure,

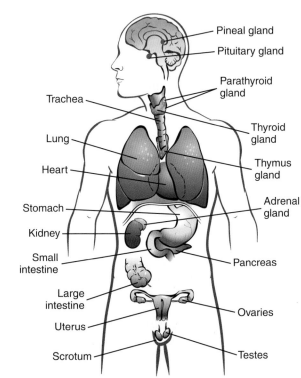

Fig. 2.18 Diagram of the human body. Glands are listed on the *right* side, and organs are listed on the *left*.

TABLE 2.4	Classification of Muscle			
Type	**Cell Shape**	**Diagrams**		**Location**
A. Skeletal wall, voluntary	Very long multinucleated fiber with cross striations composed of actin (thin) and myosin (thick) components			Bony skeleton or fascia, limbs and body, pharynx, upper esophagus
B. Smooth visceral, involuntary	Spindle-shaped fibers with a single elongated nucleus and myofilaments; nuclei located in center of fiber			Hollow organs, wall of intestines, ducts of glands, blood vessels
C. Cardiac muscle striated, involuntary	Long cross-striated fibers that branch and contain intercalated disks (junctional complexes); some muscle fibers are specialized to conduct impulses (e.g., Purkinje fibers); nuclei in center of fiber			Wall of heart, major veins opening into the heart

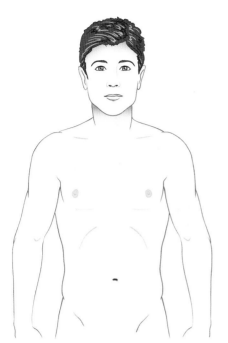

Fig. 2.19 Integumentary system. The skin is the largest organ in the body and serves to protect the body tissues from injury. The glands and nails arise from this layer of skin.

and other environmental influences. The epidermis and dermis constitute the skin. The epidermis rests on a basement membrane that separates it from the dermis (Fig. 2.20). The epithelial cells form membranes that are composed of closely associated cells with an intercellular substance between them. These varying functions are possible because of the skin's many layers of cells and the underlying layers of connective tissue that carry blood vessels, muscles, and nerves. Epithelium has five cell-type layers: a basal or germinating layer, a spinous layer called *stratum spinosum*, a layer of cells with keratohyalin granules called the *granular layer*, a clear layer called the *stratum lucidum*, and the covering layer of keratinocytes that protects all the deeper layers.

The dermis has two layers: a superficial papillary layer and a deep reticular layer. The skin also has hair follicles (Fig. 2.21), sweat glands, and sebaceous glands, which assist in the multifunctional nature of the skin.

Neural System

The neural system is composed of the CNS and the peripheral nervous system (PNS). The CNS is the control center of the nervous system and is composed of the brain and spinal cord (Fig. 2.22). The brain is located in the cranium and is connected to the peripheral tissues by cranial nerves and to the spinal cord by spinal nerves. All sensation received anywhere in the body is relayed to the brain and spinal cord, which act on the sensation. The brain continues into the spinal cord, which is within the vertebral canal. This canal is a cylindrical space extending from the brain to the lumbar vertebrae. It is composed of 31 segments, with spinal nerves coming from each. The spinal cord conveys impulses from the peripheral nervous system to the brain and from the brain to the peripheral tissues.

Nerve processes that carry information and convey it from the peripheral nervous system in skin, muscles, and glands to the CNS are called the **afferent (sensory) system**. Other neurons that convey responses from the CNS to muscles and glands are located in the **efferent (motor) system**. These two systems are further divided into the **somatic** and **autonomic nervous systems**. The nervous system is closely associated with the endocrine system, which is dependent on neural stimuli to function.

The somatic nervous system carries impulses to the voluntary muscles, the skeletal muscles, which are under conscious control. On the other hand, the efferent autonomic system carries impulses from the CNS to involuntary muscles, the smooth and cardiac muscles, and all the glands. The viscera receive most of their impulses from this system.

The autonomic system produces responses involuntarily and is further classified into the **sympathetic** and **parasympathetic divisions**. In general, these two divisions modify each other: the sympathetic division causes increased activity, and the parasympathetic division modifies or decreases activity. Fig. 2.23 outlines the nervous system.

Skeletal System

The skeletal system (Fig. 2.24) supplies the fundamental framework to which all the muscles and ligaments of the body are attached. Bone encloses the brain, spinal cord, and lungs, and offers them protection. Bone marrow is also important in producing the hematopoietic system.

Digestive System

Functions of the digestive system's alimentary canal are to absorb, transform, and extract needed components from food ingested and to excrete all unused solid waste. In addition, carbon dioxide, water, and heat are lost. A long tube (approximately 26 feet, or 8 m) starts with the mouth and oral cavity and progresses to the pharynx and esophagus, which conducts food to the stomach, a mixing and digestive chamber where food is reduced to liquid chyme (Fig. 2.25). Further digestion takes place in the small intestine, which adds glandular secretions from the liver, pancreas, and spleen. The large intestine, which absorbs nutrition, also dehydrates food and compresses it into solid waste. Digestion takes place throughout the tract through the function of salivary glands in the oral cavity; gastric glands in the stomach; the liver, gallbladder, pancreas, and spleen; and in the small intestine (Figs. 2.26 and 2.27). The walls of the tract are composed of functional layers: lining epithelium, connective tissue layers, and layers of muscle. Muscle aids in peristaltic movement of food through the tract.

Respiratory System

The function of the respiratory system is primarily to exchange gases in several phases. The process includes both inflow (inspiration) of oxygen and outflow (expiration) of carbon dioxide. The blood cells exchange oxygen and carbon dioxide with other cells in the body and with the pulmonary air sacs. The respiratory system includes the nasal chambers, in which the air is warmed by blood flowing close to the surface and becomes moist through the mucus secreted by goblet cells. These also trap dust

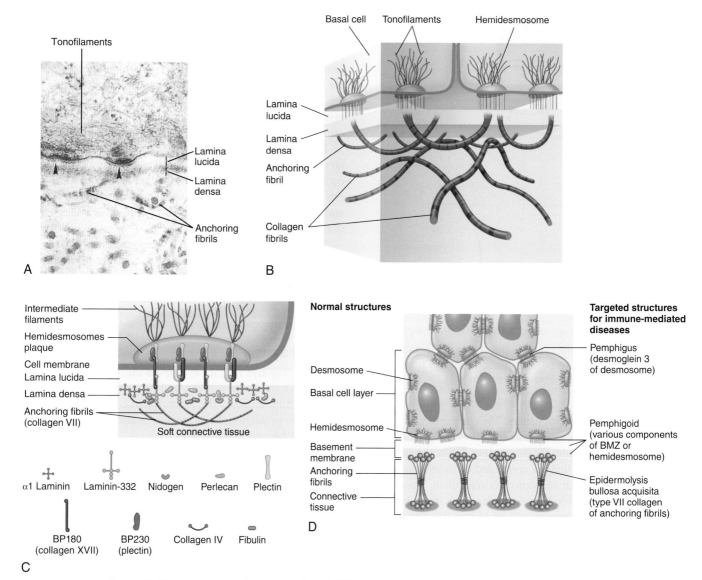

Fig. 2.20 Ultrastructure of basal lamina. **A,** High-magnification electron micrograph of the complex in oral mucosa. Hemidesmosomes *(arrowheads)* at the plasma membrane of epithelial basal cells receive bundles of intermediate filaments (tonofilaments). Adjacent to the membrane are the lamina lucida and lamina densa. Several striated anchoring fibrils loop into the lamina densa, and some contain within their loops cross sections of collagen fibrils. **B,** Schematic representation of the junction between epithelium and connective tissue. **C,** The location of principal molecular constituents of the junction. **D,** *BMZ,* Basement membrane. This figure demonstrates the complexity of the basement membrane. Figure A shows a transmission electron micrograph of the basal lamina (*basement membrane* is the term for the basal lamina at the light microscopic level) with several of the important structures labeled. Figure B is an artist's rendition of the structures in Figure A, with added dimensionality. Figure C demonstrates the molecular components of the basal lamina, as well as more of the structural components.

particles. Cilia of the lining cells of the respiratory tract move these particulate substances to the pharynx and out of the respiratory system. In addition, the system includes the pharynx, trachea, and bronchi, which function as conduction chambers, and the lungs proper, which function in respiration (Fig. 2.28).

Vascular System

The vascular system includes the heart, large elastic arteries, smaller muscular arteries, and miles of capillaries, as well as veins that carry blood from the capillaries back to the heart. It is important to address the changes in the heart during pre- and postnatal life (Fig. 2.29). The heart, which is the size of an adult's clenched fist, pumps an estimated 5 to 6 L of blood approximately 60 times a minute. The function of the bloodstream is to carry oxygen to the cells in all areas of the body and to return carbon dioxide from these cells to the lungs. The blood vascular system provides nutrition from the walls of the alimentary canal and other organs. Blood also carries waste products to the

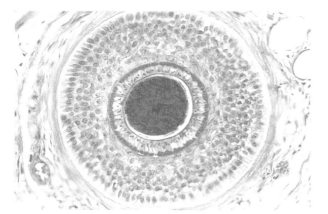

Fig. 2.21 Cross section of a hair follicle. These epithelial structures arise from the basal cells of the skin.

kidneys, the gastrointestinal tract, and other organs of excretion, such as the skin (Fig. 2.30).

Arteries function in the conduction and distribution of blood and nutrients to the entire body, capillaries are used in oxygen exchange and nutrition of the extracellular spaces, and veins return blood to the heart. The blood vascular system additionally functions in blood clotting, and some white blood cells function in phagocytosis and the immune response. Blood also conducts various hormones to their sites of action through the activities of the neuroendocrine system. Table 2.2 shows cellular and other elements of the blood.

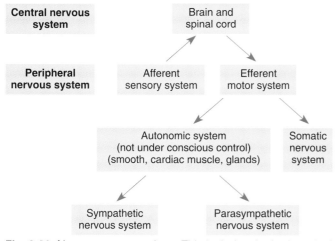

Fig. 2.22 Nervous system chart. This includes the brain, spinal cord, and all of the peripheral nervous system.

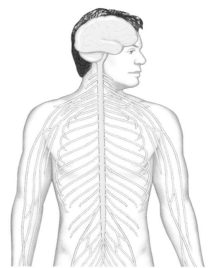

Fig. 2.23 Diagram of the nervous system. The brain, spinal cord, and peripheral nervous system function to regulate body activities. (Thibodeau GA, Patton KT. Structure and function of the body. 15th ed. St. Louis: Elsevier; 2016.)

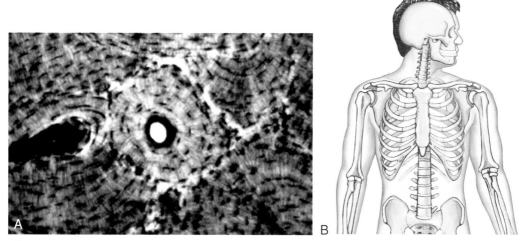

Fig. 2.24 Skeletal system. A, Cartilage and bone. **B**, The entire skeleton of the prenatal human is laid down in cartilage and gradually is transformed into bone. The last cartilage to change to bone is in the proximal and distal parts. The adult skeleton, as seen in B, allows the body to stand erect and to move, providing attachment of the muscles, whereas the bone marrow provides origin of blood cells. (B, Thibodeau GA, Patton KT. Structure and function of the body. 15th ed. St. Louis: Elsevier; 2016.)

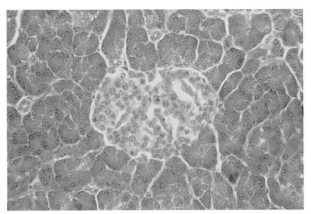

Fig. 2.27 The pancreas is a second important organ associated with the digestive tract. This highly vascularized organ controls glucose production and elimination through the islets of Langerhans, rounded groups of cells found among the renal corpuscles. This organ's secretions enter the large intestine where it attaches to the stomach.

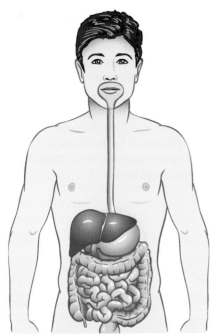

Fig. 2.25 The long tube of the digestive tract provides for physical and chemical breakdown of foods essential to bodily function. Many glands and organs are associated with and deliver their products into this tract.

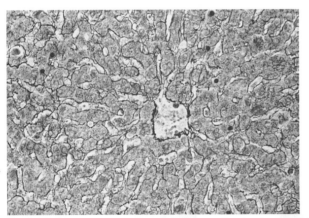

Fig. 2.26 The liver is an important organ in the body. This organ filters the blood, removing all detrimental substances. The blood enters the liver peripherally and circulates through liver cords to the central vein. Note the large oval nuclei of the liver cells. This section of the liver tissue illustrates liver cell cords radiating from a central vein. Blood filters from the periphery of each liver (hepatic) lobule. This organ filters the blood and provides a storage area. Spaces between the cell cords are termed *sinusoids.*

Lymphatic System

The lymphoid organs are part of the immune system and consist of lymph nodes, thymus, and spleen (Figs. 2.31 and 2.32). Other aggregates of lymphatic tissue composed of lymphocytes are in the bone marrow, bloodstream, tonsils, Peyer patches of the ileum in the small intestine, and other locations of the alimentary canal. A characteristic of the immune system is its ability to recognize and react specifically to macromolecules that are foreign to the body.

Muscular System

Muscle tissue is excitable, contractile, extensible, elastic, and adaptable. The striated muscles of the body represent the large muscles of the limbs, chest wall, and neck. They enable all of the actions of the body, such as standing erect, walking, and other bodily movements. Striated muscle is made up of cylindrical fibers under voluntary control of the body. Striated muscle contration functions on the "all-or-none" reaction: as long as the stimulus is above threshold, the muscle will contract and is not dependent on the strength of the stimulus. The myofibrils of muscle are arranged to permit contraction, which provides for movement of the body (see Fig. 2.14). Smooth or involuntary muscles are found in organs to help during secretion, in blood vessels larger than capillaries to control vascular diameter, and in the walls of the intestinal tract to function during peristalsis. Cardiac muscle is contained within the walls of the heart and has unique and specialized properties, including branched fibers and intercalated discs; it has properties of both striated and smooth muscle.

Endocrine System

The endocrine system includes the thyroid, parathyroid, and pituitary glands; ovaries; testes; pancreas; and adrenal medulla. A basic function of these glands is to secrete hormones into the vascular circulation. Hormones then circulate and act only on target cells through the second messenger, cyclic adenosine monophosphate (cAMP). Although 50 or more hormones traverse the bloodstream, each acts only on specific receptor cells. Hormones help regulate metabolism energy balance and aid in regulation of involuntary smooth and cardiac muscle fibers. Hormones vary body activities, regulate centers of the immune system, play a role in growth and development, contribute to the process of reproduction, and regulate volume and composition of the extracellular environment. Some organs have endocrine function but also have other functions. Examples of these organs are the salivary

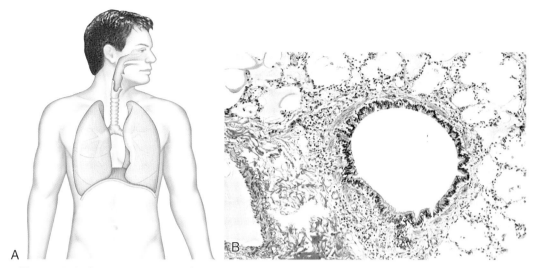

Fig. 2.28 A, Respiratory tract. Air enters the lung through the trachea, then enters the bronchi and the terminal bronchus to the air sacs seen on the left. **B**, A lung section showing a bronchiole in the left of the field and air sacs in the upper right. The bronchiole is lined with simple columnar ciliated epithelium, and signs of inflammation are seen in the cells surrounding the bronchiole. (A, Thibodeau GA, Patton KT. *Structure and function of the body.* 15th ed. St. Louis: Elsevier; 2016.)

glands, pancreas, testes, ovaries, thymus, hypothalamus, stomach, intestine, liver, kidneys, heart, and skin (Fig. 2.33). The hypothalamus is the major neural coordinating system between the nervous and endocrine systems.

Urinary System

The urinary system includes the kidneys, ureters, bladder, and urinary tract. The system filters toxic and unnecessary substances from the bloodstream and concentrates them before excretion. Kidneys excrete not only water but also nitrogenous wastes and bacterial toxins (Fig. 2.34). The major function of the urinary system is to control blood volume and pressure and the composition of urine.

This system also restores water to the blood. In this manner, renin, atrial natriuretic factor, and vasopressin help to regulate blood pressure. Other substances synthesized and secreted by the kidney include the secretion of erythropoietin, which regulates red blood cell production in the bone marrow; the secretion of renin, which is a key part of the renin–angiotensin–aldosterone system; and the secretion of the active form of vitamin D (calcitriol) and prostaglandins. Urine is stored in the urinary bladder until excreted through the external urinary meatus.

Reproductive System

The male reproductive system includes the testes, prostate, and seminal vesicles, and the female system includes the ovaries, uterus, and vagina. The female produces eggs and the male produces sperm, along with secretions of the accessory glands that produce semen. The sperm and the egg each have half the chromosome complement that enables fertilization of the egg, which produces a zygote. The uterus then provides an environment in which the embryo can develop. The testes secrete the hormone testosterone, and the female system produces estrogen and

progesterone to ensure development of the embryo and proper coordination of the menstrual cycle.

Special Senses

The special senses system permits the detection of changes in the surrounding environment. This system includes vision, hearing, equilibrium, smell, and taste.

The eye focuses a distortion-free image on the retina. The retina responds to various colors and intensities and encodes spatial and temporal parameters for transmission to the brain.

The **ear** is composed of three parts. The external ear receives sound waves, the middle ear translates these waves into mechanical vibrations, and the internal ear receives the vibrations and changes them into specific impulses that are transmitted by the acoustic nerve to the brain.

Equilibrium is controlled by the vestibular organs, which are located in the internal ear.

The **olfactory organ** is located in the olfactory epithelium, which is a pseudostratified, ciliated columnar epithelium located in the roof of the nasal cavity over the cribriform plate. The olfactory cells are bipolar nerve cells, and their axons transmit to nerve trunks in the connective tissue underlying the olfactory epithelium. From there, olfactory impulses are transmitted to the brain.

The **taste modality** is located in cells of the taste buds, which are in the circumvallate, fungiform, and foliate papillae within the specialized epithelium on the tongue's dorsal surface and other areas in the oropharyngeal region. Taste is discussed in Chapter 14.

CONSIDER THE PATIENT

A patient comes to the clinic with a puffy face and feels depressed. She describes her muscular weakness, inactivity, and need to spend much time in bed. She has a low heart rate. What do you suspect is causing her symptoms?

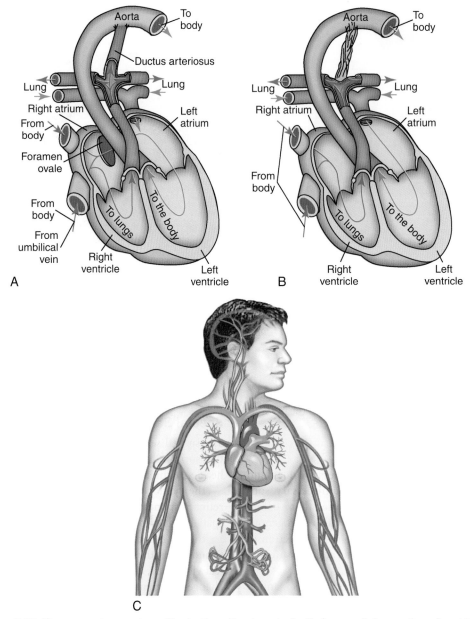

Fig. 2.29 **The vascular system illustrating the heart. A**, Before and 8 months after birth. Prenatally, oxygen comes from the placenta, and the oxygenated blood mixed with nonoxygenated blood enters the right side of the heart and is then sent to the left side of the heart, where it is pumped to the rest of the body. **B**, In the postnatal heart, the foramen ovale between the atria closes. **C**, Overview of the circulatory system, showing blood entering the right side of the heart. (C, Thibodeau GA, Patton KT. *Structure and function of the body*. 15th ed. St. Louis: Elsevier; 2016.)

CLINICAL CASE

A 31-year-old woman presented at the dentist with blistering of the oral mucosa that was not restricted to regional areas of the oral cavity, such as gingiva or under the tongue or cheeks. When asked about the history of these lesions, the patient said they appeared approximately 3 weeks earlier. Her medical history revealed that no other mucosae were affected at this time. The dentist thought that the patient could have an allergy to the specific type of toothpaste she was using and told the patient to come back in 7 days if the blistering had not cleared up. A week later, the patient came back complaining that changing toothpaste did not alleviate the blisters and now other mucosae were involved. The dentist referred the patient to an oral surgeon, who took a biopsy of the lesion, including the adjacent unaffected mucosa. The results from the pathologist diagnosed

pemphigus vulgaris. The patient was referred to an immunologist for further tests and treatment.

Pemphigus vulgaris is an acquired autoimmune disease in which antibodies attack the proteins (desmoglein 3) that form the desmosomal junctional complexes, causing disruption of the epithelium, blistering, and subsequent ulceration. The oral mucosa is likely to be the first site in the body to be affected. The disease is often difficult to diagnose since it is rare (<1 in 100,000 in most populations). The signs and symptoms are similar to other diseases, and it is paramount that the biopsy include both affected and normal tissues. Treatment will vary but usually includes steroids to reduce inflammation. Pemphigus vulgaris is a chronic disease, but if the patient is well educated on treatments, the prognosis is usually good.

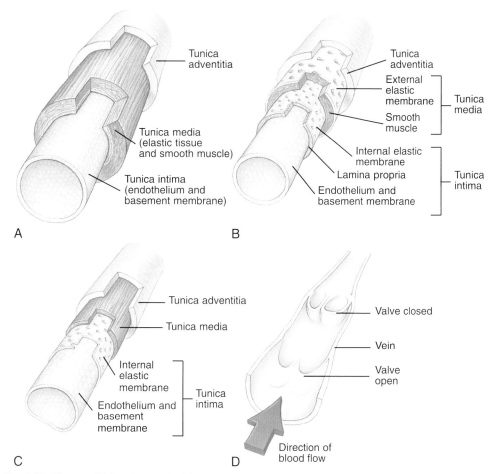

Fig. 2.30 Types of blood vessels. The structures in this figure demonstrate the anatomical characteristics of **A**, general diagram of an artery; **B**, artery; **C**, arteriole; and **D**, vein.

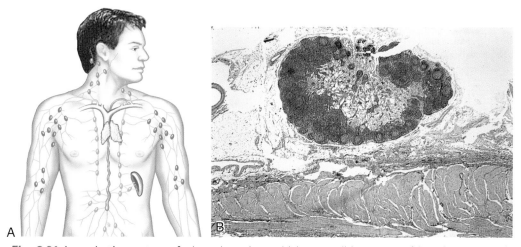

Fig. 2.31 Lymphatic system. A, Lymph nodes, which are solid masses of lymphocytes and lymph channels, are located in all parts of the body. Note the system in the head and neck, thorax, abdomen, and limbs. **B**, The composition of a lymph node, with the dense composition of lymphocytes that serve as filters to remove bacteria from lymph vessels.

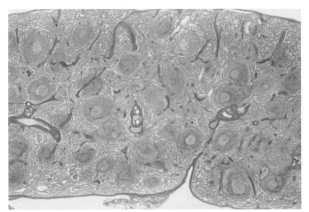

Fig. 2.32 The spleen is the largest lymphoid organ in the body. It is located in the upper left part of the abdomen. It serves as a filter for the blood and is active in destruction of old erythrocytes and in antibody production. It also produces both B and T cells.

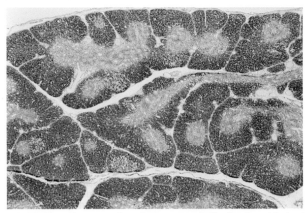

Fig. 2.33 The thymus develops prenatally in the third pharyngeal arch and functions until puberty, when it then begins to atrophy. It primarily functions in T-cell production and in instructing these cells to become immunocompetent.

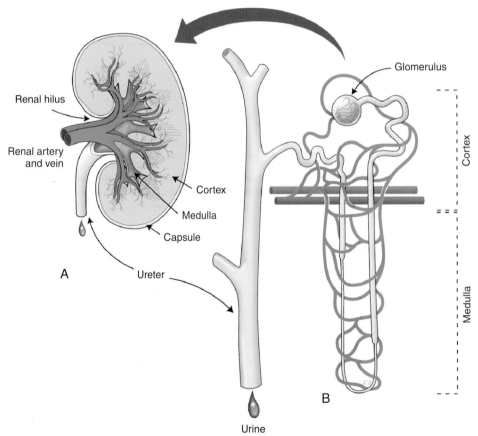

Fig. 2.34 Urinary system. A, The kidneys are filters, removing toxins but conserving water, proteins, glucose, salts, and other essential substances. The kidneys also help regulate blood pressure and acid–base balance. The kidneys then deliver the urine to the urinary bladder. **B,** Uriniferous tubules. All fluids pass through the tubule system as they carry fluid to the glomeruli and urine to the medullary area of the kidney. These highly cellular structures remove important elements and allow the urine to collect for passage to the urinary bladder. The glomeruli are important in recirculating and in toxin removal and retaining water, proteins, sugars, and other important elements.

SELF-EVALUATION QUESTIONS

1. Describe four types of loose connective tissue that have special properties.
2. Describe two types of connective tissue proper.
3. Describe three types of cartilage and their locations in the body.
4. Describe cancellous and compact bone and the location of both types.
5. Describe two types of muscle that have involuntary movement and their functions.
6. What are the simple epithelial cell types and where are they located in the body?
7. Describe the location of stratified squamous and columnar epithelium.
8. Discuss the function of the autonomic nervous system.
9. Describe how the sympathetic and parasympathetic nervous systems work together.
10. Name and briefly describe each of the nine organ systems.

SUGGESTED READING

Berman I. *Color atlas of basic histology.* 3rd ed. Stamford: Appleton & Lange; 2003.

Fawcett D, Jensh R. *Bloom and Fawcett's concise histology.* London: Hodder Arnold; 2002.

Kerr J. *Functional histology.* 2nd ed. St. Louis: Mosby; 2010.

Le Douarin NM, Kalcherin C. *The neural crest.* 2nd ed. New York: Cambridge University Press; 1999.

Tortura GJ. *Principles of human anatomy.* 7th ed. New York: Harper Collins College; 1995.

Weiss L. *Cell and tissue histology.* 5th ed. New York: Elsevier; 1983.

Weiss AT, Delcour NM, Meyer A, et al. Efficient and cost-effective extraction of genomic DNA from formalin-fixed and paraffin-embedded tissues. *Vet Pathol.* 2011;48(4):834–838.

Development of the Oral Facial Region

- Discuss the development of the oropharynx; the pharyngeal arches, including the pharyngeal pouches; and the neural and vascular muscular components.

- Describe the skeletal components and the development of the tissues of the face.

OVERVIEW

This chapter concerns development and orientation of the tissues that form the human face and neck. During the fourth week of development, the human embryo consists of a flat disk that bends down at its anterior extremity as the overlying brain expands and enlarges (Fig. 3.1). This action pushes the heart beneath the brain. A pit develops in the midline between the brain and the heart and becomes the oral cavity, or stomodeum (Fig. 3.2). Beneath this pit, the first **pharyngeal arch (branchial)**, termed the **mandibular arch**, forms. The **maxillary tissues** that form the cheeks also grow from this first arch. Below the mandibular arch, four other pharyngeal arches or bars appear during the fourth to seventh prenatal week. The second arch is called the **hyoid** (Fig. 3.3). These parallel arches are important in the development of the face and neck, and each contains blood vessels, muscles, nerves, and skeletal elements. Aortic arch blood vessels, which course through each pharyngeal arch from the heart below to the brain above, are important to craniofacial development.

The first, second, and fifth of these vessels soon disappear. The third arch vessel quickly assumes the role of supplying nutrients to the tissues of the first and second arches. This third arch vessel also shifts the blood supply to the face from the internal carotid vessels to the external carotid. Muscles arise in each of the pharyngeal arches: the mandibular arch muscles become the masticatory muscles, the second arch muscles become the facial expression muscles, and the muscles of the third and fourth arches become the constrictor muscles of the throat. Cranial nerves enter each of these muscle masses as they arise. The fifth nerve enters the mandibular arch to innervate the muscles of mastication. The seventh innervates the second arch muscle mass, and other cranial nerves, nine and ten, innervate the muscles of the neck. Cartilage also appears in each arch: **Meckel cartilage bar** in the first, the **superior hyoid** in the second, the **inferior hyoid** in the third, and the **laryngeal cartilages** in the fourth. The **cranial base cartilages** arise to support the brain, and from them come the auditory and olfactory sense capsules. All the creative events described in this chapter take place from the fourth to seventh prenatal weeks, the short time required for facial organization.

DEVELOPMENT OF THE OROPHARYNX

The oropharynx is composed of the primitive oral cavity and the area of foregut called the *pharynx*. The oral pit first appears in the fourth week of development, when the neural plate bends ventrally as the neural folds develop to form the forebrain. This cephalocaudal bend pushes the heart ventrally, and the yolk sac becomes enclosed to form an elongating tube known as the *foregut* (see Fig. 3.1).

The deepening oral pit then appears between the forebrain and the heart and eventually becomes the oral cavity (see Fig. 3.2). At its deepest extent is the **oropharyngeal membrane**, which ruptures in the fifth week, opens the oral cavity to the tubular foregut, and soon becomes the **oropharynx** (see Fig. 3.3; Fig. 3.4). The mandibular arch will grow laterally to the oral pit, developing the maxillary process, which forms the cheeks.

The enlarging heart now becomes positioned below the mandibular arch in the thorax and begins beating at the end of the fourth week (see Fig. 3.2). Blood is forced through the vessels in the pharyngeal arches supplying the face, neck, and brain. The forming face now grows away from the forebrain and presses against the chest and heart.

DEVELOPMENT OF THE PHARYNGEAL (BRANCHIAL) ARCHES

The pharyngeal arches are so termed because they bend around the sides of the pharynx as bars of tissue. Each arch is separated by vertical grooves on the lateral sides of the neck at the fifth week. Within the pharynx, grooves called **pharyngeal pouches** separate each arch. These pouches match the pharyngeal clefts on the external aspects of the neck (see Fig. 3.4).

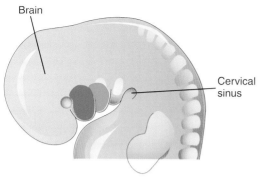

Fig. 3.1 The embryo head bends anteriorly with the growth and expansion to the head. This pushes the heart ventrally, and the oral pit (stomodeum, *see* Fig. 3.2) develops between the brain and the heart. (Moore KL, Persaud TVN, Torchia MG. *The developing human: clinically oriented embryology.* 10th ed. St. Louis: Saunders; 2016.)

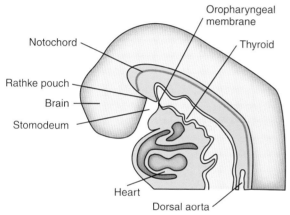

Fig. 3.2 Internal view of the oral pit at 3.5 weeks. The oropharyngeal membrane separated the oral pit (stomodeum) and the pharyngeal cavities. The membranes will then rupture, allowing the two cavities to join.

CLINICAL COMMENT

From the initial development, each pharyngeal arch has a specific cranial nerve associated with it. The nerves and the musculature of each arch emerge together and follow defined pathways to their functional positions. These events are closely regulated genetically during development, and few errors occur.

CONSIDER THE PATIENT

A patient appears with a swelling in the lateral area of the neck and states that the swelling subsides from time to time but then resumes. He asks you what you think the cause may be.

The five arches with their clefts resemble the embryonic gill slits of fish and amphibians. This is one of many similarities between human embryos and other species' embryos during early development. The first arch is termed the *mandibular arch* because it will later form the bony mandible and maxilla and

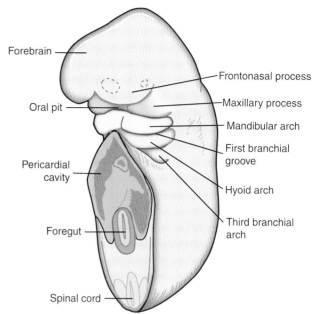

Fig. 3.3 Facial development in the fourth prenatal week. The oral pit is surrounded by the facial primordia, which are the frontonasal processes, the maxillary processes, and the mandibular arch. The pharyngeal arches are defined by grooves between each arch. The heart develops in the thorax, which is in the pericardial cavity.

the associated muscles of mastication, nerves, and blood supply. The second, or hyoid, arch forms the facial muscles, vessels, and hyoid bone. The third, fourth, and fifth arches consist of paired right and left bars that are divided before they reach the midline by the presence of the bulging heart (see Fig. 3.2). The arches become progressively smaller anterior to posterior. The outer surface of each arch is covered with ectoderm, as are the inner surface of the first arch and the covering of the anterior surface of the second. This ectoderm will become the epithelial lining of the oral cavity. The pharyngeal surface of the remaining four arches is, however, lined by endoderm, which is the same as the lining of the gastrointestinal tract (see Fig. 3.4). The cores of the arches—the blood vessels, muscles, nerves, cartilages, and bones—will differentiate and are important in the development of the adult human face.

CLINICAL COMMENT

The face develops during the embryonic period, which includes a short span of time from the end of the second week to the end of the eighth prenatal week. Environmental factors can cause a facial or pharyngeal arch defect, which would probably affect these tissues before the fourth week. This is the time to be especially careful about irradiation and chemical, hormonal, dietary, or stress-related factors.

Pharyngeal Grooves and Pharyngeal Pouches

The first pharyngeal groove deepens to become the **external auditory canal,** leading to the middle ear. The membrane at the depth of this tube becomes the **tympanic membrane.** The

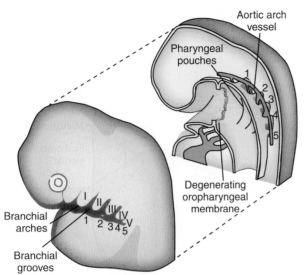

Fig. 3.4 Sagittal view of pharyngeal arches with corresponding groove between each arch. The pharyngeal arches are seen in the wall of the pharynx. The aortic arch vasculature leads from the heart through these arches to the face.

middle ear and **eustachian tube** develop from the corresponding first pharyngeal pouch. After the fifth week, no other pharyngeal grooves are seen externally as the tissues of the second and fifth arch grow over the other arches and grooves and make contact with each other (Fig. 3.5). This overgrowth obscures the tissue of both the arches and the grooves externally, although their internal structures are unaffected and play an important role in facial and body development (see Fig. 3.5).

The endodermal lining of the pharyngeal pouches differentiates into several important organs. The second pharyngeal pouch becomes the **palatine tonsils**, the third becomes the **inferior parathyroids** and **thymus**, the fourth becomes the **superior parathyroids**, and the fifth becomes the **ultimobranchial body** (see Fig. 3.5), which gives rise to the parafollicular cells of the thyroid that produce the hormone calcitonin.

The palatine tonsils function in the development of lymphocytes, which are important in the immunology of the body. The parathyroid glands regulate calcium balance throughout life. The thymus, located behind the sternum and between the lungs, is large at birth and continues to grow until puberty, during which it begins to atrophy (involute) but continues to function. Although its full importance is unknown, the thymus produces **T cells** that destroy invading microbes and are therefore important to the body's immune system. The ultimobranchial body fuses with the thyroid and contributes parafollicular cells to the thyroid. The function of the ultimobranchial body remains unknown (see Fig. 3.5).

Vascular Development

Each of the five pharyngeal arches contains a right and a left **aortic arch vessel** that leads from the heart through the arches to the face, brain, and posterior regions of the body (see Fig. 3.4). Not all of these paired aortic arches are present at the same time, however. The first and second begin to develop in the fourth week and disappear in the fifth week (Fig. 3.6). The third arch vessels then become prominent, taking over the facial area of the first two. As the fourth and fifth arch vessels arise, the fourth becomes prominent and the fifth disappears (Fig. 3.7). Next, the sixth arch vessels appear and become dominant, along with those of the third and fourth.

The third arch vessels become the **common carotid arteries**, which supply the neck, face, and brain. The fourth arch vessels become the dorsal aorta, which supplies blood to the remainder of the body, and the vessels of the sixth arch supply the lungs with **pulmonary circulation** (see Fig. 3.7).

An important feature of the common carotid arteries is the supply of blood to the face, neck, and brain from the **internal carotid** artery. However, after 7 weeks, the circulation to the face and neck shifts from the internal to the **external carotid** (Fig. 3.8). The internal carotid continues to supply the growing brain.

Muscular and Neural Development

Muscle cells in the first arch become apparent during the fifth week and begin to spread within the mandibular arch into each muscle site's origin in the sixth and seventh weeks (Fig. 3.9). By the tenth week, the muscles of the second arch (hyoid) have formed a thin sheet that extends over the face and posterior to the ear (Fig. 3.10). As these muscles grow over the face, they develop into the various groups of muscles that attach to the newly ossifying bones of the facial skeleton. The muscle masses of the mandibular arch, on the other hand, remain in the first arch and become the easily recognized muscles of mastication (see Fig. 3.9). These are the **masseter**, **medial and lateral pterygoid**, and **temporalis muscles**. They all relate to the developing mandible (Fig. 3.11).

The masseter and medial pterygoid form a vertical sling that inserts into the angle of the mandible. The temporalis muscle spreads into the infratemporal fossa that inserts into the developing coronoid process of the mandible. The lateral pterygoid extends horizontally from the neck of the condyle, and some fibers insert into the temporomandibular disk (this portion of the lateral pterygoid muscle is sometimes referred to as the sphenomeniscus muscle) (see Chapter 13). The pharyngeal constrictor muscles in the fourth arch have differentiated in the neck and function to enclose the pharynx (see Fig. 3.11).

Nerves develop in conjunction with the developing muscle fibers. By the end of the seventh week, the fibers of the fifth nerve have entered the mandibular muscle mass, as has the seventh nerve in the facial muscle mass in the second arch (Fig. 3.12). As these muscle masses develop, the nerves are present and follow or lead them as they migrate to their position of differentiation, maturation, and function. The seventh nerve supplies the stylohyoid and stapedius muscles and the posterior belly of the digastric muscle. The ninth (glossopharyngeal) nerve enters the third arch and supplies the stylopharyngeal and upper pharyngeal constrictor muscles. The tenth (vagus) nerve innervates muscles of the fourth arch, which are the inferior constrictors and laryngeal muscles. The tongue, which is primarily muscle, is innervated by branches of the

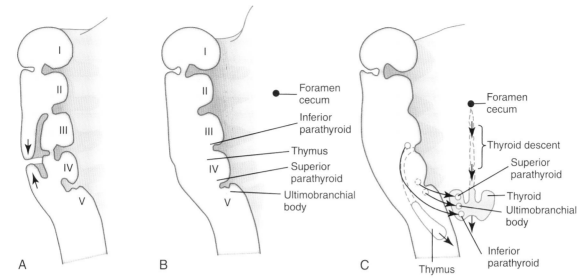

Fig. 3.5 Cross section of the pharyngeal arches. **A**, Tissues of pharyngeal arches 2 and 5 overgrow together, which results in disappearance of arches 2 to 5 and external smoothing of the neck. **B**, Resulting external appearance follows overgrowth. **C**, Contribution of the pharyngeal pouches.

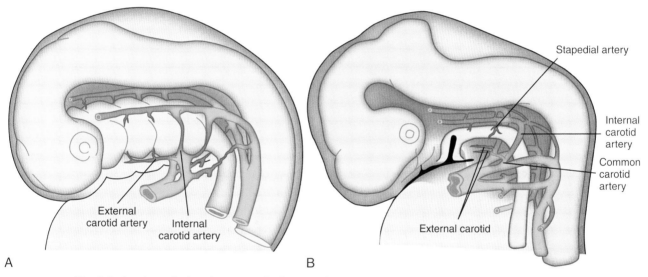

Fig. 3.6 Aortic arch development. **A**, At 4 weeks, the anterior aortic arch vessels have passed through the pharyngeal arch tissue and then disappear. The pharyngeal arch pouches project laterally between each arch. **B**, At 5 weeks, the third pharyngeal arch vessels become the right and left common carotid, which supplies the face by means of the internal carotid and stapedial arteries.

ninth nerve (IX), which carries the sensory modality of taste from the taste buds located in the posterior one-third of the tongue, and by the seventh nerve (VII), specifically the chorda tympani nerve, which carries the modality of taste from the taste buds on the anterior two-thirds of the tongue. Motor (efferent) innervation to the intrinsic muscles of the tongue is from the hypoglossal nerve (XII). The fifth nerve is the sensory nerve to the same area of the anterior tongue (see Fig. 3.12). The tongue is a good example of muscle cell migration because it originates in the occipital myotome and migrates anteriorly into the floor of the mouth. During migration, the nerves mentioned enter the muscle mass and later carry out

their functions (see Fig. 3.12). Functions and tests for cranial nerves are discussed in Table 3.1.

Cartilaginous Skeletal Development

The initial skeleton of the pharyngeal arches develops as cartilaginous bars. In the first arch, **Meckel cartilages** appear bilaterally (Fig. 3.13). The anterior aspects of these two cartilages approach each other near the midline but do not coalesce. Posteriorly, each terminates in an enlarged bulbous structure called the **malleus**. The malleus lies adjacent to a small cartilage called the **incus**. Farther posterior is a third body of cartilage, the **stapes** (see Fig. 3.13). These three bilateral cartilages later develop into bone and function in the middle ear, associated with hearing bones.

Substantial evidence shows that the contact point of the malleus and incus is the articulation of the lower jaw for the first 20 weeks of prenatal life and functions as the primary temporomandibular joint. Then the second temporomandibular joint, which is the articulation of the condyle and the temporal fossae, becomes functional (Fig. 3.14). Chapter 13 has further information about the temporomandibular joint.

The rod-shaped cartilage of the second or hyoid arch is known as *Reichert cartilage*. The stapes, styloid process, lesser horn, and upper body of the hyoid arise from this arch (see Fig. 3.13). The third arch cartilage forms the greater horn and the

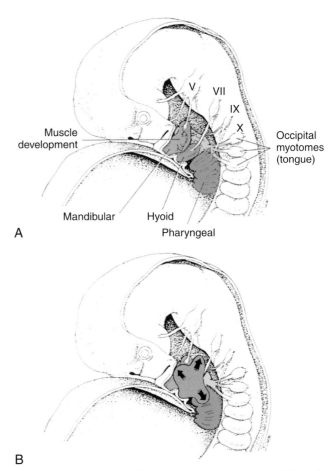

A

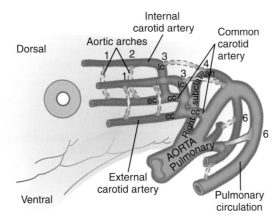

Fig. 3.7 Details of aortic arch changes during early development of 3 to 5 prenatal weeks. Aortic arch vessels numbers 1, 2, and 5 disappear as the arches modify. Arch 3 becomes the common carotid and arch 4 becomes the dorsal aorta. The dorsal aorta then enlarges so that the common carotid arises from the dorsal aorta.

B

Fig. 3.9 Development of the muscles and nerves of the pharyngeal arches. **A,** Mandibular muscle mass expands to form the muscles of mastication. **B,** At 7 weeks, the muscles of the second arch grow upward to form the muscles of the face.

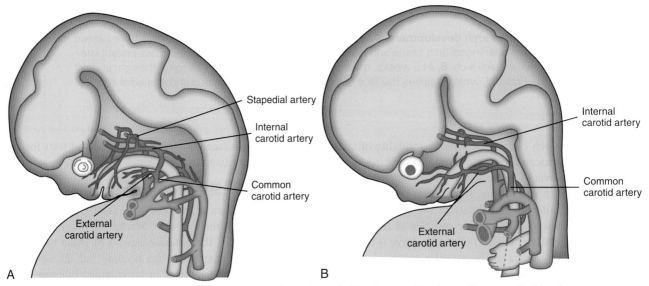

A　　　　　　　　　　　　**B**

Fig. 3.8 Shift in the vascular supply of the face. **A,** The face and brain are first supplied by the internal carotid artery. **B,** The facial vessels at 7 weeks then detach from the internal carotid artery and attach to the external carotid artery.

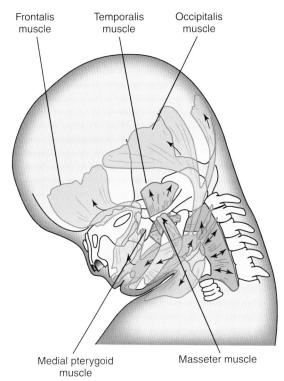

Fig. 3.10 The facial muscles grow from the second arch to cover the face, the scalp, and muscles posterior to the ear. These all become muscles of facial expression.

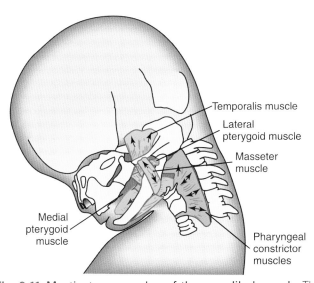

Fig. 3.11 Masticatory muscles of the mandibular arch. The medial pterygoid and masseter muscles attach as a sling at the angle of the mandible. The temporalis muscle grows from the coronoid process into the temporal fossa, and the lateral pterygoid muscle extends from the condyle anteriorly to the sphenoid bone and the pterygoid bone in the temporal fossa.

lower part of the hyoid body. The fourth arch contributes to the hyoid cartilage, which then supports the thyroid gland. The fifth arch has no adult cartilage derivatives, and the sixth arch cartilage forms the laryngeal cartilage (see Fig. 3.13).

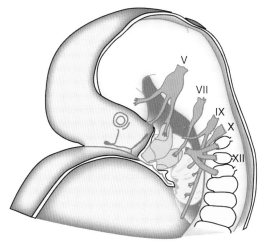

Fig. 3.12 Cranial nerves growing into the pharyngeal arches. Nerve V grows into the mandibular arch and nerve VII into the hyoid arch. Nerves V, IX, and X contribute to the tongue muscles, which are developing in the floor of the mouth.

DEVELOPMENT OF THE CRANIOFACIAL SKELETON

Cartilages of the Face

The earliest formed skeletal elements in the craniofacial area are the cartilaginous nasal capsule (**ethmoid**), the **sphenoid**, the **auditory capsules**, and the **basioccipital cartilages**. All these cartilages initially arise as a single cartilaginous continuum in the midline underlying the brain (Fig. 3.15). Anteriorly, the nasal capsule contains the organ of smell. Laterally, the auditory capsules protect the organs of hearing (Fig. 3.15). The sphenoid cartilage is posterior to the ethmoid. It later forms wings of bone that spread out under the brain laterally (Fig. 3.16). Behind the sphenoid is the occipital cartilage. Although the ethmoid capsule, sphenoid, and basioccipital cartilages are formed as a single cartilaginous unit initially, they separate later to form individual bones. These cartilages underlie and support the developing brain and are known as the **cranial base**. The cranial base is determined by drawing a line from the nasal bone (**nasion**) to the **sella turcica** of the sphenoid to the **basion**, as seen in Fig. 3.17. These cartilages are transformed into bone by endochondral bone formation.

Bones of the Face

The bony protective covering of the brain is formed by membrane (flat) bones formed by intramembranous bone formation. These bones are termed the **frontal**, **parietal**, and **squamous portions** of the **temporal** and **intraoccipital bones** (Fig. 3.18). Membrane bones form directly from connective tissue and do not initially form from cartilage.

TABLE 3.1   Cranial Nerves: Functions and Test

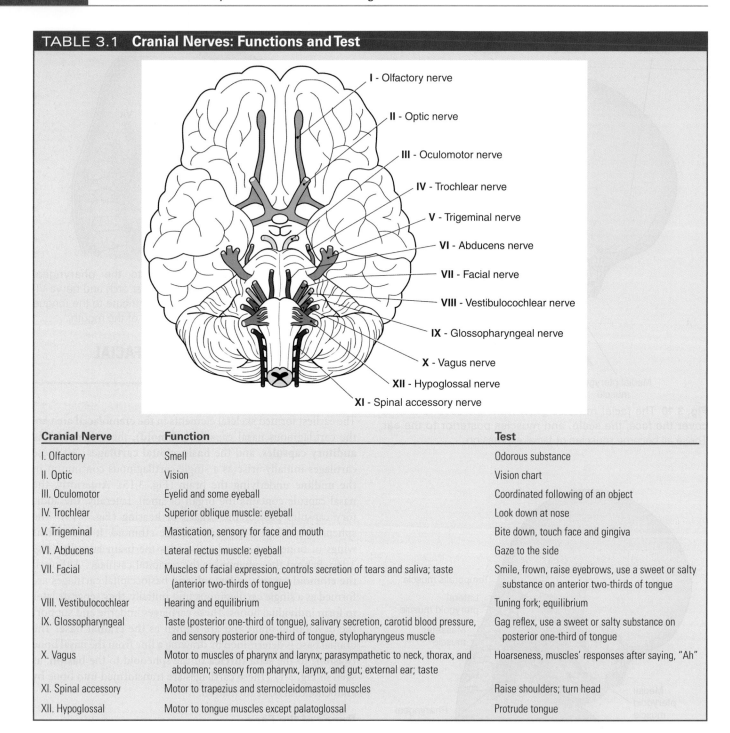

I - Olfactory nerve
II - Optic nerve
III - Oculomotor nerve
IV - Trochlear nerve
V - Trigeminal nerve
VI - Abducens nerve
VII - Facial nerve
VIII - Vestibulocochlear nerve
IX - Glossopharyngeal nerve
X - Vagus nerve
XII - Hypoglossal nerve
XI - Spinal accessory nerve

Cranial Nerve	Function	Test
I. Olfactory	Smell	Odorous substance
II. Optic	Vision	Vision chart
III. Oculomotor	Eyelid and some eyeball	Coordinated following of an object
IV. Trochlear	Superior oblique muscle: eyeball	Look down at nose
V. Trigeminal	Mastication, sensory for face and mouth	Bite down, touch face and gingiva
VI. Abducens	Lateral rectus muscle: eyeball	Gaze to the side
VII. Facial	Muscles of facial expression, controls secretion of tears and saliva; taste (anterior two-thirds of tongue)	Smile, frown, raise eyebrows, use a sweet or salty substance on anterior two-thirds of tongue
VIII. Vestibulocochlear	Hearing and equilibrium	Tuning fork; equilibrium
IX. Glossopharyngeal	Taste (posterior one-third of tongue), salivary secretion, carotid blood pressure, and sensory posterior one-third of tongue, stylopharyngeus muscle	Gag reflex, use a sweet or salty substance on posterior one-third of tongue
X. Vagus	Motor to muscles of pharynx and larynx; parasympathetic to neck, thorax, and abdomen; sensory from pharynx, larynx, and gut; external ear; taste	Hoarseness, muscles' responses after saying, "Ah"
XI. Spinal accessory	Motor to trapezius and sternocleidomastoid muscles	Raise shoulders; turn head
XII. Hypoglossal	Motor to tongue muscles except palatoglossal	Protrude tongue

The **facial bones**, which also form in membrane bone, complete the facial skeleton. They develop overlying the nasal capsule and are called the **premaxillary**, **maxillary**, **zygomatic**, and **petrous portions** of the temporal bone (see Fig. 3.18). These bones initially appear as tiny ossification centers in the face and then increase in diameter, spreading anteriorly, posteriorly, and upward into the tissues surrounding the orbit (Fig. 3.19).

The maxillary bones also grow medially into the palate to support the palatine shelf tissue (Fig. 3.20). The bones of the maxilla grow as the facial tissues continue to develop. The

height of the maxilla is due partially to the growth in length of the roots of the teeth.

The bony mandible grows laterally to the first arch cartilage as well as posteriorly to join the bony body with the cartilaginous condyle. Together, the body of the mandible and the cartilaginous condyle replace Meckel cartilage (see Fig. 3.19).

The mandible develops as several units: a **condylar** unit forms the articulation, allowing movement of the mandible; the **body** is the center of all growth and function of the mandible; the **angular process** responds to the development of the lateral pterygoid and masseter masticatory muscles; the **coronoid process** responds to the temporalis muscle development and attachment; and the **alveolar process** responds to development of the teeth (Fig. 3.21). This development produces the mature mandible (Fig. 3.22).

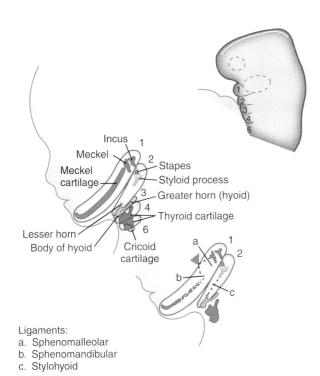

Ligaments:
a. Sphenomalleolar
b. Sphenomandibular
c. Stylohyoid

Fig. 3.13 Cartilages derived from the pharyngeal arches. Meckel cartilage, the malleus, and the incus arise from *arch 1*; stapes, styloid, and lesser horn of the hyoid form *arch 2*; the greater horn of hyoid forms *arch 3*; and thyroid and laryngeal cartilages form from *arches 4* and *6*.

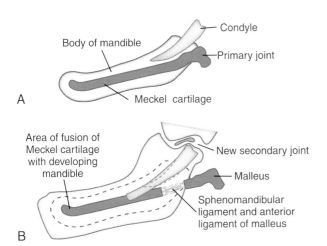

Fig. 3.14 Relationship between the primary and secondary temporomandibular joints. **A,** Meckel cartilage with its posterior malleus–incus joint, which functions in jaw movements during the first 4 months of prenatal life. **B,** A shift to the condylar–temporal articulation that occurs after that time both pre- and postnatally.

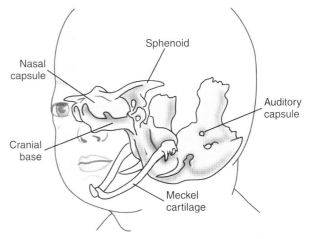

Fig. 3.15 The cartilages of the face and skull. Observe how the cranial base cartilage supports the maxillary and mandibular cartilages of the face. The locations of the nasal and auditory capsules and sphenoid are shown. All central skeletal elements arise in cartilage and later are transformed into bone.

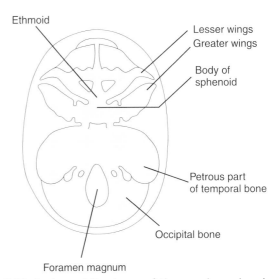

Fig. 3.16 A view of the base of the cranium showing the supporting structures of the brain. Cartilage centers initiate the formation of the cranial base bones, with growth of these bones extending outward. (Moore KL, Persaud TVN, Torchia MG. *Before we are born.* 9th ed. St. Louis: Saunders; 2016.)

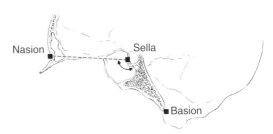

Fig. 3.17 Lateral view of the cranial base from which growth measurements are made. A dotted line drawn from sella turcica to nasion to basion is a means of measuring facial growth.

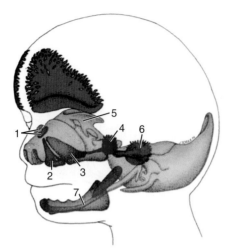

Fig. 3.18 Relationship of cranial cartilages to the membrane bones of the face at 8 weeks. The membrane bones are numbered: *1*, nasal; *2*, premaxillary; *3*, maxillary; *4*, zygomatic; *5*, sphenoid; *6*, temporal; *7*, mandible.

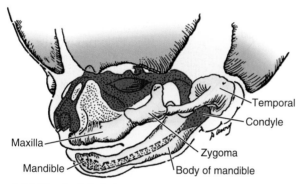

Fig. 3.19 The facial skeleton at the 12th prenatal week. This figure illustrates the relationship of the maxillary, zygomatic, and temporal bones and their articulations. The membrane bone of the body and the cartilaginous condyle of the mandible are also shown.

CLINICAL COMMENT

Many facial defects result from a lack of transformation of the pharyngeal arches to their adult derivatives. Pharyngeal cysts and fistulas contain pseudostratified ciliated columnar epithelium, with goblet cells that produce mucus and may appear along the sides of the neck because the epithelial-lined pockets remain as a result of the overgrowth of the arches. These defects may also open in the pharynx. Cysts and fistulas may result in swelling or draining of mucus from an opening on the side of the neck during an infectious process.

Sutures of the Face

A system of articulations develops between each of the major bones of the face to facilitate growth. These articulations are positioned in the direction of facial growth, which is forward, away from the brain, and downward to facilitate lengthening of the face. The articulations are termed **sutures** and are defined as fibrous joints in which the opposing surfaces are closely united. A suture develops between the **zygomatic**, **maxillary**, **frontal**,

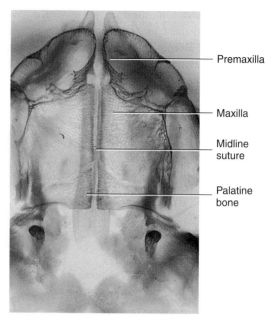

Fig. 3.20 Cleared human palate at 8 months. Sutures are seen in the midline and between the premaxillary and maxillary bones, and between the maxillary and the palatine bones in the posterior palate.

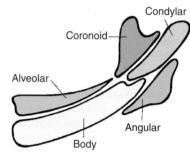

Fig. 3.21 Developing areas of the mandible and their responses to stimuli. The mandible develops from several parts. The condyle in cartilage is the articulation site; the coronoid develops in response to the temporalis muscle; the angular area is in response to the medial pterygoid and the masseter muscle; the mandible in membrane bone is the unifying structure fusing with all parts; and the alveolar process develops in response to the developing teeth.

and **temporal facial bones**. Sutures are named for the two or more bones with which they articulate. Facial sutures are named **zygomaticomaxillary**, **frontomaxillary**, and **zygomaticotemporal** (see Fig. 3.22).

These articulations are growth sites that allow the associated bones to expand and to maintain orientation at their junctions by means of the fibrous attachment that controls their relationship with the adjacent bones. Such articulations may consist of a band of connective tissue termed **syndesmosis** (Fig. 3.23). In the center of this band are osteogenic cells which, along the periphery, provide for new bone growth. The sutures of the face are of three types: **simple**, which is an uncomplicated band of tissue between bony fronts (see Fig. 3.23); **serrated**, which is an **interdigitating** type of suture (Fig. 3.24); and **squamosal**, which has a beveled or overlapping type junction (Fig. 3.25). Each connective tissue suture consists of a central zone of proliferating connective tissue cells with osteogenic cells along the peripheral bony fronts. Each suture is surrounded by a fibrous connective tissue (see Figs. 3.23 to 3.25). When the position of these sutures in the fetal skull is compared with the position of the sutures in the adult skull, the relationship of these articulations appears similar, although adult bones are larger (compare Figs. 3.26 and 3.27). When facial growth is complete, all of these sutures will fuse and become inactive, although the interface of the opposing bones remains and defines the boundary of the facial bones.

In contrast to the sutures of the external face, the articulations in the midline have interposing bands of cartilage. This

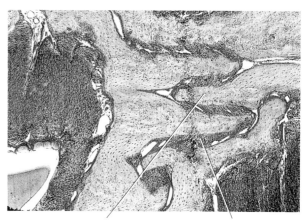

Interdigitating bone　　Connective tissue of suture

Fig. 3.24 Histology of a serrated suture of the skull. Observe the interdigitating extensions of bone from both adjacent surfaces. Connective tissue appears between these bony fronts. This is a strong suture.

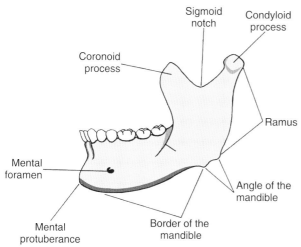

Fig. 3.22 Appearance of the adult mandible. Compare the difference of this adult mandible with the developing one in Fig. 3.21. Observe in the adult mandible that all parts have fused together to develop a strong, erect single bone.

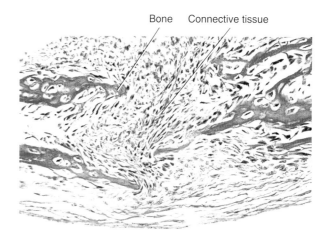

Bone　Connective tissue

Fig. 3.25 Histology of a developing squamous suture. These are overlapping sutures, and connective tissue and blood vessels appear between the bony fronts. For example, one squamous suture is between the parietal and temporal bones on the sides of the head.

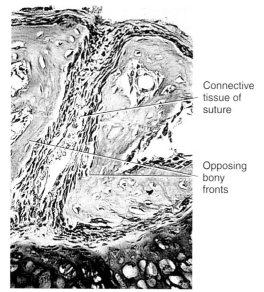

Connective tissue of suture

Opposing bony fronts

Fig. 3.23 Histology of a simple suture. Observe the opposing bony fronts with connective tissue and blood vessels between them. Osteoblasts appear along the opposing bony fronts and form bone to provide growth of this suture.

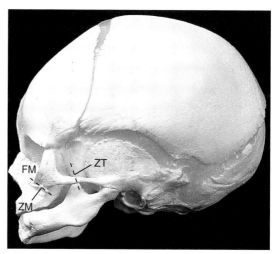

Fig. 3.26 Sutures of the developing skull of the newborn. The pterygopalatine suture is not present in the newborn but is present in the adult (see Fig. 3.25). *FM*, Frontomaxillary; *ZM*, zygomaticomaxillary; *ZT*, zygomaticotemporal.

type of articulation is termed **synchondrosis** and is located in the midline (Fig. 3.28). Synchondrosis articulations grow by forming new cartilage in the center of the suture as the cartilage is transformed into bone at the periphery of the cartilage. These

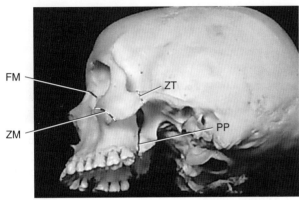

Fig. 3.27 Sutures of the adult human skull. Observe the difference in location of the sutures in the adult from those in the newborn (see Fig. 3.24). *FM*, Frontomaxillary; *PP*, pterygopalatine; *ZM*, zygomaticomaxillary; *ZT*, zygomaticotemporal.

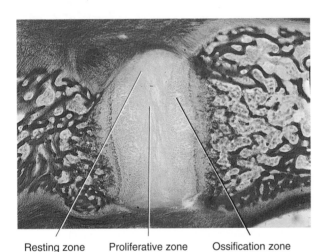

Resting zone   Proliferative zone   Ossification zone

Fig. 3.28 Histology of a cartilage suture located in the midline of the base of the skull. Observe a band of cartilage with cartilage cells differentiating in the center of it. As they migrate peripherally, the cells become osteoblasts and form bone at the peripheral surfaces of the cartilage, as seen. Bony growth thus occurs in this suture. This suture is between the ethmoid and sphenoid bone.

cartilage articulations are of only one type and exist between the ethmoid and sphenoid and the occipital bones in the midline during the period of craniofacial growth. These are known as the **ethmosphenoid** and **sphenoccipital articulations**. The **synostosis** is a type of suture in which there is a bone-to-bone union. Some sutures that were previously synchondroses of syndesmoses will fuse into a synostosis (usually after puberty). Examples include the mental and pubic symphyses and midpalatal sutures.

Table 3.2 presents a summary of all structures that develop from the pharyngeal arches, pharyngeal grooves, and pharyngeal pouches.

■ SELF-EVALUATION QUESTIONS

1. What structures are derived from the first pharyngeal arch?
2. What is the importance of Meckel cartilage?
3. Identify the structures derived from the second pharyngeal arch.
4. Rapid palatal expansion can be used by the orthodontist to increase the width of the hard palate. Why and when can the midpalatal suture be used to effect changes in the hard palate?
5. What are the contributions of the first, second, third, and fourth pharyngeal pouches?
6. Describe the origin and growth of the muscles of mastication.
7. Discuss the origin, descent, and function of the thyroid gland.
8. Discuss the origin and time of the shift in the facial blood supply.
9. Describe the cartilages of the early facial skeleton and the bones that replace them.
10. Name, locate, and describe the connective tissue sutures of the face.

CONSIDER THE PATIENT

The symptoms suggest a pharyngeal cleft and related cyst. Surgery would be recommended to correct this condition.

TABLE 3.2   Summary of Structures That Develop From Pharyngeal Arches, Pharyngeal Grooves, and Pharyngeal Pouches

Branchial Grooves		Branchial Arch Structures					Pharyngeal Pouches
	Adult derivative	Arch no.	Cranial nerve	Branchiomeric muscles	Skeletal derivative	Aortic Arch	Adult derivative
	External auditory meatus	I Mandibular	V Trigeminal	Muscles of mastication, anterior belly of digastric, mylohyoid, tensor tympani, tensor palatini	Malleus, incus, sphenomandibular ligament, sphenomalleolar ligament (Meckel cartilage)	I	1. Middle ear eustachian tube
		II Hyoid	VII Facial	Muscles of facial expression, stapedius, stylohyoid, posterior belly of digastric	Stapes, styloid process, stylohyoid ligament, lesser cornu of hyoid, upper part of body of hyoid	II	2. Palatine tonsil
		III	IX Glossopharyngeal	Stylopharyngeus	Greater cornu of hyoid, lower part of body of hyoid	III	3. Thymus, inferior parathyroid
		IV	X Vagus	Laryngeal musculature, pharyngeal constrictors	Laryngeal cartilages	IV	4. Superior parathyroid
	Cervical fistula	V	XI Spinal accessory	Sternocleidomastoid Trapezius		VI	5. Ultimobranchial body

QUANDARIES IN SCIENCE

The events occurring during the proliferative, embryonic, and fetal periods of human development are exquisitely coordinated by a series of chemical sequences determined by the genetic complement of the developing human. Each cell, tissue, and organ has to form precisely in time and space in order for it to integrate into the whole being. Some of these events take place simultaneously with other events (e.g., the migration of blood vessels and their neural innervation to vascularize a particular organ and the motor division of the trigeminal nerve [V3] innervating and migrating with the muscles of mastication), whereas other events are occur independently. When these events do not happen at precisely the correct interval, deficits can occur. Many advances have been made in understanding cellular activity at the local level, but what mechanisms synchronize the entire developmental process? Is there one signaling center, or are there multiple centers responsible for coordinating the development of the person? When is it initiated, and when is it completed? Presently, the answers to these questions are unknown, but many scientists are investigating complex biological systems such as human development in the hopes of answering some of the long-standing mysteries of science.

CLINICAL CASE

In 1957, a female infant was born with greatly shortened limbs. When the examining clinician was taking the child's medical history and the mother's history, it was discovered that the mother had experienced nausea in the first and second trimesters of her pregnancy and asked the pharmacist for a medication that would alleviate her symptoms. The drug that was recommended was thalidomide, and it was later found to result in upper and lower limb malformations in humans.

In the middle to late 1950s, the drug thalidomide was an over-the-counter drug marketed to pregnant women experiencing nausea and/or anxiety in the first and second trimesters. Thalidomide was marketed by a German company that had tested the drug on animals and found no adverse effects. However, shortly after the drug was introduced, approximately 10,000 infants were born with **phocomelia** (malformation of the limbs) to mothers who had taken this drug in West Germany and the United Kingdom. In the United States, approximately 17 children were born with limb malformations due to their mothers taking thalidomide.

The mechanism of action of thalidomide is complex and diffuse, but the consensus is that the drug interrupts angiogenesis through a myriad series of pathways and inhibits growth factors such as vascular endothelial growth factor (VEGF), NF-$\kappa\beta$, and many other proinflammatory and inflammatory cytokines and growth factors. But the primary mechanism of action of thalidomide was due to the loss of newly formed blood vessels during limb development.

SUGGESTED READING

Avery JK. *Oral development and histology*. 3rd ed. Stuttgart: Thieme Medical; 2002.

D'Amato RJ, Loughnan MS, Flynn E, et al. Thalidomide is an inhibitor of angiogenesis. *Proc Natl Acad Sci U S A*. 1994;91(9):4082–4085.

Enlow DH. *Facial growth*. 3rd ed. Philadelphia: WB Saunders; 1990.

Moore KL, Persaud TVN, Torchia MG. *The developing human: clinically oriented embryology*. Philadelphia: Saunders/Elsevier; 2008.

Sadler TW. *Langman's medical embryology*. 7th ed. Baltimore: Williams & Wilkins; 1995.

Sperber GH. *Craniofacial embryology*. 5th ed. Toronto: BC Decker; 2001.

Therapontos C, Erskine L, Gardner ER, et al. Thalidomide induces limb defects by preventing angiogenic outgrowth during early limb formation. *Proc Natl Acad Sci U S A*. 2009;106(21):8573–8578.

Vargesson N. Thalidomide-induced teratogenesis: history and mechanisms. *Birth Defects Res C Embryo Today*. 2015;105: 140–156.

4

Development of the Face and Palate

LEARNING OBJECTIVES

- Describe prenatal facial development during the fourth to seventh weeks of gestation.
- Describe palatal development during the seventh to ninth weeks of gestation.

- Explain how the tongue and thyroid develop.
- Discuss development of facial and palatal clefts and other facial defects.

OVERVIEW

This chapter describes the development of the human face and palate and developmental defects that may occur during development. An understanding of this subject is important to the dental health professional for two reasons. The professional first must understand the variability that can occur in facial form and, second, they must be aware that the human face and palate are among the areas in the body most likely to develop malformations.

The human face develops early in gestation, during the fourth through seventh weeks of the embryonic period, and the palatal processes begin to close during the eighth week. These two structures are closely related in time of development and sometimes have related malformations. The face develops from the tissues immediately surrounding the oral pit, but the forehead develops from the frontal area that lies above the pit (Fig. 4.1). The nose later develops from this area as well, so the name changes from frontal area to frontonasal area (Fig. 4.2). Below the oral pit is the mandibular arch, from which the mandible arises and articulates with the temporal bone. Lateral to the oral pit are the right and left maxillary processes, which develop from the first pharyngeal arch (mandibular arch). Cheek tissues come from these processes. Intraorally, the palate forms the mouth's roof, which separates the oral and nasal cavities. First, the medial palatal segment forms as part of the medial nasal segment. This segment provides the first separation of the oral and nasal cavities. Next, two lateral palatal shelves close anteriorly (not posteriorly) to the pharynx (see Fig. 4.12). At the same time, the tongue develops in the floor of the oral cavity but grows rapidly and expands into the nasal cavity. The tongue functions in palatine shelf closure because the shelves must override it before closure can be accomplished.

Many environmental factors can cause clefts of the face, palate, or both. These defects of the lip or palate may be unilateral or bilateral and also incomplete or complete.

FACIAL DEVELOPMENT: WEEKS 4 TO 7

Tissue Organization

The face develops primarily from tissues surrounding the oral pit. Above the oral pit is the covering of the brain termed the **frontal process**, from which develops the **forehead**. Lateral to the oral pit are the right and left **maxillary processes**, from which develop the **cheeks**, and below the oral pit is the **mandibular arch**, from which the **lower jaw** is formed. In the fourth week, when the facial tissues have just begun to organize, they measure only a few millimeters in height and width and are only as thick as a sheet of paper. Further growth of the face from this minute assembly of tissue sites is anterior to the brain. Lying inferior to the mandibular arch is the second pharyngeal or **hyoid arch**, and its muscles expand into and contribute to the face. The hyoid arch also forms part of the external and middle ear.

Development of the human face is most easily described in terms of the changes that occur at weekly intervals from the fourth to the seventh prenatal weeks.

Fourth Week

At 4 weeks of gestation, the oral pit is surrounded by several masses of tissue. Pharyngeal arches are also evident below the pit and on the sides of the neck. The frontal processes of the brain bulge forward and laterally to dominate the facial area. Below the frontal processes are two small wedge-shaped tissues, termed the *maxillary processes,* that lie lateral to the oral pit. Beneath the maxillary processes is the mandibular arch, which appears divided or constricted in the midline (see Fig. 4.1). The heart lies immediately below the face and is one of the fastest growing organs. During the fourth week, the heart begins to pump blood throughout the body.

CLINICAL COMMENT

Syndromes associated with the pharyngeal arches are seen commonly as a group of defects. They can appear as a malformed mandible; defective ear; small mouth; enlarged tongue or unequal growth of the sides of the tongue; cleft lip or palate; and swellings, cysts, or clefts of the front or sides of the neck. Usually, several or more defects appear simultaneously.

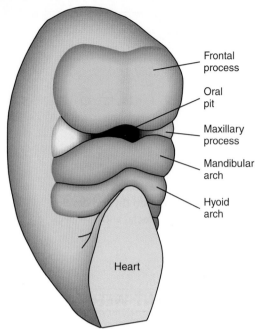

Fig. 4.1 **Human face during the fourth prenatal week.** Around the centrally located oral pit are grouped the frontal and maxillary processes and the mandibular arch. Although appearing unrelated at this time, these processes and the first arch form the human face.

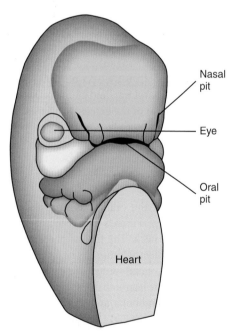

Fig. 4.2 **Human face during the fifth prenatal week.** The nasal pits develop and appear on the sides of the face. The frontal process now becomes the frontonasal process.

CLINICAL COMMENT

Environmental factors play an important role in facial and palatal malformations. The period before the fifth week is the critical time during which these factors can affect facial development.

Fifth Week

During the fifth week, the bilateral nasal placodes, or thickened areas of epithelium, appear in the upper border of the lip. They develop into nostrils as the tissues around these placodes grow, resulting in two slits opening into the oral pit. At this point, the frontal area becomes known as the **frontonasal process**. The nostrils deepen as the tissues around them continue to grow anteriorly, and the **internasal area**, the distance between the nostrils, represents the width of the face. Gradually, the frontal prominence diminishes, and the face broadens. The eyes become prominent on the sides of the head. Throughout the fifth week, the mandibular arch loses its midline constriction (see Fig. 4.2).

Sixth Week

At the beginning of the sixth week, the lateral parts of the face expand, broadening the face. This is also caused by lateral growth of the brain. The eyes and maxillary processes, which were located on the sides of the face in the fifth week, come to the front of the face. The mouth slit widens to the point at which the maxillary and mandibular tissues merge. The nasal processes are limited to the middle of the upper lip, which causes the face to appear more human. The upper lip is now composed of a medial nasal process and two lateral maxillary segments (Fig. 4.3). The medial nasal process is called the **philtrum**. A ridge of tissue surrounds each nasal pit. The tissue lateral to the pits is the **lateral nasal process**, and the tissue medial to the pits is the **medial nasal process**.

The medial nasal process is in close contact with the medial aspect of the maxillary process, and the lateral nasal process is above the maxillary process. The border of the lip consists of two maxillary processes, and the medial third is the medial nasal. A lack of contact or fusion of the medial nasal and maxillary processes results in either a unilateral or bilateral **cleft lip**. The epithelial coverings of the medial nasal and maxillary processes normally contact and create a zone of fusion termed the **nasal fin** (Fig. 4.4). This epithelial fin is soon penetrated by connective tissue growth, which binds together the two maxillary and medial nasal parts of the lip. If this penetration were not to occur, the lip could pull apart. Soon the **orbicularis oris** muscle grows around the oral pit to provide support to the upper lip. The nasal pits continue behind the nasal fin to open into the roof of the mouth at 6 weeks (see Fig. 4.4). Extending from the nostrils to the eyes is an oblique groove called the **oronasal optic groove**. In the tissue beneath this groove, the **nasolacrimal duct** develops. A modification of the first pharyngeal groove into the ear canal or **auditory tube** also appears below the corners of the mouth. Six small hillocks of tissue, termed the **auricular hillocks**, are grouped around the external ear canal. Three of these come from the mandibular arch and three from the second or hyoid arch (see Fig. 4.3; Fig. 4.5).

Seventh Week

By the seventh week, the face has a more human appearance (Fig. 4.6). The eyes approach the front of the face, and the nose represents less of the face than it did at the fourth week. The

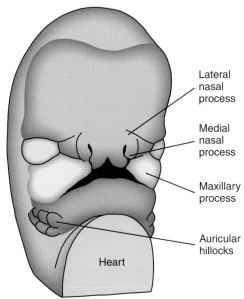

Fig. 4.3 Human face during the sixth prenatal week. Nasal pits appear more centrally located in the medial nasal process. This is the result of growth of the lateral face, which also causes the eyes to approach the front of the face. The enlarged maxillary processes are near contact with the medial nasal process. Nasal pits may be sites of cleft lips. Auricular hillocks bordering the ear canal have merged.

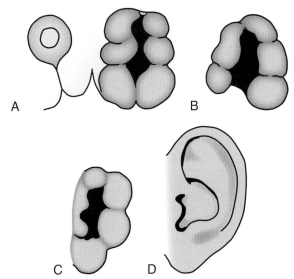

Fig. 4.5 Development of the external ear (auricles). A, The three auricular hillocks on the left are from the mandibular arch, and the three on the right are from the hyoid arch. **B,** Auricular hillocks begin to merge around the first pharyngeal groove. **C,** The hillocks merge. **D,** The ear is developed.

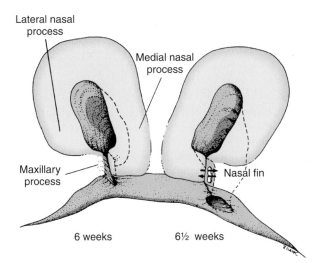

Fig. 4.4 Development of the floor of the nasal pit. On the left, the naris is in the process of closing. During this process, the medial nasal and maxillary processes fuse as connective tissue grows through this area. On the left, there is space between the maxillary and medial nasal processes, and on the right, the two areas are in contact, and the resulting nasal fin is penetrated by the connective tissue of the developing lip.

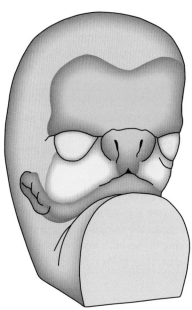

Fig. 4.6 Human face during the seventh prenatal week. The medial nasal and maxillary processes have merged. The eyes are closer to the front of the face. The nose and eyes are on the same horizontal plane, which will change with vertical growth of the face. The auricles of the ear have developed.

lateral growth of the brain, resulting in facial expansion, causes the eyes to appear on the front of the face, which makes it more recognizable as a human face. A third of the face has been added lateral to each nostril (see Fig. 4.6). The eyes are on the same horizontal plane as the nostrils, which will change after the bridge of the nose develops and lengthens. The upper lip has fused, producing a medially located **philtrum**. The mouth is limited in size with the change in facial proportions. The ear hillocks have fused and grown to form the ears (auricles). The ridges around the eyes will soon develop into eyelids (see Figs. 4.5 and 4.6). The danger of a cleft lip has passed. In just 3 prenatal weeks, separate tissue masses have enlarged, fused, and merged into a recognizable human face.

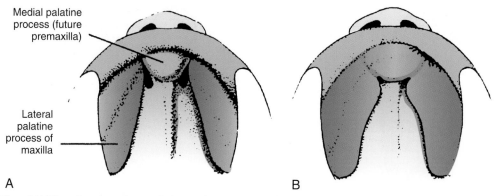

Fig. 4.7 The development of the palate. **A**, Medial and lateral palatine processes develop (enlarge). **B**, Lateral palatine processes move medially toward the midline and fuse with the medial palatine process.

CLINICAL COMMENT

Because the face develops on the surface of the brain, defects of the anterior brain may result in developmental alteration of the facial form.

PALATAL DEVELOPMENT: WEEKS 7 TO 9

Medial and Lateral Palatal Processes

The palate is the tissue that separates the oral and nasal cavities and can be divided into a hard palate, which has a bony base, and the soft palate, which has a muscular base. Both hard and soft palates are covered by epithelium. This palate, although thin, is supported by bone, which provides rigidity. The palate develops from an anterior wedge-shaped medial part and two **lateral palatine processes** (Fig. 4.7A). The medial part is also known as the **primary palate** because it develops first and is a floor to the nasal pits. Next, the lateral palatine processes develop from the maxillary tissues laterally and grow to the midline. This further limits the oral cavity from the nasal cavity posteriorly to the nasopharynx (see Fig. 4.7B). As the palatine shelves grow medially, they contact the tongue, which grows upward into the nasal cavity during the seventh week. When the palatine shelves contact the tongue, they grow downward on either side of the tongue (Fig. 4.8).

Palatal Shelf Elevation and Closure

At its posterior limits, the tongue is below the palatine shelves. This is because posteriorly the tongue is attached to the floor of the mouth, and the posterior roof of the mouth is above the tongue. During the eighth prenatal week, the posterior shelves push together, forcing the tongue forward and down (Fig. 4.9). This action causes the palatal shelves to slide over the tongue (Fig. 4.10). The process is known as **palatal shelf elevation** and is presumed to take place rapidly, about as fast as the act of swallowing. For this reason, palatal shelf elevation has never been precisely recorded.

As soon as the palatine shelves reach the resulting horizontal position, the tongue broadens and pushes upward against the shelves, which helps mold them together (Fig. 4.11). The shelves have a final growth surge until they contact in the midline; this

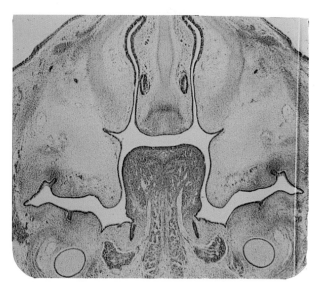

Fig. 4.8 Coronal section of facial tissue showing the tongue's growth upward into the nasal cavity during the seventh prenatal week. Palatine shelves (maxillary processes) contact the tongue during their medial growth. The tongue then grows down beside the palatal shelves. The tongue muscle begins to differentiate at this time.

contact is known as **palatine shelf closure** or **fusion** (Fig. 4.12). The first site of contact is just posterior to the medial palatine process. From this point of initial contact, the shelves merge anteriorly and posteriorly. The final step in fusion is the removal of the midline epithelial barrier between the right and left shelves. This occurs by **apoptosis**, which initiates an enzymatic action on epithelial cells resulting in self-destruction. As soon as the epithelial cells begin to break down and disappear, connective tissue grows through the midline and completes the fusion of the palate. This is the same process as the one that occurred in lip fusion with destruction of the nasal fin and is illustrated in Fig. 4.13. The fusion of the entire palate takes weeks while the palate grows in length. The palatal shelves also fuse with the overlying nasal septum in the midline of the face. This causes a complete separation of the oral and nasal cavities back to the nasopharynx. Then both the oral and nasal cavities open into the pharynx.

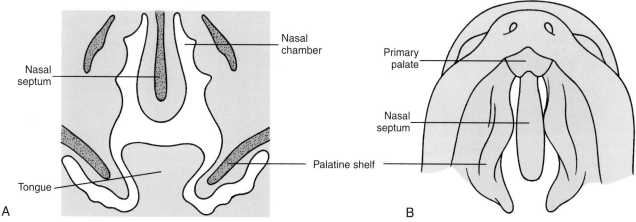

Fig. 4.9 Palatine shelves position beside the tongue anteriorly and over the tongue posteriorly. **A**, Frontal view. **B**, Intraoral/inferior view. (Hupp JR, Ellis E, Tucker MR. *Contemporary oral and maxillofacial surgery.* 6th ed. St. Louis: Mosby; 2014.)

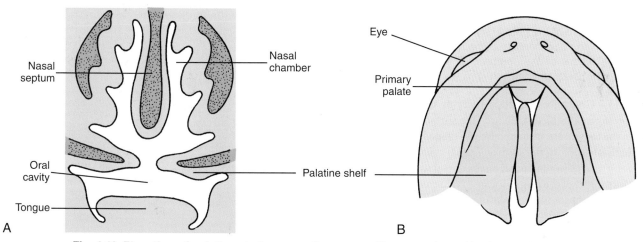

Fig. 4.10 Elevation of palatine shelves over the tongue. The tongue's position is over the palatine shelves during the elevation process early in the eighth week. **A**, Frontal view. **B**, Intraoral/inferior view. (Hupp JR, Ellis E, Tucker MR. *Contemporary oral and maxillofacial surgery.* 6th ed. St. Louis: Mosby; 2014.)

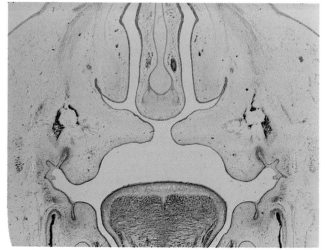

Fig. 4.11 Tongue with overlying palatal shelves at eighth week. The palatal shelves are in a near-midline position underlying the nasal septum.

Tongue Development

Body and Base

The tongue originates from the muscles of the occipital myotomes. From this posterior location, the forming muscles migrate anteriorly into the floor of the mouth and are joined by other muscles of the first and second pharyngeal arches. The tongue is innervated by the fifth, seventh, ninth, tenth, and twelfth cranial nerves. This extensive innervation is the result of the long distance the muscle cells migrate from each pharyngeal arch to reach the tongue and the varied functions the tongue performs. The muscles travel in the paths of these various nerves. The first pharyngeal arch tissue forms the anterior (movable) body of the tongue. The second and third arches form the posterior, immovable base of the tongue. Tissues of the tongue have three parts: the central **tuberculum impar** and the two **lateral lingual swellings** (Fig. 4.14). The lateral parts rapidly enlarge and merge, overgrowing the central tubercle. A U-shaped sulcus develops around the anterior part of the tongue, separating it from the jaw tissues and allowing freedom of movement

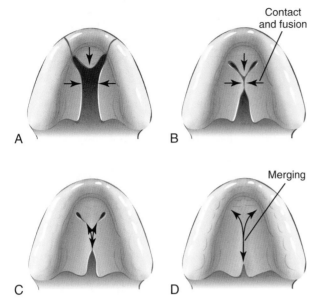

Fig. 4.12 Closure of the palatal shelves. **A,** Horizontal palatine shelf growth to attain contact in the midline. **B,** Initial contact behind the medial palatal segment. **C** and **D,** Tissues merge anteriorly and posteriorly from the point of initial contact.

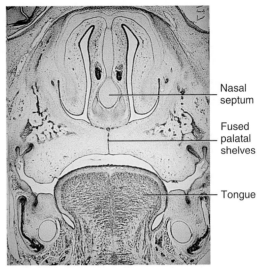

Fig. 4.13 Coronal section of facial tissue showing palatal shelf fusion in the midline. After contact, the epithelial seam breaks down between the palatal shelves and the overlying nasal septum.

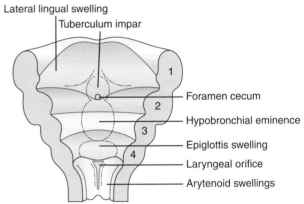

Fig. 4.14 Early tongue development. The body of the tongue develops from two lateral lingual swellings and a centrally located tuberculum impar. The base of the tongue develops from the second and third pharyngeal arches. (Coburne MT, DiBiase AT. *Handbook of orthodontics.* 2nd ed. St. Louis: Elsevier; 2016.)

(Fig. 4.15). Gradually, the three parts of the anterior tongue merge to form a unified structure. The surface of the body and base of the tongue are separated by a V-shaped groove called the **terminal sulcus**. Posterior to the terminal sulcus, the base of the tongue forms the **lingual tonsil** on the dorsal surface. The lingual tonsil forms part of the ring of tonsils (Waldeyer tonsillar ring) in the pharynx, along with the **palatine** and **pharyngeal tonsils**. In the later stages of development, several types of papillae differentiate on the oral mucosa of the tongue's dorsal body. The lingual tonsil differentiates on the surface of the tongue's base.

Thyroid Gland

The thyroid gland develops as an epithelial proliferation from the **foramen cecum** on the surface of the tongue at the junction of the body and base. Cells arise and migrate ventrally in the throat, thus creating the thyroid gland (see Fig. 4.15; Fig. 4.16). Then the cells from the foramen cecum rim descend in the midline floor of the pharynx past the hyoid cartilages to the level of the laryngeal cartilage. Finally, by the seventh week, the thyroid descends to the front of the trachea. During this long migration, the thyroid gland remains attached to the tongue by an epithelial cord or duct termed the **thyroglossal duct**, which later becomes solid and eventually disappears (see Fig. 4.16).

Cysts, sinuses, and fistulas are occasionally found along the route of descent of the thyroid tissue. A **thyroglossal cyst** is a blind pocket lined most commonly by pseudostratified columnar epithelium with goblet cells or stratified squamous and/or thyroid gland tissue and located at the midline. During diagnoses, ultrasound, computed tomography, or magnetic resonance imaging can be used to visualize the cyst. When the clinician suspects that thyroid gland tissue was left in the tract during the thyroid gland descent, a radioactive solution of iodine technetium will be injected into the patient and imaged. If ectopic thyroid tissue is found, then postsurgical treatment could include

replacement therapy. This cyst appears as a midline swelling and is commonly found in the area of the hyoid bone. A **thyroglossal fistula** appears as a swelling that has an opening on the surface of the neck (Fig. 4.17). The gland finally acquires two lateral lobes joined by a thin central isthmus of cells. By the end of the third month of prenatal life, the gland becomes functional.

CLINICAL COMMENT

Occasionally, after an infant has a cold, the parents discover a swelling in the midline of the neck. This swelling can be located along the tract that is formed as the thyroid gland descends from the foramen cecum to reside in the neck and is a result of secretions from the pseudostratified ciliated epithelium with goblet cells lining the duct. At times, thyroid tissue can be found along the tract and can be rapidly diagnosed with an injection of iodine (needed by the thyroid gland to function properly). The iodine will be taken up by the ectopic thyroid tissue and can be imaged. The usual treatment is surgical resection of the sinus, duct, or cyst.

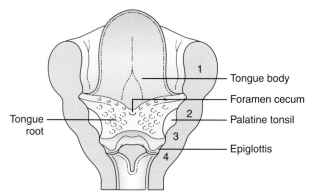

Fig. 4.15 Late tongue development illustrating body and base of the tongue. The foramen cecum is the initial site of the descent of the tubular downgrowth resulting in the thyroid gland. (Coburne MT, DiBiase AT. *Handbook of orthodontics.* 2nd ed. St. Louis: Elsevier; 2016.)

Labels: 1, Tongue body; Foramen cecum; Palatine tonsil; 2; 3; Epiglottis; 4; Tongue root

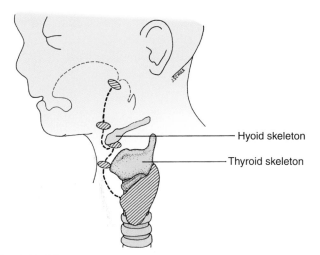

Fig. 4.16 Migratory path down front of neck of thyroid gland tissue. Epithelial cysts and fistulas may arise anteriorly in the midline along path of descent as well as remnants of thyroid tissue along path of descent. The site may be in the region of the thyrohyoid skeleton.

Labels: Hyoid skeleton; Thyroid skeleton

MALFORMATIONS

Facial and palatal clefts usually occur because of a combination of environmental and genetic factors. An individual's susceptibility to stress is one factor that can have adverse effects.

Cleft lip is the most common facial malformation. Genetic factors play a role, as shown by the differences among racial groups. In the White population of the United States, the incidence of cleft lip is 1 in every 700 births. Proportionately, significantly fewer Blacks have clefts, the incidence being only 1 in 2000 newborns. In the Asian population, the incidence is 3 in 2000 births. Asians with one child born with a cleft palate have a 1 in 25 chance of having a second child with the defect. The disparity is not surprising because congenital malformation affects races in different ratios. Evidence shows

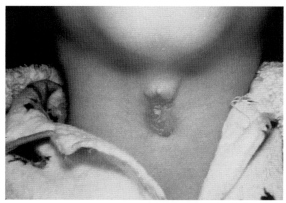

Fig. 4.17 Clinical view of thyroglossal fistulas appearing in the anterior midline of the neck. These fistulas typically appear in the region of the thyrohyoid skeleton.

that a hereditary role exists, along with various environmental susceptibility factors.

The incidence of clefts in male and female infants differs according to type of cleft. White boys have nearly twice the number of cleft lips or cleft lips and palates as girls. However, more White girls have cleft palates, which occur at the rate of about 1 in every 2000 births. Overall, cleft palate is less common than cleft lip or a combination of cleft lip and palate.

> **CLINICAL COMMENT**
>
> Clefts of the lips and palate usually occur early in development. These clefts vary in size and shape and usually occur along fusion lines. Most clefts today are corrected by surgical intervention in early life and give the patient an improved quality of life, thus allowing the baby to nurse and feed in an appropriate manner.

Facial Clefts

Facial clefts are classified according to position and extent. A cleft may affect one or both sides of the lip (unilateral or bilateral) and can be either incomplete or complete (Figs. 4.18 to 4.20). An incomplete cleft lip ranges in size from a notch to a deep groove in the upper lip but does not involve an opening of the nostril into the oral cavity (see Fig. 4.18). A true "harelip" is a midline cleft of the maxilla. The term *harelip* is used because a rabbit's upper lip develops with a midline cleft. The rabbit does not develop a medial nasal process, so the two maxillary processes meet in the midline. This condition, which is rare in humans, involves a notch in the medial nasal tissue that may be minute or may extend as a cleft into the nose (Fig. 4.21).

A cleft of the mandible may appear in the midline, although this also is rare (Fig. 4.22). A midline constriction in the mandible is observed during the fourth week. In this case, the early constriction did not disappear and later resulted in a separation of the mandible's halves. This condition is believed to occur because of pressure from the adjacent enlarged heart, which begins beating before the mandible's midline fusion.

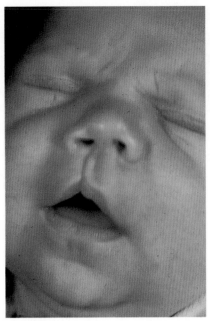

Fig. 4.18 Clinical view of a unilateral cleft of the lip. This partial cleft is located in the line of fusion of the medial nasal and maxillary processes.

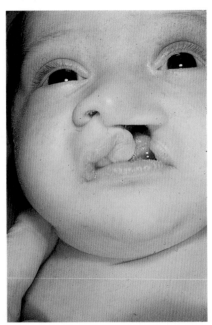

Fig. 4.19 Clinical view of a unilateral complete cleft lip. In this case, the maxillary and medial nasal processes did not fuse and then pulled apart during facial growth.

> **CLINICAL COMMENT**
>
> Cleft lip and cleft palate are among the most common congenital malformations. They appear in 1 of every 700 births in the White population and in 1 of 2000 births in the Black population in the United States.

Palatal Clefts

All the preceding facial clefts involve the lip, but some may extend into the palate as unilateral and bilateral cleft lip and

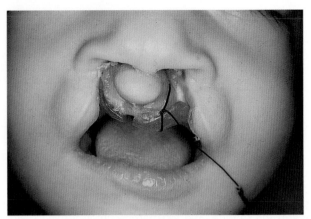

Fig. 4.20 Clinical view of bilateral complete cleft of the lip. The medial labial process did not fuse on either side of the developing maxillary processes. This results in anterior extrusion of the medial labial process.

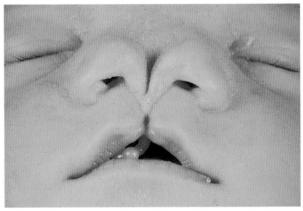

Fig. 4.21 Clinical view of a midline cleft of the lip. This rare cleft occurs when the two parts of the medial nasal process fail to merge. The etiology of this condition can be seen in Fig. 4.3.

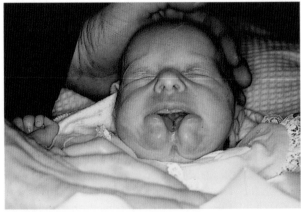

Fig. 4.22 Clinical example of a midline cleft of the mandible. The two parts of the first pharyngeal arch, including the bony mandible, are separated at birth in this rare condition.

palate defects (Fig. 4.23). Because the palatine shelves meet in the midline, both unilateral and bilateral clefts of the palate are in the midline clefts. Clefts must, however, extend around the medial palatal segment before they proceed in the midline

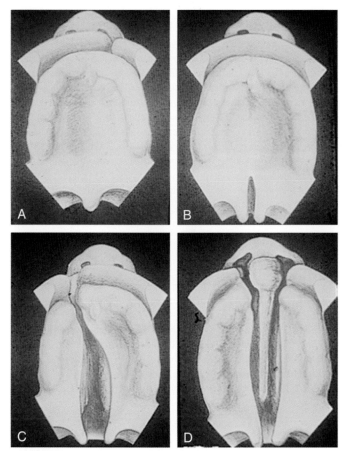

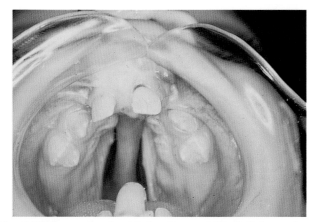

Fig. 4.25 Example of a bilateral complete cleft lip and palate. This bilateral cleft extends lateral to the medial palatal process and then posteriorly in the midline.

Fig. 4.23 Examples of cleft lip and palate. **A**, Cleft lip only. **B**, Cleft palate only. **C**, Unilateral complete cleft lip and palate. **D**, Bilateral complete cleft lip and palate.

locations. However, most cleft palates occur in combination with cleft lips (Figs. 4.24 and 4.25).

CONSIDER THE PATIENT

A patient tells you she heard that prenatal surgery has been developed in the past 10 years to correct life-threatening malformations. In this procedure, the fetus is removed from the uterus, corrections are made, and the fetus is returned to the uterus until proper delivery time. One advantage is a lack of scarring. She asks whether any prenatal surgeries in the area of dentistry may be of interest.

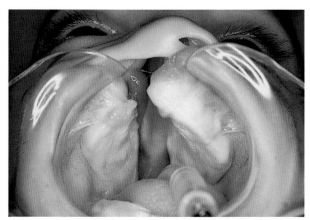

Fig. 4.24 Example of a unilateral complete cleft lip and palate. Ventral view of a cleft of the palate developed lateral to the medial palatal segment, then posteriorly in the midline between the two palatal processes. This cleft occurs along the fusion lines of the palatal processes. The nasal tissue is also malformed.

(see Fig. 4.23). Just as clefts of the lip can occur alone, clefts of the palate may occur as isolated defects (see Fig. 4.23B). These palatal clefts can extend just a short distance into the posterior of the palate, can appear in the anterior, or can appear in both

Other Defects

Numerous other facial deformities appear clinically, some common and others rare. The most common defects are various malocclusions of the teeth. Midfacial hypoplasia—such as Apert and Crouzon syndromes—is a less common abnormality.

▌SELF-EVALUATION QUESTIONS

1. From what four embryonic processes does the face arise?
2. During which 3 prenatal weeks does the face develop human characteristics?
3. When do the palatine shelves elevate and begin closure?
4. Name the upper lip's three segments. When do they begin to coalesce into one unit?
5. From what structure does the nasal fin arise, and why is its disappearance important?
6. What is the origin of the auricles of the ear? From what pharyngeal arches do they arise?
7. Define the primary and secondary palates, explain when each appears, and discuss their relative importance.
8. Describe the process of palatal elevation and the tissues that are believed to contribute to this event.
9. Compare the ratios of facial and palatal defects in the Asian, White, and Black populations.
10. From what three masses does the body of the tongue arise? What is the origin of the tongue base?

CLINICAL CASE

Two White parents and their newborn male child present at the pediatrician's for their first postnatal visit at 4 weeks. The child appears healthy but has a cleft lip on the left aspect of the face between the medial nasal and maxillary processes. After a thorough genetic background history, it was determined that this congenital malformation was nonsyndromic. Appointments were made with a plastic surgeon to repair the cleft, and this was accomplished without complication at 7 weeks to facilitate nursing.

The causes of cleft lip and palate are variable and many. Problems with genes from one or both parents, as well as alcohol, drugs, viruses, or other toxins, all can cause these birth defects. Nonsyndromic cleft lip and palate may occur along with other syndromic or birth defects, depending on the causative factor(s). Some agents that cause syndromic conditions will affect similar structures in addition to those located in the head and neck. Other agents, such as those that inhibit neural crest migration, will affect all neural crest–derived structures that are developing at the same time. For example, many times, hearing problems are associated with cleft lip and/or palate since the affected structures are also derived from the first pharyngeal arch and are developing at the same time that the medial and lateral nasal processes are fusing with the maxillary process.

Surgical closure of cleft lip and/or palate is usually done when the child is between 6 and 9 weeks old so the child can nurse efficiently and so that speech develops correctly. On occasion, an obturator appliance is fitted to close off the nasal cavity from the oral cavity so the child can develop suction.

The majority of these babies will heal without incident. As the child's primary and permanent dentition develop and erupt into the oral cavity, the child may require intervention by an orthodontist, and a speech therapist sometimes is also needed.

CONSIDER THE PATIENT

Prenatal surgery could correct defects such as cleft lip and cleft lip and palate without leaving scars.

QUANDARIES IN SCIENCE

The development of the head and neck, including the face and palate, requires a high degree of precision and integration to ensure that no malformations occur. When malformations do occur, they can vary from lethal to minimal. Scientists are beginning to understand the origin of many craniofacial defects, but many are still unknown. Deficits in the face are often visible and affect a person's quality of life. Formation of many of the structures of the face requires multiple processes to form, migrate, and fuse, with little room for variation and timing. For example, how does the thyroid anlage know when to descend into the neck and when and where to stop? How do the signals get to a specific cell or set of cells? Are the signals released from adjacent cells (paracrine) or is the signal sent through the developing vascular system (endocrine) from a distant cell? Or do electrical signals and neurotransmitters regulate and coordinate these activities? Presently, we have many questions but few answers.

SUGGESTED READING

Avery JK. *Oral development and histology.* 3rd ed. Stuttgart: Thieme Medical; 2002.

Moore KL, Persaud TVN, Torchia MG. *The developing human: clinically oriented embryology.* 10th ed. St. Louis: Elsevier; 2016.

Sadler TW. *Langman's medical embryology.* 13th ed. Baltimore: Lippincott Williams & Wilkins; 2015.

Sperber GH. *Craniofacial embryology.* 5th ed. Toronto: BC Decker; 2002.

5

Development of Teeth

- Describe the origin of the tooth formative cells and the role of induction in tooth formation.
- Describe the stages of tooth formation and the mineralization of enamel and dentin.

- Describe the development of the tissues that surround the developing teeth.

OVERVIEW

The human is a species with two sets of dentition (diphyodont) that normally include 20 primary and 32 permanent teeth that develop from the interaction of the oral ectodermal cells and the underlying mesenchymal cells. Each developing tooth grows as an anatomically distinct unit, but the basic developmental process is similar for all teeth.

Each tooth develops through successive bud, cap, and bell stages (Fig. 5.1A–C). During these early stages, the tooth germs grow and expand, and the cells that are to form the hard tissues of the teeth differentiate. Differentiation takes place in the bell stage, setting the stage for enamel and dentin formation (Fig. 5.1D and E). As the crowns are formed and mineralized, the roots of the teeth begin to form. After the roots calcify the supporting tissues of the teeth, the cementum, periodontal ligament, and alveolar bone begin to develop (Fig. 5.1F and G). This formation occurs whether the tooth is an incisor with a single root, a premolar with several roots, or a molar with multiple roots. Subsequently, the completed tooth crown erupts into the oral cavity (Fig. 5.1G). Root formation and cementogenesis continue until a functional tooth and its supporting structures are fully developed (Fig. 5.1G and H).

CLINICAL COMMENT

Developmentally missing permanent teeth can be a result of a genetic abnormality. When fewer than six teeth are missing, it is termed *hypodontia*, and when more than six teeth are missing, it is called *oligodontia*.

INITIATION OF TOOTH DEVELOPMENT

Teeth develop from two types of cells: oral ectodermal cells form the enamel organ, and ectomesenchymal cells (neural crest cells) form the dental papilla. Enamel develops from the enamel organ, and dentin forms from the dental papilla. The interaction of these epithelial and mesenchymal cells is vital to the initiation and formation of the teeth. In addition to these cells, the **neural crest cells** contribute to tooth development. The neural crest cells arise and begin their migration from the mesencephalic portion of the developing neural tube at an early stage of development and migrate into the jaws, intermingling with mesenchymal cells. They function by integrating with the dental papillae and epithelial cells of the early enamel organ, which aids in the development of the teeth. The cells also function in the development of the salivary glands, bone, cartilage, nerves, and muscles of the face. Chapter 1 discussed neural crest cells and explained the cell's migration (see Fig. 1.18).

The first sign of tooth formation is the proliferation of ectodermal cells overlying specific areas of the oral ectoderm where the homeobox gene *MSX-1* can be localized. The resultant proliferation and downgrowth of the ectoderm result in the development of the **dental lamina**. The dental lamina develops into a sheet of epithelial cells that pushes into the underlying mesenchyme around the perimeter of both the maxillary and mandibular jaws beginning at the midline (Fig. 5.2). At the leading edge of the lamina, 20 areas of enlargement appear that form tooth buds for the 20 primary teeth (see Fig. 5.2). At this early stage, the tooth buds have already determined their crown morphology of an incisor or molar. This is the result of a complicated series of gene expressions that alternates between the epithelium and the mesenchymal tissue. After primary teeth develop from the buds, the leading edge of the lamina continues to grow to develop the permanent teeth, which succeed the 20 primary teeth. This part of the lamina is thus called the **successional lamina** (Fig. 5.3). The lamina continues posteriorly into the elongating jaw, and from it come the posterior teeth (first, second, and third molars), which form behind the primary teeth. In this manner, 20 of the permanent teeth replace the 20 primary teeth, and 12 posterior permanent molars develop behind the primary dentition (see Fig. 5.3). The last teeth to develop are the third molars, which develop about 15 years after birth. Because the permanent molars do not succeed the primary teeth, they do not form from the successional lamina but

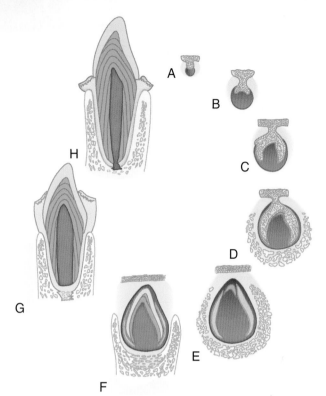

Fig. 5.1 Stages of tooth development. **A**, Bud. **B**, Cap. **C**, Bell. **D** and **E**, Dentinogenesis and amelogenesis. **F**, Crown formation. **G**, Root formation and eruption. **H**, Function.

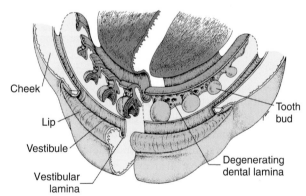

Fig. 5.2 Development of tooth buds in the alveolar process. Anterior teeth are more advanced in development than posterior teeth. Anterior lamina has begun to degenerate as posterior lamina forms. When tooth buds have differentiated, lamina is no longer needed and degenerates.

from the general lamina and are termed *accessional teeth*. The initiating dental lamina that forms both the successional and general lamina begins to function in the sixth prenatal week and continues to function until the 15th year, producing all 52 teeth. In general, the teeth develop anteroposteriorly, beginning at the mesial of the mandible and maxilla, which relates to the growing jaws. The posterior molars do not develop until space is available for them in the posterior jaw area. The permanent dentition does not develop until after the primary teeth are formed

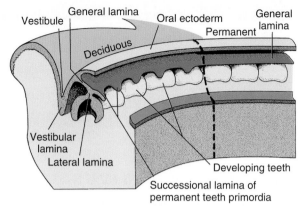

Fig. 5.3 Dental lamina formation shown in relation to the general lamina. From the successional lamina come permanent teeth, which replace the primary teeth except for the permanent molars.

and functioning. Gradually, the permanent teeth form under the primary crowns and later, posteriorly to the primary molars.

STAGES OF TOOTH DEVELOPMENT

Although tooth formation is a continuous process, it is characterized by a series of easily distinguishable stages known as the **bud**, **cap**, and **bell stages**. Each stage is defined according to the shape of the ectodermally derived enamel organ, which is a part of the developing tooth. The initial stage, the bud stage, is a rounded, localized growth of ectodermal cells surrounded by proliferating mesenchymal cells (Fig. 5.4). Gradually, as the rounded epithelial bud enlarges, it gains a concave surface, which begins the cap stage (Fig. 5.5). The ectodermal structure then differentiates to become the enamel organ and remains attached to the lamina. The ectomesenchyme forms the **dental papilla**, which becomes the dental pulp when surrounded by mineralized tissue. The tissue surrounding these two structures is the dental follicle, which is bounded by the walls of the bony crypt protecting the developing tooth organ.

After further growth of the papilla and the enamel organ, the tooth reaches the morphodifferentiation and histodifferentiation stage, also known as the *bell stage* (Fig. 5.6). At this stage, the inner enamel epithelial cells are characterized by the shape of the tooth they form (see Fig. 5.6). Also, the cells of the enamel organ have differentiated into the **outer enamel epithelial cells**, which cover the enamel organ, and **inner enamel epithelial cells**, which become the **ameloblasts** that form the enamel of the tooth crown. Between these two cell layers are the **stellate reticulum cells**, which are star-shaped, with cytoplasmic processes attached to each other. The stellate reticulum contains glycosaminoglycans in the extracellular matrix, which are hydrophilic and help maintain space for the developing crown. The stellate reticulum also has been reported to contain various growth factors and may function with the enamel knot (see later discussion) to direct the growth of the crown. A fourth layer in the enamel organ is composed of **stratum intermedium cells**. These cells lie adjacent to the inner enamel epithelial cells. They assist the ameloblast in the formation of enamel by allowing molecules into or out of the ameloblasts layer, depending on

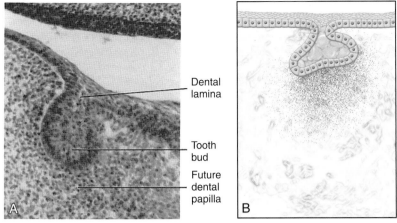

Fig. 5.4 **Initiation of tooth development. A**, Histology of the bud stage. **B**, Diagram of the bud stage. (B, Hargreaves KM, Cohen S. *Cohen's pathways of the pulp.* 10th ed. St. Louis: Mosby; 2011.)

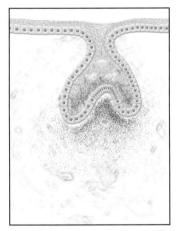

Fig. 5.5 **Cap stage of tooth development.** The enamel organ is outlined in blue, indicating that it is of ectodermal origin. The mesenchyme of the dental papilla surrounds the enamel organ. (Hargreaves KM, Cohen S. *Cohen's pathways of the pulp.* 11th ed. St. Louis: Mosby; 2016.)

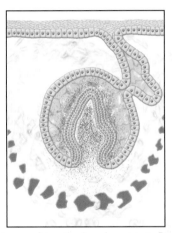

Fig. 5.6 **Bell stage of tooth development.** During this stage of tooth development, both odontoblasts and ameloblasts have fully differentiated in the cuspal region(s). Blood vessels develop in the dental papilla, whereas the only vascularized structure in the enamel organ is the outer enamel epithelium that contains a capillary plexus. (Hargreaves KM, Cohen S. *Cohen's pathways of the pulp.* 11th ed. St. Louis: Mosby; 2016.)

the functional state of the ameloblasts. The function of the outer enamel epithelial cells is to organize a network of capillaries that will bring nutrition to the ameloblasts by diffusion through the stellate reticulum and stratum intermedium.

From the outer enamel epithelium, nutrients will percolate through the stellate reticulum to the ameloblasts. During the bell stage, cells in the periphery of the dental papilla become **odontoblasts**. These cells differentiate from neural crest cells or, synonymously, ectomesenchymal cells. After the odontoblasts elongate, become columnar, and polarize, they form an extracellular matrix of 90% type I collagen fibers and 10% noncollagenous proteins termed **predentin**. After 24 hours, this increment of matrix calcifies and becomes **dentin**. When several increments of dentin have formed, the differentiated ameloblasts deposit an enamel matrix. Dentinogenesis always precedes amelogenesis. After the enamel organ is differentiated, the dental lamina begins to degenerate by undergoing autolysis. The dental lamina disappears in

the anterior part of the mouth, although it remains active in the posterior region for many years (see Figs. 5.2 and 5.3).

Cells interact through a system of effectors, modulators, and receptors, a process called **cell signaling**. An example of such a system is epithelial–mesenchymal interaction in tooth development. The precursor cells, odontoblast and ameloblast, establish a positional relationship by means of effectors and receptors that are on the cell surface. The ameloblast differentiates first, causing the precursor odontoblast (neural crest cell) to locate itself adjacent. Then the odontoblast differentiates, establishing with the ameloblast a basement membrane that then forms a predentin/dentinal matrix. After this formation occurs, the ameloblast forms the enamel matrix. Thus it is not only cells but also basal lamina and dentin matrix that contain substances that cause cell changes and position.

DEVELOPMENT OF THE DENTAL PAPILLA

Densely packed ectomesenchymal cells characterize the dental papilla. This is evident even in the early bud stage, during which cells proliferate around the enlarging tooth buds at the leading edge of the dental lamina (Fig. 5.7). The papilla cells are believed to be significant in furthering enamel organ bud formation into the cap and bell stages. This cell density is maintained as the enamel organ grows. Cells of the dental papilla are found on close examination to morphologically resemble fibroblasts and appear to be in a delicate reticulum (Fig. 5.8). Blood vessels appear early in the dental papilla, initially in the central region along with postganglionic sympathetic nerve fibers associated with these vessels. The vessels bring nutrition to the rapidly growing organ. As the papilla grows, smaller vessels are also seen in the periphery of the organ, bringing nutrition to the elongating odontoblasts (see Fig. 5.6). Cellular changes result in formation of a mineralized tissue around the central papilla. As this occurs, the papilla becomes known as the **dental pulp**.

DENTINOGENESIS

As the odontoblasts elongate, they gain the appearance of a protein-producing cell with a basally placed nucleus and a well-developed rough endoplasmic reticulum and Golgi apparatus. A process develops at the proximal end of the cell, adjacent to the dentinoenamel junction. Gradually, the cell moves pulpward, and the cell process, known as the **odontoblast process,** elongates (Fig. 5.9). The odontoblast becomes active in dentinal matrix formation, similar to an osteoblast when it moves away from a spicule of bone. Increments of dentin are formed along the dentinoenamel junction. The dentinal matrix is first a meshwork of type I collagen fibers, but within 24 hours it becomes calcified. It is called *predentin* before calcification and *dentin* after calcification. At that time, the dental papilla becomes the dental pulp as dentin begins to surround it. The odontoblasts maintain their elongating processes in dentinal tubules (see Fig. 5.9).

When the odontoblasts are functioning, their nuclei occupy a more basal position in the cell, and the organelles become more evident in the cell cytoplasm. The appearance of granular endoplasmic reticulum, the Golgi complex, and mitochondria indicates the protein-producing nature of these cells (Fig. 5.10C–E). The odontoblasts then secrete protein externally via vesicles at the apical part of the cell and along the cell processes (see Fig. 5.10). The collagenous dentinal matrix is laid down in increments like bone or enamel, which is indicative of a daily rhythm for hard tissue formation. The site of initial formation is at the cusp tips (see Fig. 5.8), and, as further increments are formed, more odontoblasts are activated along the dentinoenamel junction (see Fig. 5.9). As the odontoblast migrates toward the developing pulp, a process forms and elongates, a tubule is formed in the dentin, and an extracellular matrix is formed around this tubule and maintained by the cell as well as the dentinal fluid that is derived from the blood plasma and is also included in the dentinal tubule (Fig. 5.10C and D).

Dentinogenesis takes place in two phases. First is type I collagen matrix formation, followed by the deposition of calcium phosphate (calcium hydroxyapatite) crystals in the matrix. The initial calcification appears as crystals that are in small vesicles on the surface and within the collagen fibers (Fig. 5.11). The crystals grow, spread, and coalesce until the matrix is completely calcified. Only the newly formed band of dentinal matrix along the pulpal border is uncalcified (Fig. 5.12). Matrix formation and mineralization therefore are closely related. Mineralization proceeds by an increase in mineral density of the dentin. As each daily increment of predentin forms along the pulpal boundary, the adjacent peripheral increment of predentin formed the previous day calcifies and becomes dentin (see Figs. 5.10 and 5.12; Fig. 5.13).

AMELOGENESIS

Ameloblasts begin enamel deposition after a few micrometers of mineralized dentin have been deposited at the dentinoenamel junction (Fig. 5.14). Enamel synthesis, secretion, and

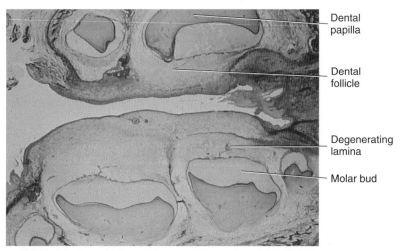

Dental papilla

Dental follicle

Degenerating lamina

Molar bud

Fig. 5.7 **Histology of tooth development.** Sagittal view of the human maxillary and mandibular molar tooth buds.

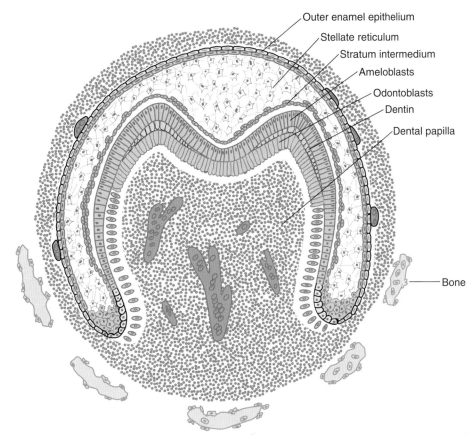

Outer enamel epithelium
Stellate reticulum
Stratum intermedium
Ameloblasts
Odontoblasts
Dentin
Dental papilla
Bone

Fig. 5.8 Dentinogenesis stage of tooth development. The initial formation of dentin (yellow) at the cuspal tips and the vascularized pulp organ are characteristic of the dentinogenesis stage. The dental follicular cells are differentiating around the enamel organ, and alveolar bone proper is beginning to define the dental crypt.

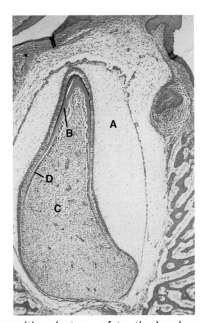

Fig. 5.9 Appositional stage of tooth development. During this stage of tooth development, both enamel and dentin are actively secreted until the crown is complete. **A**, Enamel organ. **B**, Developing dentin. **C**, Dental papilla. **D**, Odontoblast layer. (Berkovitz BKB, Holland GR, Moxham BJ. *Oral anatomy, histology, and embryology.* 4th ed. St. Louis: Mosby; 2009.)

subsequent mineralization is a complex process involving the structural proteins amelogenin, **ameloblastin**, and enamelin, and two proteinases, kallikrein-4 and enamelysin. At the bell stage, cells of the inner enamel epithelium differentiate. They elongate and are ready to become active secretory ameloblasts. The ameloblasts then exhibit changes as they differentiate and pass through five functional stages: (1) morphogenesis, (2) organization and differentiation, (3) secretion, (4) maturation, and (5) protection (see Fig. 5.10). The Golgi apparatus appears centrally in the ameloblasts, and the amount of rough endoplasmic reticulum (RER) increases in the apical area (see Fig. 5.10D and E). The row of ameloblasts maintains orientation by cell-to-cell attachments (desmosomes) at both the proximal and distal ends of the cell. This maintains the cells in a row as they move peripherally from the dentinoenamel junction, depositing enamel matrix (see Fig. 5.9).

Short, conical processes (**Tomes processes**) develop at the apical end of the ameloblasts during the secretory stage (see Fig. 5.10E; Fig. 5.15). Junctional complexes called the **terminal bar apparatus**, consisting of a series of desmosomes, appear at the junction of the cell bodies and Tomes processes and maintain contact between adjacent cells (see Fig. 5.10E). As the ameloblast differentiates, the matrix is synthesized within the RER, which then migrates to the Golgi apparatus, where it is condensed and packaged in membrane-bound granules. Vesicles migrate to the

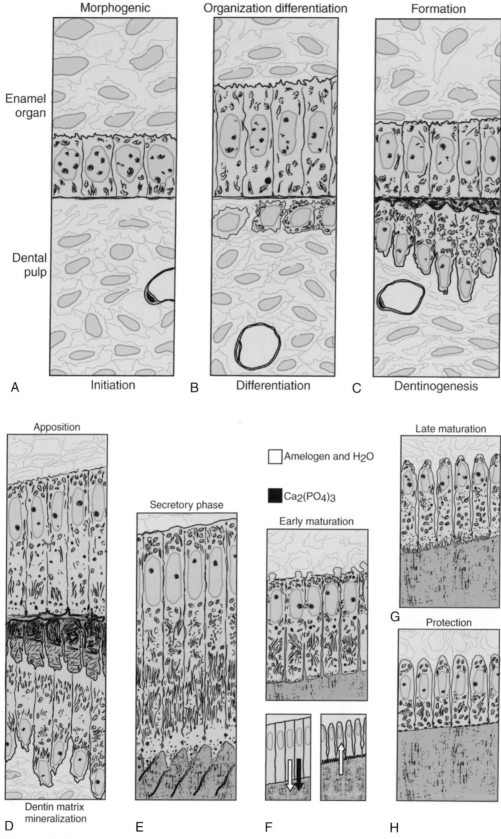

Fig. 5.10 Diagram of enamel and dentin formation. **A**, Initiation. **B**, Differentiation. **C**, Dentinogenesis. **D**, Apposition of enamel and dentin. **E** to **H**, Stages of enamel formation. **E**, Secretory stage of enamel formation. **F**, Early maturation. **G**, Late maturation. **H**, Protective stage in which the ameloblasts secrete the developmental cuticle. During maturation of enamel, an influx of mineral is accompanied by a loss of organic matter and water from the enamel matrix.

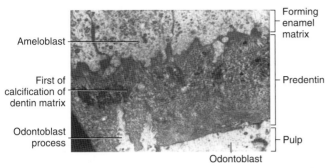

Fig. 5.11 Initiation of dentinogenesis. A transmission electron micrograph of a band of predentin, dentin, and enamel at the dentinoenamel junction. This initially secreted dentin is mantle dentin and is significantly different from the dentin that is formed by incremental deposition later in development. Calcification of the predentin will spread from nucleation sites within the matrix vesicles.

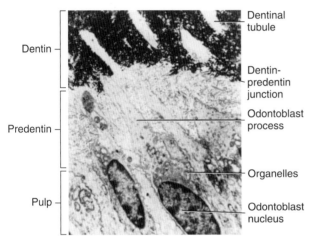

Fig. 5.12 Calcification of dentin at the mineralization front.

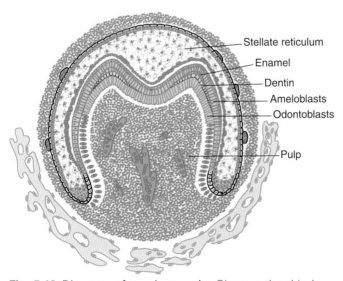

Fig. 5.13 Diagram of amelogenesis. Observe the thin layer of enamel secreted by the overlying ameloblasts at the cusp tips. Underlying the enamel is a layer of dentin formed by the odontoblasts. Observe the two layers of hard tissue that lie in apposition and form first at the cusp tips.

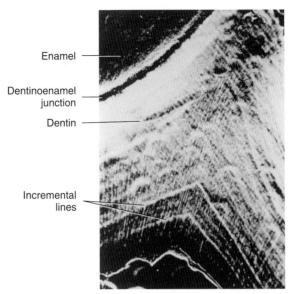

Fig. 5.14 Microradiograph of dentin illustrating incremental lines in dentin and showing the deposition of dentin in increments.

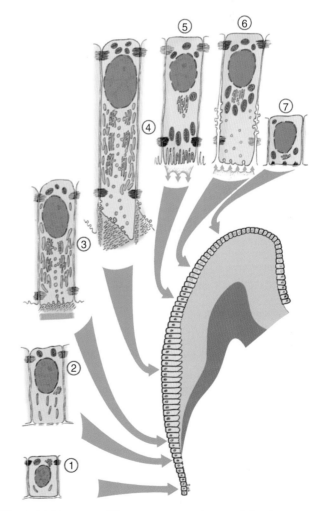

Fig. 5.15 Diagram of Tomes process, the specialized secretory process of the ameloblast during enamel formation. (Nanci A. *Ten Cate's oral histology.* 8th ed. St. Louis: Mosby; 2013.)

apical end of the cell, where their contents are secreted by exocytosis and are deposited first along the junction of the enamel and dentin (Fig. 5.16). This first enamel deposited on the surface of the dentin establishes the dentinoenamel junction. Fig. 5.17 is an electron micrograph of young enamel matrix formed along the dentinoenamel junction. The Tomes process of the ameloblast indents the surface of the enamel (see Figs. 5.10E, 5.15, and 5.16). This is because the center of the rod does not form at the same rate as the rod walls; this can best be seen in Fig. 5.17. As the enamel matrix develops, it forms in continuous rods from the dentinoenamel junction to the surface of the enamel.

When ameloblasts begin secretion, the overlying cells of the stratum intermedium change in shape from spindle to pyramidal (see Fig. 5.10B–F). As amelogenesis proceeds, both of these cell layers, ameloblasts and stratum intermedium, are held together by cell junctional complexes termed **desmosomes**, with synthesis of enamel occurring in both cells. Substances needed for enamel production arrive via the blood vessels and pass through the stellate reticulum to the stratum intermedium and ameloblasts. In this manner, the protein **amelogenin** is produced. Only a few

ameloblasts at the tip of the cusps begin to function initially (see Fig. 5.13). As the process proceeds, more ameloblasts become active, and the increments of enamel matrix become more prominent. At each cusp tip, an *enamel knot*, or a condensation of cells, forms that coordinates crown development. In teeth with multiple cusps, there is an enamel knot for each cusp.

Growth of individual cusps by incremental deposition continues until tooth eruption. This occurs in posterior multicuspid teeth as the ameloblasts continue to differentiate from the inner enamel epithelium and form enamel. Cusps then coalesce in the intercuspal region of the crown (Fig. 5.18). In radiographs, cusps initially appear separated and are joined together as growth progresses. The inner enamel epithelium forms the blueprint for the shape of the developing crown.

CLINICAL COMMENT

Amelogenesis imperfecta is a genetic problem in which the enamel is poorly developed and mineralized. This can be the result of cellular error resulting in defective enamel matrix formation. Multiple genes have been reported to be the cause of amelogenesis imperfecta, including *AMELX*, *AMBN*, *ENAM*, *MMP20*, and *KLK4*, and the defect is due to the malformation of their protein products, including amelogenin, ameloblastin, tuftelin, and enamelin.

CROWN MATURATION

As amelogenesis is completed and amelogenin is deposited, the matrix begins to mineralize (see Fig. 5.10F–H). As soon as the small crystals of mineral are deposited, they begin to grow in length and diameter. The initial deposition of mineral amounts to approximately 25% of the total enamel. The other 70% of mineral in enamel is a result of growth of the crystals (5% of enamel is water). The time between enamel matrix deposition and its mineralization is short. Therefore the pattern of mineralization closely follows the pattern of matrix deposition. The first matrix deposited is the first enamel mineralized, occurring along the dentinoenamel junction. Matrix formation and mineralization continue peripherally to the tips of the cusps and then laterally on the sides of the crowns, following the enamel incremental deposition pattern (Fig. 5.19). Finally, the cervical region of the

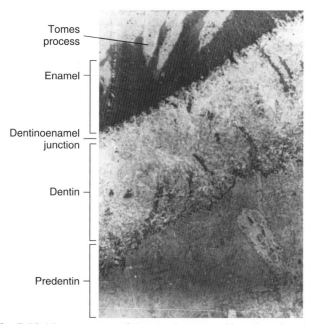

Tomes process

Enamel

Dentinoenamel junction

Dentin

Predentin

Fig. 5.16 Ultrastructure of the dentinoenamel junction showing early enamel and dentin matrix formation.

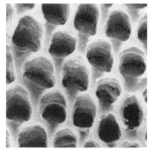

Human deciduous molar

Developing enamel surface

Height of field, 15-18 μm

Fig. 5.17 Scanning electron micrograph showing the interface between ameloblast and enamel matrix during amelogenesis. Pits are a result of the presence of the Tomes process.

Growth of cusps to predetermined point of completion

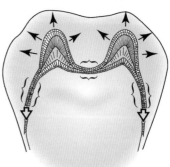

Fig. 5.18 Diagram of growth areas of developing crown. Growth occurs at cusp tips, then intercuspal zones and the cervical zone.

crown mineralizes. During this process, protein of the enamel changes or matures and is termed **enamelin**.

The mineral content of enamel is approximately 95% as it rapidly surpasses that of dentin (69%) to become the most highly calcified tissue in the human body. Because of the high mineral content of enamel, almost all water and organic material are removed during maturation (see Fig. 5.10E–H).

As the ameloblast completes the matrix deposition phase, its terminal bar apparatus disappears, and the surface enamel becomes smooth (see Fig. 5.10F and G). This phase is signaled by a change in the appearance of the cell, as well as by a change in the function of the ameloblast. The apical end of this cell becomes ruffled along the enamel surface to increase the surface area for the physiologic process of resorption. The length of the ameloblast decreases, as does the number of organelles within it. The enamel has now reached the maturation phase, and the ameloblast becomes more active in absorption of the organic matrix and water from enamel, which allows mineralization to proceed (see Fig. 5.10F–H).

The increased mineral content in enamel is dependent on the removal of fluid and protein. This process of exchange occurs throughout much of enamel maturation and is not limited to the final stage of mineralization. Even after the teeth erupt, mineralization of enamel continues.

Finally, after the ameloblasts have completed their contributions to the mineralization phase, they secrete an organic cuticle on the surface of the enamel, which is known as the **developmental** or **primary cuticle**. The ameloblasts then attach themselves to this organic covering of the enamel by **hemidesmosomes** (see Fig. 5.10H). A hemidesmosome is half of a desmosome-attachment plaque, whereas a desmosome functions in attaching a cell to an adjacent cell and requires both adjacent cells each producing a hemidesmosome. A hemidesmosome relates to the attachment of a cell to a surface membrane. The hemidesmosome-attachment plaque is developed by the ameloblast, and this stage of plaque formation and attachment

is known as the **protective stage** of ameloblast function. The ameloblasts shorten and contact the stratum intermedium and outer enamel epithelium, which fuse together to form the **reduced enamel epithelium**. At this point, the four layers of the fused reduced enamel epithelium, plus the added developmental cuticle, cover and protect the still-maturing enamel matrix, and this cellular organic covering remains on the enamel surface until the tooth erupts into the oral cavity.

With mineralization of enamel complete and its thickness established, the crown of the tooth is formed (Fig. 5.20). The nearly completed crown with the reduced enamel epithelium is seen in Fig. 5.21. Meanwhile, dentin formation proceeds. The next stage of development will be root formation.

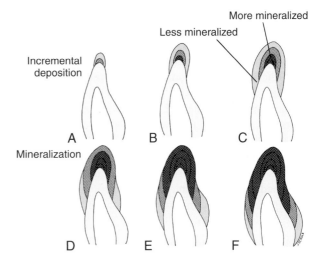

Fig. 5.20 Summary of enamel mineralization stages. A, Initial enamel is formed. **B**, Initial enamel is calcified as further enamel is formed. **C**, More increments are formed. **D**, Matrix deposition and mineralization proceeds. **E** and **F**, Matrix is formed on the sides and cervical areas of the crown.

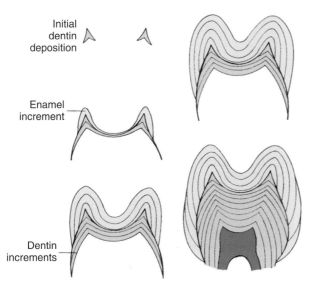

Fig. 5.19 Incremental pattern of enamel and dentin formation from initiation to completion. Development is shown vertically, proceeding from upper left to lower right.

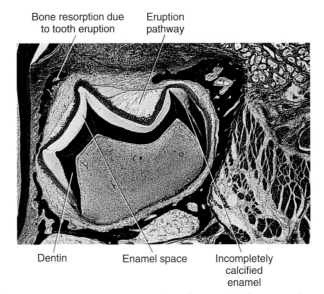

Fig. 5.21 Demineralized section of enamel of crown showing loss of mineralized enamel. Enamel matrix is present only at the cervical region, where the matrix still contains developmental enamel proteins.

DEVELOPMENT OF THE TOOTH ROOT

Root Sheath

As the crown develops, cell proliferation continues at the cervical region or base of the enamel organ, where the inner and outer enamel epithelial cells fuse to form the root sheath (Fig. 5.22). When the crown is completed, the cells in this region of the enamel organ continue to grow, forming a double layer of cells termed the **epithelial root sheath** or **Hertwig epithelial root sheath (HERS)** (see Fig. 5.22A). The inner cell layer of the root sheath forms from the inner enamel epithelium or ameloblasts in the crown, and enamel is produced. In the root, these cells induce odontoblasts of the dental papilla to differentiate and form dentin. The root sheath originates at the point that enamel deposits end. As the root sheath lengthens, it becomes the architect of the root. The length, curvature, thickness, and number of roots are all dependent on the inner root sheath cells. As the initial formation of the root dentin takes place, cells of the inner root sheath function in the deposition of **intermediate cementum**, a thin layer of acellular cementum composed of a keratin-like protein of epithelial origin that covers and seals the open ends of the dentinal tubule and seals the root surface. Then, the root sheath cells disperse into small clusters and move away from the root surface as **epithelial rests** (see Fig. 5.22B). As the cells of the follicle and dental pulp are induced to differentiate into odontoblasts on the side of the pulp and alveolar bone proper osteoblasts, periodontal ligament (PDL) fibroblasts, and cementoblasts on the side of the follicle, the root sheath breaks down and forms epithelial rests. When the root sheath fails to break down and remains attached to the dentin, it can induce enamel pearls as the root sheath. If the root sheath breaks down prematurely and then reforms, accessory or lateral canals are formed, with direct communication from the PDL to the dental pulp. Enamel pearls can be seen in Fig. 5.23.

At the proliferating end, the root sheath bends at a nearly 45-degree angle. This area is termed the **epithelial diaphragm** (see Fig. 5.22). The vertical part of the root sheath is called the root trunk. The epithelial diaphragm encircles the apical opening of the dental pulp during root development. It is the proliferation of these cells that allows root growth to occur.

As the odontoblasts differentiate along the pulpal boundary, root dentinogenesis proceeds and the root lengthens. Dentin formation continues from the crown into the root (Fig. 5.24). The dentin tapers from the crown into the root to the apical epithelial diaphragm. In the pulp adjacent to the epithelial diaphragm, cellular proliferation occurs. This is known as the **pulp proliferation zone** (see Fig. 5.22). It is believed that this area produces new cells needed for root lengthening. Dentinogenesis continues until the appropriate root length is developed. The root then

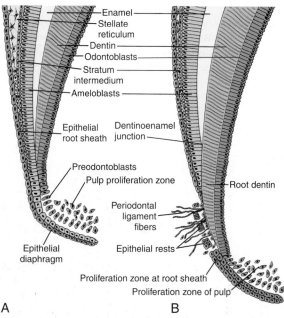

Enamel
Stellate reticulum
Dentin
Odontoblasts
Stratum intermedium
Ameloblasts
Epithelial root sheath
Dentinoenamel junction
Preodontoblasts
Pulp proliferation zone
Root dentin
Periodontal ligament fibers
Epithelial diaphragm
Epithelial rests
Proliferation zone at root sheath
Proliferation zone of pulp

A   B

Fig. 5.22 Root formation, showing root sheath and epithelial diaphragm. **A**, Time of epithelial root sheath formation showing fusion of outer and inner enamel epithelium to form the epithelial root sheath, which includes the vertical epithelial root trunk and inward-bending epithelial diaphragm. **B**, Later stage of root sheath development. Root dentin has formed below the cervical enamel on the surface of the pulp organ. Cementoblasts, periodontal ligament fibers, and epithelial rests are present in the ligament.

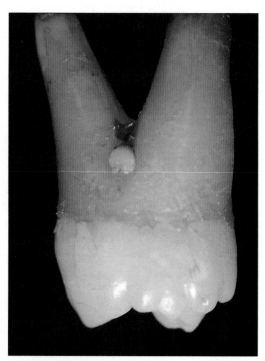

Fig. 5.23 An enamel pearl is caused by failure of the root sheath to break down and instead remains adherent to the root surface, inducing this developmental defect. (Courtesy Dr. Rudy Melfi. In: Ibsen O, Phelan J. *Oral pathology for the dental hygienist.* 7th ed. St. Louis: Saunders; 2017.)

thickens until the apical opening is restricted to approximately 1 to 3 mm, which is sufficient to allow neural and vascular communication between the pulp and the periodontium.

When the crown is complete and with the increase in root length, the tooth begins eruptive movements, which provide space for further lengthening of the root. The root lengthens at the same rate as the tooth eruptive movements occur (Fig. 5.25).

CLINICAL COMMENT

The presence of the epithelial root sheath determines whether a root will be curved or straight, short or long, or single or multiple.

Single Root

The root sheath of a single-rooted tooth is a tubelike growth of epithelial cells that originates from the enamel organ, enclosing a tube of dentin and the developing pulp (see Fig. 5.23). As soon as the root sheath cells deposit the intermediate cementum, the root sheath breaks up, forming epithelial rests (see Fig. 5.22B; Fig. 5.26). The epithelial rests persist as they move away from the root surface into the follicular area. Mesenchymal cells from the tooth follicle move between the epithelial rests to contact the root surface. There, they differentiate into cementoblasts and begin the appositional secretion of **cementoid** on the surface of

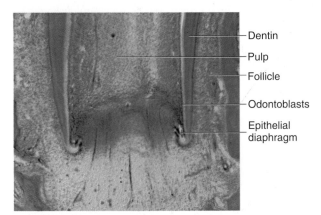

Fig. 5.24 Histology of root formation, showing root sheath and epithelial diaphragm. The highly cellular pulp proliferative zone is shown in the apical pulpal zone.

(Labels: Dentin, Pulp, Follicle, Odontoblasts, Epithelial diaphragm)

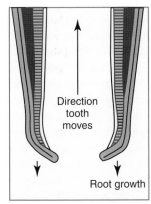

Fig. 5.25 Direction of root growth versus eruptive movements of the tooth.

(Labels: Direction tooth moves, Root growth)

the intermediate cementum. Cementoid is noncalcified cementum that soon calcifies into mature cementum (Fig. 5.27). The root sheath is never seen as a continuous structure because its cell layers break down rapidly once the root dentin forms. However, the area of the epithelial diaphragm is maintained until the root is complete; then it disappears.

Multiple Roots

The roots of multirooted teeth develop in a fashion similar to those of single-rooted teeth until the furcation zone begins to form (Fig. 5.28). Division of the roots then takes

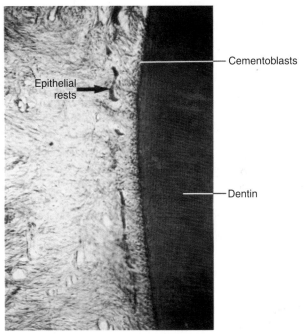

Fig. 5.26 Epithelial rests resulting from breakup of epithelial root sheath.

(Labels: Cementoblasts, Epithelial rests, Dentin)

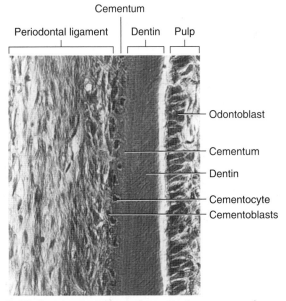

Fig. 5.27 Cementum formation on the root surface after breakup of the epithelial root sheath. Cementocytes can be seen on the surface and within the cementum.

(Labels: Cementum, Periodontal ligament, Dentin, Pulp, Odontoblast, Cementum, Dentin, Cementocyte, Cementoblasts)

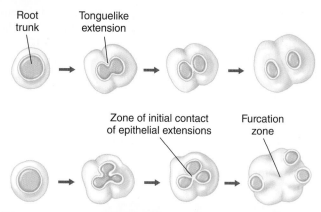

Fig. 5.28 Development of multirooted teeth. As the epithelial diaphragm grows, it may make contact and fuse to develop one-, two-, or three-rooted teeth.

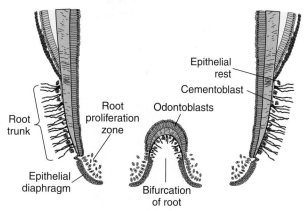

Fig. 5.29 Bifurcation root zone in multiple root formation. The root trunk is the junction area between the crown and the root bifurcation area.

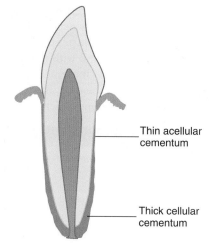

Fig. 5.30 Location of thin cementum on cervical area of root (younger individual) and additional apical cementum in an older individual.

DEVELOPMENT OF PRIMARY AND PERMANENT TEETH

Primary and permanent teeth develop very similarly, although the time needed for development of primary teeth is much less than for the permanent teeth. Primary teeth begin development in utero and the crown undergoes complete mineralization before birth, whereas the permanent teeth begin formation at or after birth. Any prenatal systemic disturbance will affect mineralization of the primary tooth crowns, whereas postnatal disturbances may affect the permanent tooth crowns.

Primary teeth function in the mouth approximately 8.5 years. This time may be divided into three periods: crown and root development, root maturation and root resorption, and shedding of the teeth. The first period extends for about a year, the second for about 3.75 years, and the final stage of resorption and shedding lasts for about 3.5 years. In contrast, some of the permanent teeth may be in the mouth from the fifth year until death. One must also consider the permanent molars, which may be in the mouth only from the 25th year on until they are lost or death occurs. The permanent teeth may function seven or eight times as long as the primary teeth. This time of function of permanent teeth includes 12 years of development, 3 years longer than the primary teeth.

Many separate events occur within a few millimeters during development of the dentition. For a single primary tooth and its successor, an example of two possibly simultaneous events could be eruption with root formation of the primary tooth and mineralization of the crown of the permanent tooth. Other examples of complex events during this mixed dentition stage are root resorption of the primary tooth root and formation of the root of the permanent tooth. In a 6-year-old child, one or more of these formative processes may be occurring in up to 28 of 32 permanent teeth, while some degree of resorption is occurring in the 20 primary teeth. Timing and coordination of myriad events allow continual function within the growing jaws.

In addition to the formative events, the primary teeth undergo root resorption and pulp degeneration.

place through differential growth of the root sheath. The cells of the epithelial diaphragm grow excessively in two or more areas until they contact the opposing epithelial extensions. These extensions fuse, and then the original single opening is divided into two or three openings. The epithelial diaphragm surrounding the opening to each root continues to grow at an equal rate. When a developing molar is sectioned through the center of its root, it shows the root sheath as an island of cells (Fig. 5.29).

As the multiple roots form, each one develops by the same pattern as a single-rooted tooth. After the root is complete and the sheath breaks up, the epithelial cells migrate away from the root surface as they do in a single-rooted tooth. Cementum then forms on the surface of the intermediate cementum surface. The cementum usually appears cellular, although the cementum near the cementoenamel junction is less cellular than that at the apices of the root (Fig. 5.30). Because the apical cementum is thicker, it is said to require more cells to maintain vitality. The primary function of this cementum involves the attachment of the principal periodontal ligament fibers.

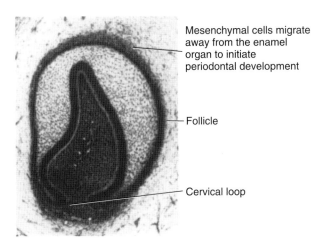

Fig. 5.31 Histology of enamel organ at time of cervical loop development. At this time, mesenchymal cells develop adjacent to the enamel organ on the external surface of the developing enamel organ and differentiate into follicular cells.

DEVELOPMENT OF SUPPORTING STRUCTURES

The mesenchymal cells surrounding the teeth are known as the *dental follicle (dental sac)* (see Fig. 5.7). Some of these follicular cells, which lie immediately adjacent to the enamel organ, migrate during the cap and bell stages from the enamel organ peripherally into the follicle to develop the alveolar bone and the periodontal ligament (Fig. 5.31). These cells have been traced from this origin to the site where they differentiate into cementoblasts, osteoblasts that form the alveolar bone proper, or fibroblasts that form the principal fibers of the periodontal ligament. After tooth eruption, these tissues serve to support the teeth during function.

Periodontal Ligament

Cells of the dental follicle differentiate into collagen-forming fibroblasts of the ligament and cementoblasts, which synthesize and secrete cementum on the surface of the tooth roots. Some cells of the ligament invade the root sheath as it breaks apart. Other cells of the ligament area form delicate fibers that appear along the forming roots near the cervical region of the crown. These are probably the stem cell fibroblasts that form the principal fiber groups, which appear as the roots elongate (Fig. 5.32). As these fibers become embedded in the cementum of the root surface, the other end attaches to the forming alveolar bone proper. Evidence suggests that these fibers turn over rapidly and are continually renewed as the location of origin is established. Collagen fiber turnover takes place throughout the ligament, although the highest turnover is in the apical area and the lowest is in the cervical region. Maturation of the ligament occurs when the teeth reach functional occlusion. At this time, the density of fiber bundles increases notably, as does the final orientation of the principal fiber groups.

Alveolar Process

As the teeth develop, so does the alveolar bone, which keeps pace with the lengthening roots. At first, the alveolar process forms labial and lingual plates between which a trench is formed

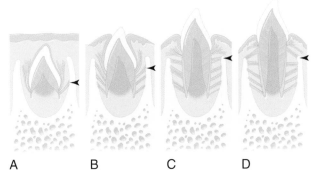

Fig. 5.32 Development of principal fibers of the periodontal ligament. **A**, Initial fiber development during preeruptive movements. **B**, Secondary fiber development below alveolar crest as the tooth moves into prefunctional occlusion. **C**, Further fiber development and maturation of the principal fibers and the gingival group of fibers occurs when the tooth reaches toward functional occlusion. **D**, Although the apical foramen is still open at this point, the principal fibers of the periodontal ligament (PDL) and gingival group are fully formed, enabling the tooth, the PDL, and the alveolar bone proper to react to the stresses of the maturing individual, including the development of larger muscles of mastication and concomitant increased occlusal forces.

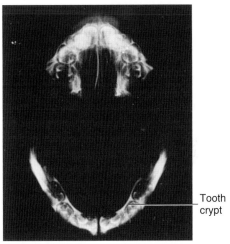

Fig. 5.33 Microradiograph of maxillary and mandibular arches showing alveolar bone and primary tooth crypts enclosing developing teeth.

where the tooth organs develop. As the walls lining this trench increase in height, bony septa appear between the teeth to complete the crypts (Fig. 5.33). When the teeth erupt, the alveolar process and intervening periodontal ligament mature to support the newly functioning teeth (Fig. 5.34). Bone that forms between the roots of the multirooted teeth is termed **interradicular bone**. In the mature form, alveolar bone is composed of **alveolar bone proper** and **supporting bone**. Alveolar bone proper lines the tooth socket, has the principal fibers of the periodontal ligament inserted into the matrix, and is sustained by supporting bone, which is composed of both spongy and dense or compact bone (Fig. 5.35). Supporting bone forms the cortical plate, which covers the mandible. The interactions of the tooth

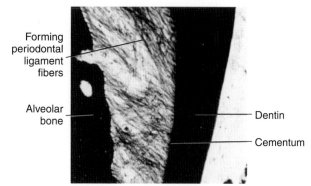

Fig. 5.34 Developing periodontal ligament fibers. Density of fibers similar to **C** in Fig. 5.32.

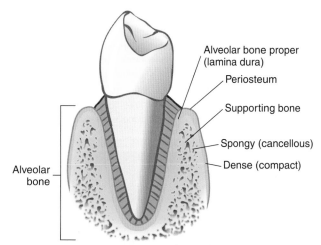

Fig. 5.35 Tooth in alveolar bone. Alveolar bone is composed of alveolar bone proper, which lines the socket, and supporting bone, which consists of spongy or cancellous bone and compact bone.

with the surrounding alveolar bone are necessary, because if the tooth is lost, the bone will resorb. The exact biological mechanisms are unknown.

In summary, tooth development involves the interactive events of several types of tissues: epithelial, mesenchymal, and ectomesenchymal. These tissues develop through the soft tissue stages of bud, cap, and bell. This level is followed by the hard tissue formative stages of dentinogenesis, amelogenesis, and appositional growth. Root formation logically follows crown development. Each developmental progression includes morphologic changes in shape and size that are coordinated with microscopic changes in cell shape and function. Most of these relationships are seen in Fig. 5.36.

CLINICAL COMMENT

Accessory root canals may connect the pulp with the periodontal ligament at any point along the root, although they usually appear near the root apex in permanent teeth. Pulp or periodontal infection can spread by means of this route to the adjacent tissue. A periodontal pocket that is resistant to treatment could be caused by this defect.

CLINICAL COMMENT

Dentinogenesis imperfecta is an autosomal dominant genetic disorder of tooth development that often makes the teeth susceptible to excessive wear. It can affect the primary and permanent teeth, with an incidence of between 1 in 6000 and 1 in 8000 people. Current evidence suggests that this disorder is caused by a mutation in the gene that produces dentin sialoprotein and dentin phosphoprotein, both of which are necessary for the proper mineralization of dentin by the odontoblasts. Improper mineralization of the dentin extracellular matrix causes the dentin to be compressible and results in the enamel chipping off. The dentinoenamel junction is much less scalloped, and this also contributes to the enamel chipping. Restoration of these primary teeth is usually accomplished with a stainless steel crown to preserve the tooth, which usually has an intact and vital pulp, and to allow the permanent tooth to erupt in the correct manner and space.

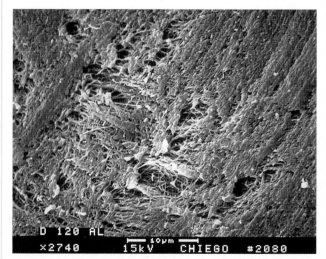

Dentinogenesis imperfecta type II: Unmineralized globular dentin extracellular matrix containing type III collagen.

CONSIDER THE PATIENT

White, chalky areas in the cervical enamel of some crowns are caused by a lack of mineralization of the enamel. The chalkiness occurs in this location because this is the last area of the crown to calcify, and sometimes the crown erupts before the cervical enamel has completely mineralized.

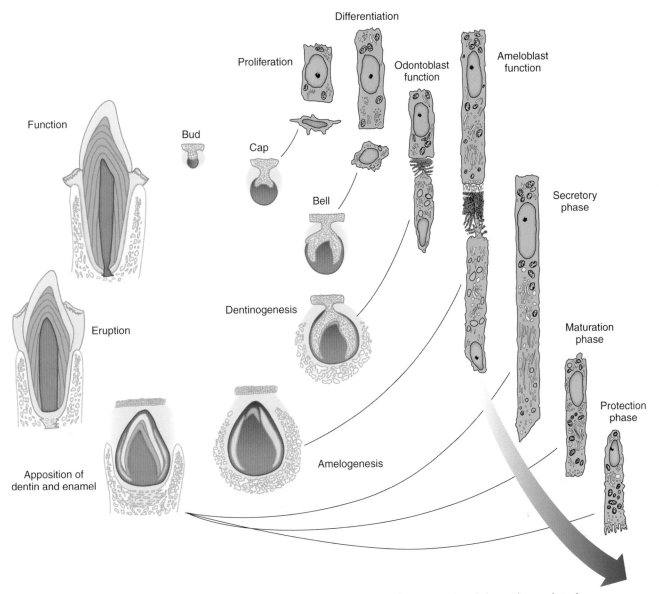

Fig. 5.36 Changes in formative cells of developing teeth shown on the right and correlated with morphologic changes of tooth organ on the left. Cell proliferation relates to the cap stage, whereas cell differentiation relates to the bell stage. Odontoblast function relates to dentinogenesis and ameloblast function to amelogenesis. The labels *secretory phase, maturation phase,* and *protection phase* relate to ameloblast function.

SELF-EVALUATION QUESTIONS

1. What two cell types interact in tooth development?
2. Describe two characteristics of the bell stage of tooth development.
3. List and describe each stage of tooth development.
4. Describe the dental papilla. When does it become the dental pulp organ?
5. Describe the differentiation of the odontoblast and the initiation of dentin formation.
6. Why is dentinogenesis called *the two-phases process?*
7. What are the five phases of enamel production?
8. What structures enable the ameloblasts to move in a row rather than individually during enamel production?
9. What areas of enamel are first and last to calcify in the crown?
10. Which two processes signal enamel completion?

ACKNOWLEDGMENTS

Dr. Nicholas P. Piesco and Dr. Nagat M. ElNesr contributed to the production of chapters in Avery JK, *Oral development and histology*, 3rd ed., Stuttgart, Thieme Medical, 2002. Some of the figures in that text have been used in preparation of this chapter.

QUANDARIES IN SCIENCE

Neural crest cells (NCCs) contribute to many structures in the oral–facial complex from development through adulthood and have a major role in tooth development. Before the neural tube fuses to form the spinal cord, NCCs begin to migrate along predetermined pathways to aggregate under specific areas of the oral ectoderm that have high concentrations of specific homeobox genes, where they interact with the ectoderm to initiate tooth development through a complex series of well-orchestrated epithelial–mesenchymal interactions and end in a functional tooth and supporting apparatus. However, at times, deficits can occur such that the teeth do not develop or there are multiple copies of the same tooth. Science is just beginning to understand the genetic basis for many of the anomalies associated with tooth development, but many developmental processes are still enigmatic. For example, the sequence of growth factors, transcription factors, and genes needed to induce tooth development is the same as for inducing hair, mammary and salivary glands, and more. The type of molecule or signaling event critical for just tooth induction is still an unsolved mystery, although many candidates have been suggested.

CASE STUDY

A family makes a dental appointment for their child because they have noticed the enamel chipping off his primary teeth. Because the enamel is no longer protecting the teeth, the child is experiencing intermittent pain. After a comprehensive medical history, the dentist does a complete oral exam with radiographs and makes the diagnosis of dentinogenesis imperfecta type II. Teeth present are bulbous and constricted at the cervical region and appear bluish and translucent. In areas where the enamel has chipped off the dentin, the dentin appears smooth and glassy, suggesting that sclerotic dentin has formed under the affected area. Radiographically, the pulp chambers are greatly reduced or obliterated, as are the root canals. Since there are no other symptoms or manifestations of the disease, the dentist restores the affected teeth with stainless steel crowns to maintain space for the developing permanent dentition to erupt and to maintain functional occlusion.

Dentinogenesis imperfecta is caused by mutations of the gene coding for dentin sialophosphoprotein (DSPP). This gene codes three important noncollagenous proteins found in the extracellular matrix of dentin: (1) dentin sialoprotein, (2) dentin glycoprotein, and (3) dentin phosphoprotein. There are many types of dentinogenesis imperfecta, including dentinogenesis imperfecta type I, dentinogenesis imperfecta type II, dentinogenesis imperfecta type III, dentine dysplasia type I, and dentine dysplasia type II. Some types of dentinogenesis imperfecta are nonsyndromic, such as dentinogenesis imperfecta type II. However, others are syndromic, such as dentinogenesis imperfecta type I associated with osteogenesis imperfecta, and are associated with other clinical conditions. Understanding a patient's complete medical, dental, and genetic history is paramount to a correct diagnosis and subsequent treatment.

SUGGESTED READING

Bartlett JD, Simmer JP. Kallikrein-related peptidase-4 (KLK4): role in enamel formation and revelations from ablated mice. *Front Physiol.* 2014;5:240.

Harrison JW, Roda RS. Intermediate cementum. Development, structure, composition, and potential functions. *Oral Surg Oral Med Oral Pathol Oral Radiol Endod.* 1995;79(5):624–633.

Kallenbach E, Piesco NP. The changing morphology of the epithelium–mesenchyme interface in the differentiation of growing teeth of selected vertebrates and its relationship to possible mechanisms of differentiation. *J Biol Buccale.* 1978;6:229–240.

Larmas M, Sándor GKB. Enzymes, dentinogenesis and dental caries: a literature review. *J Oral Maxillofac Res.* 2014;5(4):e3.

Marks SC, Gorski JP, Cahill DR, et al. Tooth eruption, a synthesis of experimental observations. In: Davidovich Z, ed. *The biological mechanisms of tooth eruption and root resorption.* Birmingham, AL: EBSCO Information Services; 1988.

McKnight DA, Simmer JP, Hart PS, et al. Overlapping DSPP mutations cause dentin dysplasia and dentinogenesis imperfecta. *J Dent Res.* 2008;87(12):1108–1111.

Robinson C, Kirkham J. Dynamics of amelogenesis as revealed by protein compositional studies. In: Butler W, ed. *The chemistry and biology of mineralized tissues.* Birmingham, AL: EBSCO Media; 1985.

Thesleff I, Vaahtokari A. The role of growth factors in the determination of the odontoblastic cell lineage. *Proc Finn Dent Soc.* 1992;88(suppl 1):357–368.

Warshawsky H, Josephsen K, Thylstrup A, et al. The development of enamel structure in the rat incisor as compared to the teeth of monkey and man. *Anat Rec.* 1981;200:371–399.

Wise GE, Marks Jr SC, Cahill DR. Ultrastructural features of the dental follicle associated with formation of the tooth eruption pathway in the dog. *J Oral Pathol.* 1985;14:15–26.

6

Eruption and Shedding of the Teeth

LEARNING OBJECTIVES

- Describe the three phases of tooth eruption: preeruption, prefunctional, and functional.

- Describe the initial growth of the tooth and the compensational changes that occur in the surrounding overlying and underlying tissues.

OVERVIEW

Tooth eruption is the process by which developing teeth emerge through the soft tissue of the jaws and the overlying mucosa to enter the oral cavity, contact the teeth of the opposing arch, and function in mastication. The movements related to tooth eruption begin during crown formation and require adjustments relative to the forming bony crypt. This is the **preeruptive phase**. Tooth eruption is also involved in the initiation of root development and continues until the tooth's emergence into the oral cavity, which is the **prefunctional eruptive phase**. The teeth continue to erupt until they reach incisal or occlusal contact. Then they undergo functional eruptive movements, which include compensation for jaw growth and occlusal wear of the enamel. This stage is the **functional eruptive phase**. Eruption is actually a continuous process that ends only with the loss of the tooth. Each dentition, primary and permanent, has various problems during eruption and in the sequencing of eruption in the oral cavity. Teeth differ extensively in their eruptive schedules as well. This chapter describes these events. Finally, the process of tooth shedding or exfoliation of the primary dentition is discussed (Boxes 6.1 and 6.2). Primary tooth loss results from three fundamental causes: root resorption, bone resorption, and size of crown being too small to withstand mastication.

PREERUPTIVE PHASE

The preeruptive phase includes all movements of primary and permanent tooth crowns from the time of their early initiation and formation to the time of crown completion. Therefore this phase is finished with early initiation of root formation. The developing crowns move constantly in the jaws during the preeruptive phase. They respond to positional changes of the neighboring crowns and to changes in the mandible and maxilla as the face develops outward, forward, and downward away from the brain in its maturing growth path. During the lengthening of the jaws, primary and permanent teeth make mesial and distal movements. Eventually the permanent tooth crowns move within the jaws, adjusting their position to the resorptive

roots of the primary dentition and the remodeling alveolar processes, especially during the mixed dentition period from 8 to 12 years of age.

Early in the preeruptive period, the permanent anterior teeth begin developing in the mandible lingual to the incisal level of the primary teeth (Figs. 6.1 and 6.2). Later, however, as the primary teeth erupt, the permanent successors are positioned lingual to the apical third of their roots. The permanent premolars shift from a location near the occlusal area of the primary molars to a location enclosed within the roots of the primary molars (see Fig. 6.2). This change in relative position is the result of the eruption of the primary teeth and an increase in height of the supporting structures. On the other hand, the permanent molars, which have no primary predecessors, develop without this type of relationship (Fig. 6.3). Maxillary molars develop within the tuberosities of the maxilla with their occlusal surfaces slanted distally. Mandibular molars develop in the mandibular rami with their occlusal surfaces slanting mesially (see Fig. 6.3). This slant is the result of the angle of eruption as the molars arise from the curvature of the condyle of the posterior mandible. All movements in the preeruptive phase occur within the crypts of the developing and growing crown before root formation begins.

PREFUNCTIONAL ERUPTIVE PHASE

The prefunctional eruptive phase starts with the initiation of root formation and ends when the teeth reach occlusal contact. Four major events occur during this phase:

1. **Root formation** requires space for the elongation of the roots. The first step in root formation is proliferation of the epithelial root sheath, which in time causes initiation of root dentin and formation of the pulp tissues of the forming root. Root formation also causes an increase in the fibrous tissue of the surrounding dental follicle (Fig. 6.4).
2. **Movement** occurs incisally or occlusally through the bony crypt of the jaws to reach the oral mucosa. The movement is the result of a need for space in which the enlarging roots

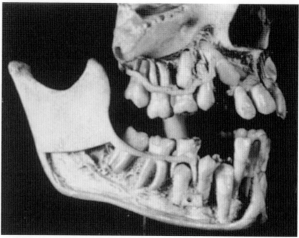

Fig. 6.3 Human jaws at 8 to 9 years of age, during the mixed dentition period. Permanent teeth are replacing primary teeth, and positions of each are shown. The permanent mandibular molar has not emerged from the coronoid process.

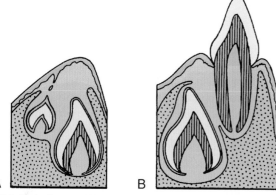

Fig. 6.1 Relative position of primary and permanent incisor teeth. **A**, Preeruptive period. **B**, Prefunctional eruptive period.

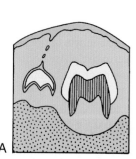 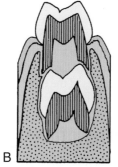

Fig. 6.2 Relative position of primary and permanent molar teeth. **A**, Preeruptive period. **B**, Prefunctional eruptive period.

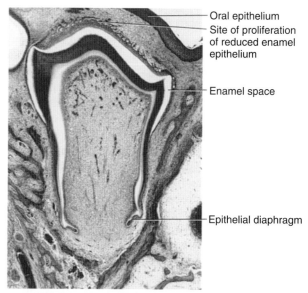

Oral epithelium
Site of proliferation of reduced enamel epithelium

Enamel space

Epithelial diaphragm

Fig. 6.4 Histology of the prefunctional eruptive phase. The root develops, and reduced epithelium overlying the crown approaches oral mucosa. Reduced enamel epithelium proliferates, anticipating fusion.

can form. The reduced enamel epithelium, along with the developmental cuticle, next contacts and fuses with the oral epithelium (Fig. 6.5). Both of these epithelial layers proliferate toward each other, their cells intermingle, and fusion occurs. A reduced epithelial layer overlying the erupting crown arises from the reduced enamel epithelium (Fig. 6.6).

3. **Penetration** of the tooth's crown tip through the fused epithelial layers allows entrance of the crown enamel into the oral cavity. Only the organic developmental cuticle (primary), secreted earlier by the ameloblasts, covers the enamel (Fig. 6.7).

4. **Intraoral occlusal** or **incisal movement** of the erupting tooth continues until clinical contact with the opposing crown occurs. The crown continues to move through the mucosa, causing gradual exposure of the crown surface with an increasingly apical shift of the gingival attachment (see Fig. 6.7). The exposed crown is the clinical crown, extending from the cusp tip to the area of the gingival attachment. In contrast, the anatomic crown is the entire crown, extending from the cusp tip to the cementoenamel junction.

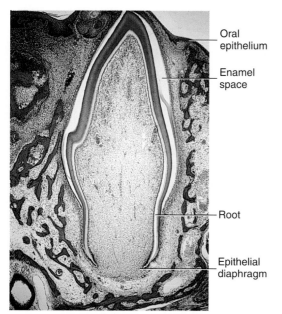

Oral epithelium

Enamel space

Root

Epithelial diaphragm

Fig. 6.5 Histology of an erupting cuspid tooth. The crown tip is in contact with oral epithelium.

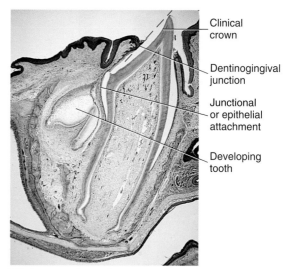

Clinical crown

Dentinogingival junction

Junctional or epithelial attachment

Developing tooth

Fig. 6.7 An erupting primary tooth appears in the oral cavity. The permanent tooth's position is shown on the left. The dashed line indicates cuticle overlying the enamel surface of the erupting tooth.

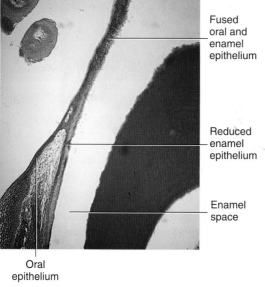

Fused oral and enamel epithelium

Reduced enamel epithelium

Enamel space

Oral epithelium

Fig. 6.6 Fused reduced enamel epithelium and oral epithelium overlie the enamel of the crown. Enamel space occurs as enamel is dissolved in preparation of slide.

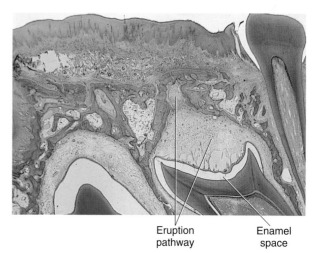

Eruption pathway

Enamel space

Fig. 6.8 Histology of a prefunctional erupting tooth. Observe the appearance of the eruption pathway developed overlying the crown.

CLINICAL COMMENT

Hypereruption occurs with the loss of an opposing tooth. This condition allows the tooth or teeth to erupt farther than normal into the space provided.

Changes in Tissues

The prefunctional eruptive phase is characterized by significant changes in the **tissues overlying, surrounding**, and **underlying** the erupting teeth.

Overlying the Teeth

The dental follicle changes and forms a pathway for the erupting teeth. A zone of degenerating connective tissue fibers and cells

immediately overlying the teeth appears first (Figs. 6.8 and 6.9). During the process, the blood vessels decrease in number, and nerve fibers break up into pieces and degenerate. The altered tissue area overlying the teeth becomes visible as an inverted triangular area known as the **eruption pathway**. In the periphery of this zone, the follicular fibers, regarded as the **gubernaculum dentis** or **gubernacular cord** (Fig. 6.10), are directed toward the mucosa. Some scientists believe that these fibers guide the teeth in their movements to ensure complete tooth eruption.

Macrophages appear in the eruption pathway tissue. These cells cause the release of hydrolytic enzymes that aid in the destruction of the cells and fibers in this area with the loss of blood vessels and nerves. Osteoclasts are found along the borders of the resorptive bone overlying the teeth. This bone loss adjacent to the teeth keeps pace with the eruptive movements of

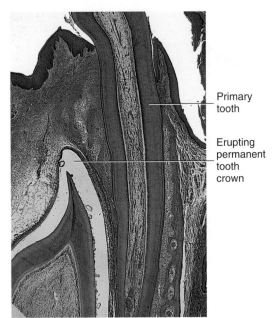

Fig. 6.9 Observe the relation of the functional primary tooth root on the right to the permanent prefunctional erupting crown on the left.

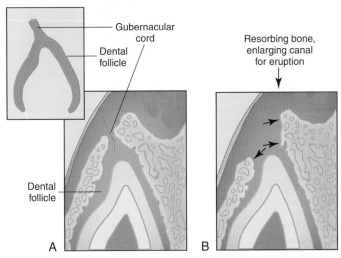

Fig. 6.10 Diagram of a developing eruption pathway. **A,** Early developing eruption pathway. **B,** Resorption of bone in eruption pathway.

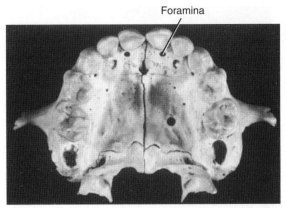

Fig. 6.11 Foramina palatal to maxillary primary incisors. These are sites of eruption for permanent incisors.

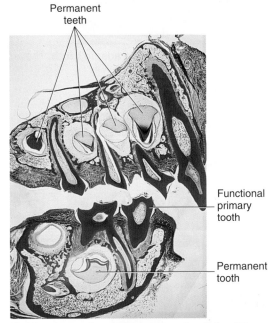

Fig. 6.12 Histology of maxilla in the mixed dentition period. Roots of erupted primary teeth are undergoing resorption. Crowns of developing permanent teeth appear below primary teeth.

the teeth (see Fig. 6.9). **Osteoclasts** and **osteoblasts** constantly remodel the alveolar bone as the teeth enlarge and move forward in the direction of the growing face.

Although the process of eruption for permanent teeth is similar to that of the primary teeth, the presence of roots from primary teeth poses a problem. The resorption of their roots is similar to the process of bone resorption for the emergence of primary teeth. Permanent teeth establish an eruptive path lingual to the primary anterior teeth and the premolars under the primary molars. Permanent molars erupt into the alveolar free space behind primary teeth (see Fig. 6.9). Small foramina just posterior to the primary tooth row are evidence of the eruption

sites of the anterior permanent teeth (Fig. 6.11). As the roots resorb, the primary crowns are lost or shed (Fig. 6.12). Dentin resorption is similar to bone resorption (see Fig. 6.10).

The resorptive process of primary and permanent teeth results from action of osteoclasts that arise from monocytes of the circulating bloodstream. These monocytes appear and fuse with others to form the giant multinucleated osteoclasts. Their function is to resorb the hard tissue. They do so by first separating the mineral from the collagen matrix through the action of the hydrolytic acids and enzymes secreted by the osteoclasts. This enzymatic action is believed to occur within lacunae, which are developed by the osteoclasts. The osteoclast's cell membrane is in contact with the bone and becomes modified by an enfolding process termed the **ruffled border** (Figs. 6.13 and 6.14). This border greatly increases the surface area of the osteoclast

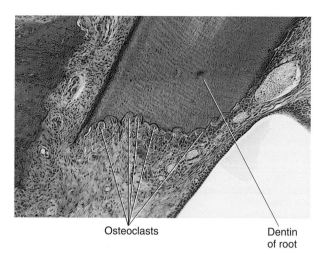

Fig. 6.13 Histology of active resorption sites on primary tooth roots. Osteoclasts appear in lacunae in root cementum and dentin.

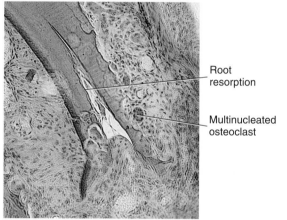

Fig. 6.14 Histology of osteoclasts in advancing resorption lacunae. Observe the large multinucleated cells shown within the lacunae.

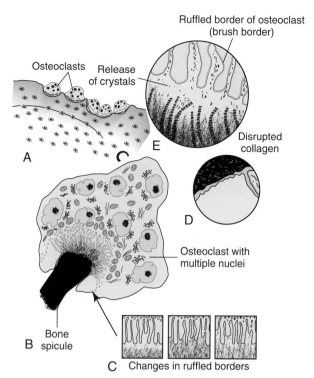

Fig. 6.15 Osteoclast activity. **A**, Osteoclasts in lacunae on bone surface. **B**, Large multinucleated osteoclasts with brush border in contact with bone spicule. **C**, High magnification of ruffled border of osteoclast showing mineral crystals passing into spaces between cell extensions. Unmasked collagen fibers are nearby. **D**, Clear zone on osteoclast surface. **E**, Ruffled border of osteoclast in constant motion or change.

and allows the cell to function maximally in bone resorption (Fig. 6.15).

Hard tissue resorption is believed to occur in two phases: the **extracellular phase**, in which the mineral is separated from the collagen and is broken into small fragments (see Fig. 6.15), and the **intracellular phase**, in which the osteoclast ingests these mineral fragments and continues the dissolution of this mineral. Crystals appear in cytoplasmic vacuoles of the osteoclast and are gradually digested within them. Resorption of mineral occurs at the ruffled border interface outside the cell, and the mineral is then taken within the cell (Fig. 6.16). Osteoclasts and special **fibroblast** cells are believed to destroy the remaining collagen fibers secondarily by ingesting them in an intracellular phagolysosome system (Fig. 6.17). Amino acids resulting from this breakdown are used in the formation of collagen within this same cell and can be used in this same area for bone formation. Only the posterior permanent molars, which have no primary predeciduous teeth, erupt through alveolar bone (Fig. 6.18). Fig. 6.19 summarizes what happens in the tissues overlying the teeth

during their prefunctional eruptive phase. Bone loss occurs as the tooth approaches the oral epithelium and forms an eruption pathway while the reduced enamel epithelium fuses with the oral ectoderm to form the junctional epithelium, which attaches to the developmental cuticle by hemidesmosomes formed by the gingival keratinocytes and helps prevent oral bacteria and other substances present in the oral cavity from entering the body (see Fig. 6.19A). The tooth organ epithelium makes contact with the oral mucosa (see Fig. 6.19B and C). This contact causes stretching and thinning of the oral membrane and finally its rupture and penetration by the tooth (see Fig. 6.19D and E). Only a thin developmental cuticle then covers the tooth (see Fig. 6.19E and F). As the tooth emerges farther into the mouth, more crown is exposed, and as clinical contact with the opposing tooth is made, the epithelial attachment shifts to the cervical area (see Fig. 6.19G). Clinically, tooth eruption is seen as a blanching of the mucosa, and this condition may persist for several days because the eruptive process is neither rapid nor continuous. Each eruptive movement, however, results in greater exposure of the crown. With successive eruptive movements, the area of attached epithelium becomes lower on the clinical crown.

Surrounding the Teeth

The tissues around the teeth change from delicately fine fibers lying parallel to the surface of the tooth to bundles of fibers attached to the tooth surface and extending toward the

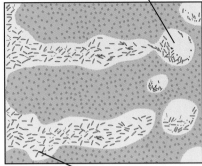

Crystal uptake by vacuoles

Breakdown of bone into
A   collagen fibers and crystals   B

Crystals visible within
ruffled border

Fig. 6.16 Diagram of ruffled border of an osteoclast. **A**, High magnification of unmasked collagen fibers. Mineral crystals are near the osteoclast surface. **B**, Diagram of uptake of crystals into osteoclast vacuoles.

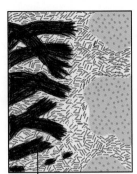

Fig. 6.17 Fibroblasts are capable of simultaneous synthesis of collagen and its breakdown. Collagen fibers are phagocytosed into cells and are broken down to release amino acids (AA). These amino acids are then used to form new collagen molecules.

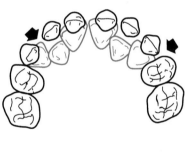

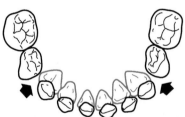

Fig. 6.18 The relationship between primary and permanent teeth during the mixed dentition period. (Berkovitz BKB, Holland GR, Moxham BJ. *Oral anatomy, histology, and embryology.* 5th ed. St. Louis: Elsevier; 2017.)

periodontium. The first fibers to appear are those in the cervical area as root formation begins (Fig. 6.20A). As the root elongates, bundles of fibers appear on the root surface (see Fig. 6.20B and C). Fibroblasts are the active cells in both the formation and the degradation of the collagen fibers. With tooth eruption, the

alveolar bone crypt increases in height to accommodate the forming root. After the teeth attain functional occlusion, the fibers gain their mature orientation (see Fig. 6.20C). Special fibroblasts have been found in the periodontium around the erupting teeth. These fibroblasts have contractile properties. During eruption, collagen fiber formation and fiber turnover are rapid, occurring within 24 hours. This mechanism enables fibers to attach and release and attach in rapid succession. Some fibers may detach and reattach later while the tooth moves occlusally as new bone forms around it. Gradually, the fibers organize and increase in number and density as the tooth erupts into the oral cavity. Blood vessels then become more dominant in the developing ligament and exert additional pressure on the erupting tooth (Fig. 6.21).

CLINICAL COMMENT

Teeth are considered submerged when eruption is prevented because of crowding or tipping of the adjacent teeth into the space created by the missing primary tooth. Retained primary teeth may be caused by the lack of development of the permanent successor.

Underlying the Teeth

As the crown of a tooth begins to erupt, it gradually moves occlusally, providing space underlying the tooth for the root to lengthen (Fig. 6.22). In the fundic region, these changes in the soft tissue and the bone surrounding the root apex are believed to be largely compensatory for the lengthening of the root. During root formation, the dentin of the root apex tapers to a fine edge that terminates in the epithelial diaphragm (Fig. 6.23). Fibroblasts form collagen around the root apex, and these fiber bundles become attached to the cementum as it begins to form on the apical dentin. Fibroblast-like cells appear in great numbers in the fundic area, and some of these fibers form strands that mature into calcified trabeculae. These trabeculae form a network, or bony ladder, at the tooth apex. This is believed to fill the space left behind as the tooth begins eruptive movement (see Fig. 6.23). Gradually, this delicate bony ladder becomes denser as additional bony plates appear (Fig. 6.24). The bony plates remain until the teeth are in functional occlusion at the end of

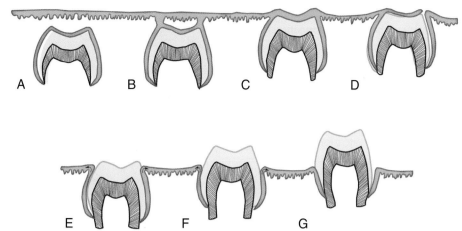

Fig. 6.19 Stages of tooth eruption. A, Tooth crown approaching oral epithelium in preeruptive stage. **B,** Contact of reduced enamel epithelium, including the developmental cuticle fusing with oral epithelium. **C,** Fusion of reduced enamel epithelium, including the developmental cuticle and oral epithelia. **D,** Thinning of fused epithelia. **E,** Rupture of oral epithelium, formation of the attached gingiva, and emergence. **F,** Clinical crown appearance into the oral cavity (prefunctional stage). **G,** Tooth erupting into functional occlusion.

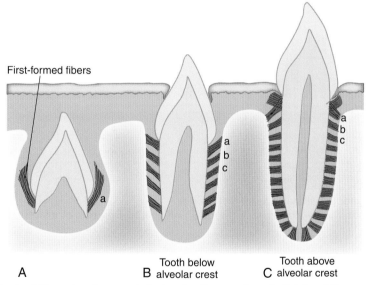

Fig. 6.20 Principal fiber development during tooth eruption. A, Origin of fibers at the cervical root area of crown. **B,** Fiber development with root growth. *a,* Initial fiber formation; *b,* development of secondary fibers; *c,* further fiber development. **C,** Change in orientation of the fibers with occlusal function. Initial fiber groups (*a, b,* and *c*) change direction with function.

this phase. Dense bone then forms around the tooth's apex, and bundles of fibers attach to the apical cementum and extend to the adjacent alveolar bone to provide more support (Fig. 6.25).

FUNCTIONAL ERUPTIVE PHASE

The final eruptive phase takes place after the teeth are functioning and continues as long as the teeth are present in the mouth. During this period of root completion, the height of the alveolar process undergoes a compensating increase. The fundic alveolar plates resorb to adjust for formation of the root tip apex. The root canal narrows as a result of root tip maturation, during which the apical fibers develop to help cushion the forces of occlusal impact. Root completion continues for a considerable length of time, even after the teeth begin to function. This process takes about 1 to 1.5 years for deciduous teeth and 2 to 3 years for permanent teeth.

The most marked changes occur as occlusion is established. At that time, the mineral density of the alveolar bone increases, and the principal fibers of the periodontal ligament increase in dimension and change orientation to their mature state. These fibers separate into groups oriented about the gingiva, the alveolar crest, and the alveolar surface around the root. Such fibers stabilize the tooth to a greater degree, and the blood vessels become more highly organized in the spaces between the bundles of fibers (see Fig. 6.25). Later in life, attrition and abrasion may wear down the occlusal or incisal surface of the teeth, causing the teeth to erupt slightly to compensate for this loss of tooth structure. Any such change results in deposition of cementum on the root's apex (Fig. 6.26). Cementum is also deposited in the furcation area of a two- or three-rooted tooth. Because of

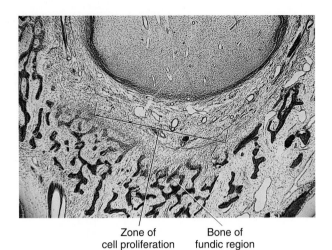

Zone of cell proliferation   Bone of fundic region

Fig. 6.23 Histology of changes in fundic region during tooth eruption. Fine trabeculae of new bone appear near tooth apices that will aid in stabilizing the tooth during eruption.

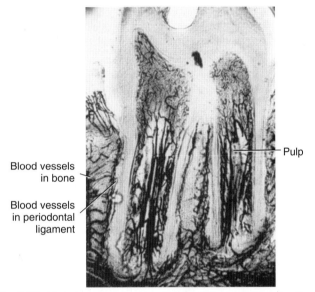

Pulp

Blood vessels in bone

Blood vessels in periodontal ligament

Fig. 6.21 Histology of erupting tooth with vascular injection. An outline of the blood vessels in the periodontium and tooth pulp is shown.

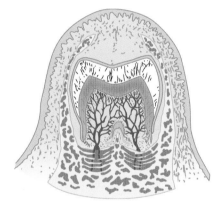

Fig. 6.24 Diagram of a later stage of tooth eruption. The fundic region further develops a bony ladder.

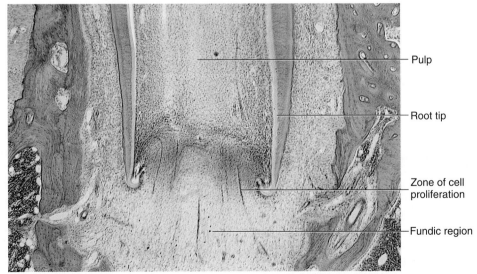

Pulp

Root tip

Zone of cell proliferation

Fundic region

Fig. 6.22 Histology of erupting tooth with immature roots and open apex. As the tooth erupts, the roots will develop and fill in the wide pulpal tooth apex.

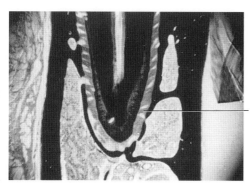

Fig. 6.25 Histology of tooth in functional occlusion to show density of functioning periodontal fibers. Areas between fiber bundles are for blood vessels and nerves.

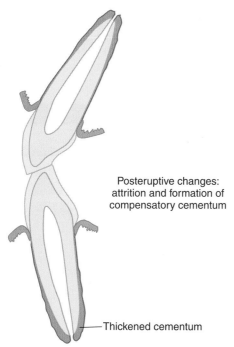

Posteruptive changes: attrition and formation of compensatory cementum

Thickened cementum

Fig. 6.26 Functional eruptive changes illustrating attrition of the incisal surface of enamel. Observe the compensatory deposition of cementum on the apical region of the root surface.

the different biologic properties of the tissues comprising the periodontium, cementum is the last to reorganize after the periodontal ligament and the alveolar bone proper.

> **CLINICAL COMMENT**
>
> Lack of eruption resulting from failure of root formation may be caused by crowding of teeth, crown-to-root fusion, and lack of development of the pulp proliferative zone.

POSSIBLE CAUSES OF TOOTH ERUPTION

Of the numerous causes of tooth eruption, the most frequently cited are root growth and pulpal pressure. Other important causes are cell proliferation, increased vascularity, and increased bone formation around the teeth. Additional possible

causes that have been noted are endocrine influence, vascular changes, and enzymatic degradation. Probably all these factors have an influencing role, not necessarily independent of one another.

Although not all factors associated with tooth eruption are known, elongation of the root and modification of the alveolar bone and periodontal ligament are thought to be the most important ones. These events are coupled with changes overlying the tooth that produce the eruption pathway. Blood vessels in this area are compressed by the influence of the advancing crown and become nonfunctional. Connective tissue in the eruption pathway gradually disappears as the tooth epithelium and the oral epithelium fuse. In summary, the erupting tooth moves from an area of increased pressure to an area of decreased pressure.

> **CLINICAL COMMENT**
>
> The 6/4 rule for primary tooth emergence means that from birth, 4 teeth emerge for each 6 months of age. Thus 6 months, 4 teeth; 12 months, 8 teeth; 18 months, 12 teeth; 24 months, 16 teeth; and 30 months, 20 teeth.

SEQUENCE AND CHRONOLOGY OF TOOTH ERUPTION

The formula for the eruptive sequence of the primary and permanent dentition appears in Box 6.3. Table 6.1 shows the chronologic development and eruption of the primary dentition, and Table 6.2 shows the development and eruption of the permanent dentition.

> **CLINICAL COMMENT**
>
> A lack of eruption may be related to fusion of tooth roots to the bony socket or to the crown of a permanent tooth. The condition is known as *ankylosis* (Fig. 6.27) because the cementum of the tooth root fuses with the alveolar bone proper surrounding the alveolus (socket).

> **CONSIDER THE PATIENT**
>
> A patient complains about a retained primary tooth. She notes the absence of the permanent successor. How could you determine what has occurred?

BOX 6.3	Sequence of Tooth Eruption			
Primary				
CI	LI	$_1$M	Cu	$_2$M
L	U	U	U	L
U	L	L	L	U
Permanent								

U_1M	LCI	UL	LCU	U_1Pre	U_2Pre	UCu	L_2M	L_3M
L_1M	UCI	LL		L_1Pre	L_2Pre		U_2M	U_3M

TABLE 6.1   Chronology of Development of the Primary Dentition[a]

Primary Teeth Listed in Order of Eruption (Sequence)	Beginning Calcification (Mo in Utero)	Crown Completed Postnatally (Mo)	Appearance in the Oral Cavity (Eruption Time) (Mo)	Root Completed (Yr)
Lower central incisor	3–4	2–3	6–8	1–2
Upper central incisor	3–4	2	7–10	1–2
Upper lateral incisor	4	2–3	8–11	2
Lower lateral incisor	4	3	8–13	1–2
Upper first molar	4	6	12–15	2–3
Lower first molar	4	6	12–16	2–3
Upper canine	4–5	9	16–19	3
Lower canine	4–5	9	17–20	3
Lower second molar	5	10	20–26	3
Upper second molar	5	11	25–28	3

[a]The normal range of eruption times indicates a wide variation in eruption times. It is important to know that a difference of 1 or 2 months on either side of the normal range does not necessarily indicate that a child's eruption time schedule is abnormal. Only deviations considerably out of this range should be considered abnormal.

TABLE 6.2   Chronology of Development of the Permanent Dentition

Permanent Teeth Listed in Order of Eruption (Sequence)	Beginning Calcification	Crown Completed (Yr)	Appearance in the Oral Cavity (Eruption Time) (Yr)	Root Completed (Yr)
Lower first molar	Birth	3–4	6–7	9–10
Upper first molar	Birth	4–5	6–7	9–10
Lower central incisor	3–4 mo	4	6–7	9
Upper central incisor	3–4 mo	4–5	7–8	10
Lower lateral incisor	3–4 mo	4–5	7–8	9–10
Upper lateral incisor	10–12 mo	4–5	8–9	10–11
Lower canine	4–5 mo	5–6	9–10	12–13
Upper first premolar	1–2 yr	6–7	10–11	12–14
Lower first premolar	1–2 yr	6–7	10–11	12–14
Upper second premolar	2–3 yr	7–8	10–12	13–14
Lower second premolar	2–3 yr	7	11–12	14–15
Upper canine	4–5 mo	6–7	11–12	14–15
Lower second molar	2–3 yr	7–8	11–12	14–15
Upper second molar	2–3 yr	7–8	12–13	15–16
Lower third molar	8–10 yr	12–16	17–20	18–25
Upper third molar	7–9 yr	12–16	18–20	18–25

SHEDDING OF PRIMARY TEETH

Humans are considered **diphyodonts** because they possess two dentitions, primary and permanent. Teeth in the primary dentition are smaller and fewer in number than the permanent dentition to conform to the smaller jaws of the young person. Teeth in the permanent dentition are larger, longer, and more numerous, which the larger jaws of the adult can accommodate.

The primary dentition functions from about 2 to 8 years of age. Teeth from both dentitions are present in the **mixed dentition period**, which extends from about 8 to 12 years of age. This is an interesting period because only part of the primary teeth roots are present while they undergo resorption, and only part of the permanent roots are present while they are in the formative stage. In this way, nearly 50 teeth can be accommodated in the jaws during this 4-year span (see Fig. 6.12).

The period of tooth shedding follows the mixed dentition period. **Shedding** is the loss of the primary dentition caused by the physiologic resorption of the roots, the loss of the bony

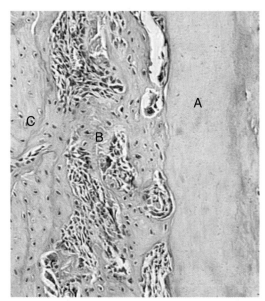

Fig. 6.27 Ankylosis. This photomicrograph demonstrates anky-losis between the cementum on the root surface **A**, the alveolar bone proper **C**, and the area that was the periodontal ligament **B**, which is now filled in with bone and connective tissue and fused with the cementum and the alveolar bone proper.

supporting structures, and therefore the inability of these teeth to withstand the masticatory forces.

The degeneration of primary pulp tissue is similar to that of the tissues in the eruption pathway with a loss of cells, nerves, and blood vessels. When a primary tooth is extracted, blood is still likely to be in the crown, although only the oral epithelium holds the tooth in the socket. Fig. 6.28 shows the correlation between root growth and eruption. It illustrates changes that occur in the preeruptive (Fig. 6.28A and B), prefunctional (Fig. 6.28C and D), and functional eruptive (Fig. 6.28E) stages of the tissues overlying and around the root surface as the tooth develops functionally.

COMPARISONS OF THE PRIMARY AND PERMANENT DENTITIONS

This section compares the morphology and histology of the primary and permanent dentition and describes some clinical problems in the developing jaw of the growing child as compared with the jaw of the adult and related characteristics of the developing primary and permanent teeth and their supporting structures (Table 6.3).

Tooth Number and Size

The main difference between the primary and permanent denti-tions is the number of teeth—20 in the primary dentition and 32 in the permanent dentition. The permanent teeth replacing the primary teeth are called *successional*. There are 12 perma-nent teeth, the permanent molars, that have no predecessors. They are called *accessional*. As the permanent molars are added, arch length and occlusal surface are increased (see Fig. 6.18). Primary and permanent teeth differ in size and form. Several of these differences influence decisions about clinical treatment.

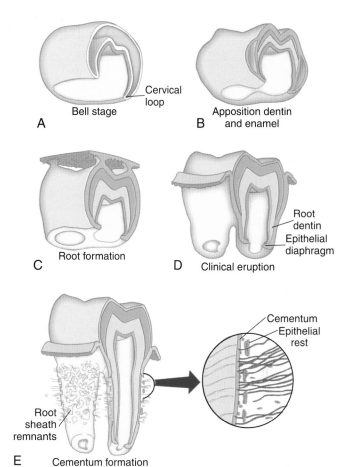

Fig. 6.28 Summary of tooth eruption. **A**, Early preeruptive changes in enamel organ at the bell stage. **B**, Late preerup-tive changes as enamel and dentin form. **C**, Early prefunctional changes as the tooth moves to oral epithelium. **D**, Late pre-functional changes as the tooth emerges into the oral cavity. **E**, Functional eruptive phase with clinical contact. Root growth is shown with the root sheath detaching from the root surface. Epithelial rests and cementum formation by cementoblasts are now occurring.

Crowns of primary teeth are smaller than the crowns of their successors, with only a few key exceptions. Crowns of perma-nent incisors and canines are larger than their primary coun-terparts in all dimensions (see Fig. 6.3). The difference between the cumulative mesiodistal diameters of the primary molars and canines and those of the permanent molars and canines is called the *leeway space*, which totals 1.3 mm in the maxillary arch and 3.1 mm in the mandibular arch.

Primary teeth resemble permanent teeth. Both permanent and primary incisors have single roots and incisal edges. Both primary and permanent canines also have single roots and a single cusp. Primary molars, however, bear no resemblance to the premolars that will succeed them. The crowns of the perma-nent molars are larger than crowns of primary molars; the latter have a larger mesiodistal diameter than crowns of the succeed-ing premolars. This difference has clinical significance in caries patterns on approximal surfaces and in cavity design for caries removal. Interproximal lesions will be cervical to the contact areas and of similar shape.

TABLE 6.3   Brief Outline of the Comparison of Primary and Permanent Teeth

	Primary	Permanent
Number of teeth	20	32
Enamel and dentin	Thinner	Thicker
Lifespan	Develop quicker: span ≈ 8.5 yr	Develop slower: span ≈ 6 yr to?
Size	Smaller, except MD width of molars	Larger
Crown shape	Greater contour, especially at cervical area	Curved M/D/B/L
Contact areas	Flat	Point
Root shape	Curved molar roots	Straighter roots
Pulp chamber	Larger in relation to rest of tooth	Smaller
	Ribbon-like pulp in root	
	MB pulp horn large in molars	Oval shape in root
Accessory canals	More in bifurcation area than permanent teeth	More in apical area
MD width of incisors (difference is named *incisors liability*)	Smaller (incisors are more erect)	Larger (incisors have greater angulation)
MD width of primary molars and permanent premolars (difference is named *leeway space*)	Larger	Smaller (1.3 mm in maxillary, 3.1 mm in mandibular)
Root resorption	Normal	Pathologic
Dentin hardness	Peripheral dentin ≈same	≈Same
Central dentin	Softer	Harder
Pulpal dentin	Softer	Harder

MB, Mesiobuccal; *MD*, mesiodistal; *M/D/B/L*, mesial/distal/buccal/lingual.

Roots

The roots of primary teeth are shorter than roots of permanent teeth and are more divergent. The flat curved roots of primary teeth permit development of the crown of the permanent successor (see Fig. 6.18). As the permanent teeth erupt, the roots of the primary teeth are resorbed. Root shape dictates the shape of the root pulp and is correlated with two important clinical considerations. First, curved roots with thin walls make mechanical access of root canals more difficult in primary molars than in permanent molars. Second, the flat ribbon-shaped root canals of the primary teeth are in sharp contrast to the tube-like canals of the permanent teeth. Significant developmental differences occur in the root canals of the primary molars; the root canal fills in unevenly with secondary dentin, which leaves calcified bridges, making endodontic instrumentation difficult.

Tooth Structure

Primary and permanent teeth have a similar enamel prism structure, except at the tooth surface. Primary teeth are more likely to have a prismless surface, and this reflects on the clinician's ability to etch the surface and provide an interface for attachment of sealants and other restorative procedures. Enamel is about twice as thick in permanent teeth as in primary teeth and is more highly pigmented. Primary tooth dentin is slightly softer than the permanent teeth.

Pulp Shape and Size

The coronal pulps of primary teeth are relatively larger than in permanent teeth. The largest pulp horn in primary molars is the mesiobuccal pulp horn, and the second largest is the mesiolingual pulp horn. These differences are used in the design of dental restoration. Primary and permanent teeth are similar in basic histologic architecture and vasculature; connective tissue and odontoblastic and subodontoblastic zones are similar in appearance. Permanent teeth have a larger number of nerves than primary teeth. The usual location of accessory canals in primary teeth is in the furcation zone and in permanent teeth at the apical one-third of the completed root.

Arch Shape

Arch shape is similar in the anterior portion of the two dentitions, but the permanent dentition extends further distally. Tooth-size differences are critical in assessment of potential space for permanent teeth to erupt into alignment.

The succession of smaller primary incisors with larger permanent incisors is called *incisor liability*, and the difference in the mesial distal dimension between the primary molars and permanent premolars is called the *leeway space*.

Root Resorption and Pulp Degeneration

The primary tooth roots have a higher susceptibility to resorption than do permanent teeth. The process of resorption is accompanied by gradual changes in the pulp. The first sign is a reduction in the number of cells in the pulp; nerve trunks degenerate, and some fibrosis occurs. Blood vessels remain until the tooth is exfoliated.

During root formation, the primary tooth pulp is highly cellular. As the roots are completed, fewer cells and more fibers are evident. The proliferation of fibers continues during the root resorption phase, with fiber bundles becoming more prominent.

CONSIDER THE PATIENT

To answer this question, the dentist takes a radiograph of the area to determine whether the permanent tooth is missing or displaced. In either case, the primary tooth is retained in position while the dentist determines the status of the permanent tooth and, if the tooth is present, aids its eruption into the proper place.

Nerve fibers gradually organize in the pulp chamber of the primary tooth. As the tooth reaches functional occlusion, the nerve fibers form a parietal plexus. These nerve fibers are lost during resorption of the primary tooth roots, which makes teeth insensitive to pulpal pain at the time of exfoliation.

The periodontal support of primary and permanent teeth is similar in basic architecture.

SELF-EVALUATION QUESTIONS

1. Define tooth eruption and each of its phases.
2. Describe the changes overlying the tooth during eruption.
3. Describe the changes occurring around the tooth during eruption.
4. Describe the significant changes in the area underlying the teeth that relate to eruption.
5. What are the three fundamental causes of tooth shedding?
6. Give the sequence of eruption of the primary and permanent teeth.
7. What is the origin of osteoclasts?
8. Give the sequence of events that occur in hard tissue resorption.
9. Give the chronology of eruption for the primary teeth.
10. Give the chronology of eruption for the permanent teeth.

ACKNOWLEDGMENTS

Dr. N.M. EL Nesr contributed to the production of chapters in Avery JK, *Oral development and histology*, 3rd ed., Stuttgart, Thieme Medical, 2002. Some of the figures in that text have been used in preparation of this chapter.

QUANDARIES IN SCIENCE

The processes of tooth eruption and shedding of the primary teeth are almost as much a mystery now as they were in the distant past when scientists first started to hypothesize about the biologic sequence of events culminating in a functional tooth. Many theories have been suggested and are under active investigation, but none has been proven. Because the entire process requires many steps, including tooth development, bone remodeling, tooth movement, and induction of many cell types, and because each step is complicated, intricate, and exquisitely timed, it is extremely difficult to form a complete picture of this multifactorial event. This chapter discusses the theories, but ultimately why, how, and when teeth erupt is still to be scientifically determined. It may be that scientists should be asking different questions to get to the right answer; for example, why don't teeth erupt?

CASE STUDY

During an initial dentist office visit, the dentist observes that his patient, a 16-year-old boy, has retained his maxillary lateral and central incisor primary teeth, which should have been shed by this age. He asks the patient about any injuries or predisposing factors that could have resulted in the retained teeth. Other than falling while skiing and bumping his central incisors on a tree branch, the patient could not recall any other factors that could have resulted in the retained teeth. After taking diagnostic radiographs, the dentist could not define a periodontal ligament space, which strongly indicated that the teeth were ankylosed. To complete the examination, the dentist ordered blood chemistry and a vitamin study. The patient was referred to an oral and maxillofacial surgeon who extracted the "impacted" teeth without complications, allowing the underlying permanent teeth the access needed to complete eruption and enter prefunctional occlusion.

There are many reasons for retained teeth, but the most common is ankylosis due to a previous injury. Other reasons could be failure of the underlying tooth to develop or a systemic disease that would prevent the necessary bone remodeling to occur for the erupting tooth to form an eruption pathway. Diabetes mellitus, cleidocranial dysplasia, and osteopetrosis are diseases that prevent bone remodeling, and are common causes of retained teeth.

SUGGESTED READING

Frost HM. A 2003 Update of bone physiology and Wolff's Law for clinicians. *Angle Orthod.* 2004;74(1):3–15.

Gorski JP, Marks Jr SC. Current concepts of the biology of tooth eruption. *Crit Rev Oral Biol Med.* 1992;3:185–206.

Marks Jr SC, Gorski JP, Cahill DR, et al. Tooth eruption: a synthesis of experimental observations. In: Davidovich Z, ed. *The biological mechanisms of tooth eruption and root resorption.* Birmingham, AL: EBSCO Media; 1988.

Moxham BJ. The role of the periodontal ligament in tooth eruption. In: Davidovich Z, ed. *The biological mechanism of tooth eruption and root resorption.* Birmingham, AL: EBSCO Media; 1988.

Proffit WR. The effect of intermittent forces on eruption. In: Davidovich Z, ed. *The biological mechanism of tooth eruption and root resorption.* Birmingham, AL: EBSCO Media; 1988.

Sarrafpour B, Swain M, Li Q, et al. Tooth eruption results from bone remodelling driven by bite forces sensed by soft tissue dental follicles: a finite element analysis. *PLoS One.* 2013;8(3):e58803.

Wise GE, Marks Jr SC, Cahill DR. Ultrastructural features of the dental follicle associated with formation of the tooth eruption pathway in the dog. *J Oral Pathol.* 1985;14:15–26.

7

Enamel

- Describe the physical features of enamel, such as the structure of the enamel rods, incremental lines, lamellae, tufts, and spindles.
- Discuss how these affect the permeability of enamel.
- Discuss the surface characteristics and the etching of enamel.

OVERVIEW

Enamel, the hard protective substance that covers the crown of the tooth, is the hardest biologic tissue in the body. It consequently is able to resist fractures during the stress of mastication. Enamel provides shape and contour to the crowns of teeth and covers the part of the tooth that is exposed to the oral environment.

Enamel is composed of interlocking rods that resist masticatory forces. Enamel rods are deposited in a keyhole shape by the formative ameloblastic cells. Groups of ameloblasts migrate peripherally from the dentinoenamel junction as they form these rods. Ameloblasts take variable paths, which produces a bending of the rods. These cells maintain a relationship as they travel in different directions and produce adjacent rods. The enamel rod configuration viewed in incidental light appears as light and dark bands of rod groups termed Hunter-Schreger bands. Because these rods bend in an exaggerated, twisted manner at the cusp tips, they are called gnarled enamel.

All enamel rods are deposited at a daily appositional rate or increment of 4 µm. Such increments are noticeable, like rings in a cross section of a tree, and appear as dark lines known as striae of Retzius or lines of Retzius. The growth lines become apparent on the surface of enamel as ridges, known as perikymata. Two structures are noticeable at the dentinoenamel junction: spindles, the termination of the dentinal tubules in enamel, and tufts, hypocalcified zones caused by the bending of adjacent groups of rods.

Because enamel is composed of bending rods, which in turn are composed of crystals, minute spaces or gaps exist where crystals did not form between rods. This feature causes enamel to be variable in its density and hardness. Therefore some areas of enamel may be more prone to penetration by small particles. This characteristic leads to tooth destruction by dental caries.

After enamel is completely formed, no more enamel can be deposited.

CLINICAL COMMENT

Perikymata are surface manifestations of the incremental lines usually found at the cervix of the crown. During scaling, some perikymata are more prominent and present difficulties to the novice clinician, who may confuse them with calculus.

PHYSICAL PROPERTIES

Because enamel is very hard, it is also brittle and subject to fracture. Fracture is especially likely to occur if the underlying dentin is carious and has weakened the enamel's foundation.

Enamel is about 96% inorganic mineral in the form of hydroxyapatite and 4% water and organic matter. Hydroxyapatite is a crystalline calcium phosphate that is also found in bone, dentin, and cementum. The organic component of enamel is the protein enamelin, which is similar to the protein keratin that is found in the skin. The distribution of enamelin between and on the crystals aids enamel permeability. Enamel is grayish white but appears slightly yellow because it is translucent and the underlying dentin is yellowish. Enamel ranges in thickness from a knifelike edge at its cervical margin to about 2.5 mm maximum thickness over the occlusal incisal surface.

ROD STRUCTURE

Enamel is composed of rods that extend from their site of origin at the dentinoenamel junction to the enamel outer surface (Fig. 7.1). Each rod is formed by four ameloblasts. One ameloblast forms the rod head, a part of two ameloblasts forms the neck, and the tail is formed by a fourth ameloblast. Fig. 7.2 shows the six-sided design that is the shape of the ameloblast in contact with the forming keyhole- or racquet-shaped rod, which is columnar in its long axis. The head of the enamel rod is the broadest part, at 5 µm wide, and the elongated thinner portion, or tail, is about 1 µm wide. The rod, including both head and tail, is 9 µm long. The enamel rod is about the same size as a red blood cell (7 to 10 micrometers) (Fig. 7.3).

Each rod is filled with crystals. Those in the head follow the long axis of the rod, and those in the tail lie in the cross axis to the head (Figs. 7.4 and 7.5). The upper right rod head of Fig. 7.4 indicates how the mineral is oriented during the rod's development, which forms the rod head and tail as seen on the left side of the figure. The architecture of the mineral orientation

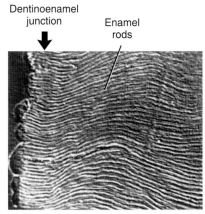

Fig. 7.1 Enamel rods appear wavy in section of enamel as they extend from the dentinoenamel junction on the left to the enamel surface on the right. This figure is possible because the section is etched and viewed with a scanning electron microscope. (Avery JK. *Oral development and histology*. 3rd ed. Stuttgart: Thieme Medical; 2002.)

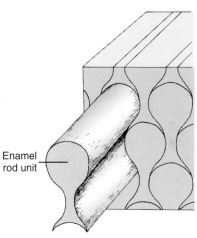

Fig. 7.3 One rod is pulled out to illustrate how individual enamel rods interdigitate with neighboring rods. (Avery JK. *Oral development and histology*. 3rd ed. Stuttgart: Thieme Medical; 2002.)

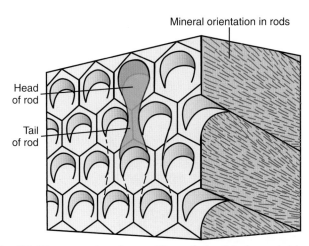

Fig. 7.2 Diagram showing outline of six-sided ameloblasts overlying keyhole-shaped enamel rods. Parts of four cells form each enamel rod. Crystal orientation of three rods can be seen on the right side of the model. (Avery JK. *Oral development and histology*. 3rd ed. Stuttgart: Thieme Medical; 2002.)

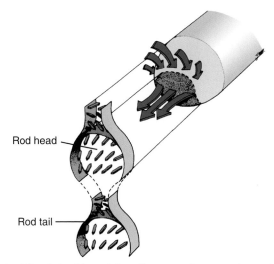

Fig. 7.4 The left side of the diagram shows orientation of crystals in the forming rod head and tail. The right part shows how forming crystals pack in the rod from the cell complex *(arrows)*.

is complex, especially when viewed in any direction other than cross section (see Fig. 7.5).

Rods form nearly perpendicular to the dentinoenamel junction and curve slightly toward the cusp tip. This unique rod arrangement also undulates throughout the enamel to the surface. Each rod interdigitates with its neighbor, the head of one rod nestling against the necks of the rods to its left and right (see Fig. 7.3). The rods run almost perpendicular to the enamel surface at the cervical region but are gnarled and intertwined near the cusp tips (Fig. 7.6). The surface of each rod is known as the rod sheath, and the center is the core. The rod sheath contains slightly more organic matter than the rod core (Fig. 7.7).

Groups of rods bend to the right or left at a slightly different angle than do adjacent groups (see Fig. 7.6). It is believed that this feature provides the enamel with strength for mastication and biting. When light is projected at the surface of a thin slab of enamel, light and dark bands appear. These bands are seen because the light transmits along the long axis of one group of rods but not along the adjacent rods, which lie at right angles. This is known as the Hunter-Schreger bands phenomenon (Fig. 7.8). These bands are named after John Hunter, the dental

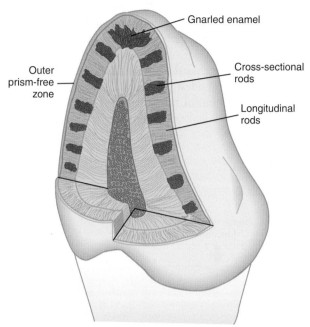

Fig. 7.6 Diagram of enamel rod orientation as shown in both longitudinal and cross section of the crown. Enamel rods are intertwined at the cusp tip; this is called gnarled enamel. Groups of outer enamel rods all run nearly perpendicular to the surface of the enamel, whereas inner groups of enamel rods alternate. Some appear in cross section, and adjacent groups appear longitudinal. (Avery JK. Oral development and histology. 3rd ed. Stuttgart: Thieme Medical; 2002, with modifications.)

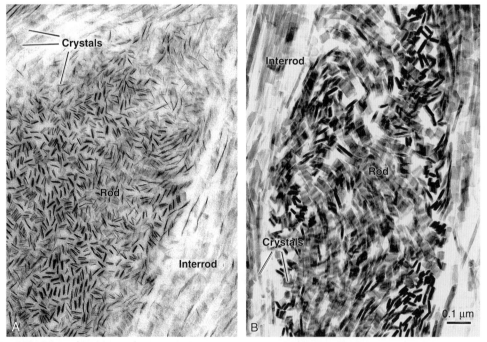

Fig. 7.5 Orientation of enamel crystals in mature enamel as seen in this transmission electron micrograph of a sagittal section at low **A**, and high **B**, magnification. (Nanci A. Ten Cate's oral histology. 8th ed. St. Louis: Mosby; 2013.)

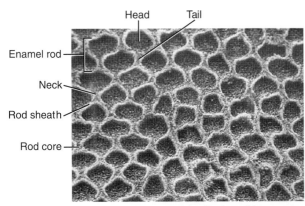

Fig. 7.7 Enamel rods in cross section. Each rod has a sheath and core. The rod sheath surrounds rod head and tail. This enamel sample has been etched to reveal organic matrix.

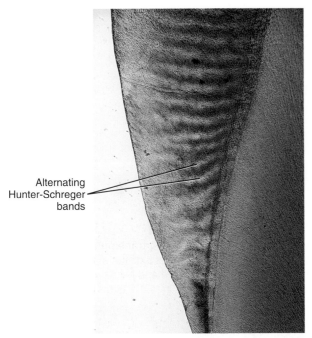

Fig. 7.8 Photomicrograph of enamel taken by reflected light and illustrating phenomena of light and dark (Hunter-Schreger) bands.

scientist who first noted the Schreger band effect microscopically. The repeating pattern from the cervical area to the incisal or occlusal areas can be seen along the long axis of the tooth. Hunter-Schreger bands extend through one-half to two-thirds of the thickness of enamel, as shown in Fig. 7.6 (diagram) and Fig. 7.8 (a tooth section).

CONSIDER THE PATIENT

A patient has attrition of cusp tips in the enamel of the crowns. What do you expect when you look at the root length radiographically? Why would you see this?

CLINICAL COMMENT

The rods that form enamel are woven during formation into a mass that resists average masticatory impact of 20 to 30 pounds per tooth. Enamel is thin in the cervical areas, where masticatory impact is the least, and thickest over the areas of crown cusps, where impact is greatest.

INCREMENTAL LINES

The incremental lines in enamel are the result of the rhythmic recurrent deposition of the enamel. As the enamel matrix mineralizes, it follows the pattern of matrix deposition and provides the growth lines in enamel (Fig. 7.9). These lines may be accentuated because of a variation in the mineral deposited at the point of enamel hesitation in deposition. In some cases, the incremental lines are not visible. With enamel development, a row of ameloblasts covering the crown hesitates during deposition. These hesitation lines mark the path of amelogenesis. The spaces between the crystals entrap air molecules, accentuating these lines. Dr. Retzius, who first noted these "growth lines," termed them the striae of Retzius.

Part of the enamel of most deciduous teeth is formed before birth, and part is formed after birth. Because environment and nutrition change abruptly at birth, a notable line of Retzius occurs at that time. This is known as the neonatal line (Fig. 7.10). Although the neonatal line is an accentuated incremental line, it can be seen microscopically that this line is prominent for another reason. The enamel internal to this line is of a different consistency from that external to it because it was formed before birth, and the external was formed after birth. The prenatal enamel has fewer defects than the postnatal. The postnatal enamel has numerous minute spaces that are stained with pigment.

CLINICAL COMMENT

Enamel is composed of calcium hydroxyapatite, mineral crystals that are the same as those found in dentin, cementum, and bone. Unlike bone and cementum, the mineral crystals in enamel are not replaced once deposited.

ENAMEL LAMELLAE

Enamel lamellae are cracks in the surface of enamel that are visible to the naked eye (see Fig. 7.9 and Fig. 7.11). Lamellae extend from the surface of enamel toward the dentinoenamel junction. Some lamellae form during enamel development, creating an organic pathway or tract. Spaces between groups of rods are another example of lamellae and may be caused by stress cracks that occur because of impact or temperature changes. Breathing cold air or drinking hot or cold beverages may cause small checks to occur in enamel, especially enamel weakened by underlying caries. Lamellae are not tubular defects but appear leaflike, extending around the crown (see Fig. 7.11). Lamellae are a possible avenue for dental caries.

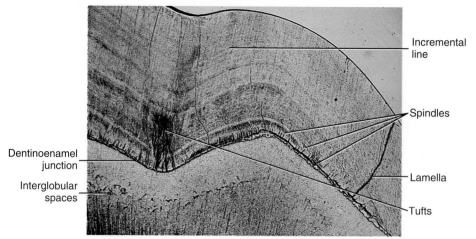

Fig. 7.9 Photomicrograph of dentinoenamel junction showing dentin below and enamel above this junction. Enamel exhibits incremental lines, tufts, spindles, and lamella. Within dentin, a band of primary dentin is just below the dentinoenamel junction. At the lower border of this band of primary dentin is a row of interglobular spaces.

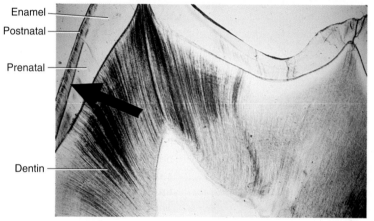

Fig. 7.10 Photomicrograph of section of enamel and dentin of primary tooth by transmitted light. The neonatal line is at the point of the arrow. Enamel to the left of this line is a darker stain than enamel to the right of it. The enamel formed before birth is less pigmented and has fewer defects than postnatal enamel. Dentin exhibits numerous dead tracts as dark lines. Dead tracts are tubules filled with air; hence, they appear black in transmitted light.

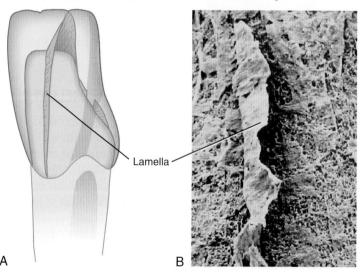

Fig. 7.11 Enamel lamellae. **A**, Diagram of possible location of leaflike enamel lamellae extending from the cervical to incisal enamel. **B**, Scanning electron micrograph of lamellae in enamel. (Enamel was decalcified away, and lamellar space was impregnated with resin for its maintenance.) (Avery JK. *Oral development and histology*. 3rd ed. Stuttgart: Thieme Medical; 2002, with modifications.)

Temperature changes from breathing cold air or drinking hot or cold beverages may cause small checks or cracks to develop in enamel. This is especially evident in enamel weakened by underlying caries but can also appear in otherwise normal enamel.

ENAMEL TUFTS

Another developmental defect in enamel is enamel tufts, which are filled with the organic protein amelogenin. They are located at the dentinoenamel junction and appear at right angles to it. They can extend one-fifth to one-tenth of the distance from the dentinoenamel junction to the occlusal surface of the tooth (Figs. 7.12 and 7.13). Tufts form between groups of enamel rods, which are oriented in slightly different directions at the dentinoenamel junction. These spaces are thus developed between adjacent groups of rods, which are filled with organic material termed amelogenin. The interface of the junction of dentin and enamel is scalloped, and often tufts arise from these scalloped peaks (see Fig. 7.12).

ENAMEL SPINDLES

Spindles arise at the dentinoenamel junction and extend into enamel during development. These spindles are extensions of dentinal tubules that pass through the junction into enamel (see Fig. 7.13). Because dentin forms before enamel, the odontoblastic process occasionally penetrates the junction, and enamel forms around this process, forming a tubule. These small tubules may contain a living process of the odontoblast, possibly contributing to the vitality of the dentinoenamel junction. Tubules are found singularly or in groups and are shorter than tufts, at only a few millimeters in length. The fingerlike spindles appear quite different from the broader and longer tufts.

SURFACE CHARACTERISTICS

The enamel surface may be smooth or have fine ridges. Such ridges result from the termination of the striae of Retzius on the surface of enamel (Fig. 7.14). These surface manifestations are ridges called **perikymata** or **imbrication** lines. Perikymata are produced by the ends of rod groups accentuated by hesitation

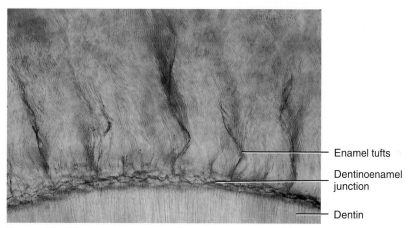

Fig. 7.12 Transmitted light micrograph of the dentinoenamel junction area showing enamel tufts. In addition to tufts, scalloped dentinoenamel junction and fine enamel rod structure can be seen between tufts. Below the junction are dentinal tubules. (Avery JK. *Oral development and histology.* 3rd ed. Stuttgart: Thieme Medical; 2002.)

Enamel tufts

Dentinoenamel junction

Dentin

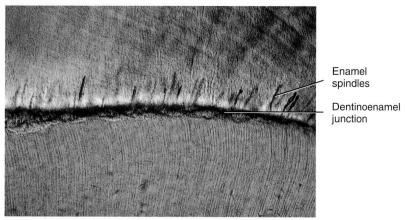

Enamel spindles

Dentinoenamel junction

Fig. 7.13 Enamel spindles at the dentinoenamel junction are extensions of dentinal tubules that may contain odontoblastic processes in enamel. (Avery JK. *Oral development and histology.* 3rd ed. Stuttgart: Thieme Medical; 2002.)

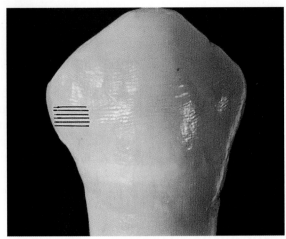

Fig. 7.14 Fine ridges on the enamel surface of the crown are perikymata or imbrication lines. (Avery JK. *Oral development and histology.* 3rd ed. Stuttgart: Thieme Medical; 2002.)

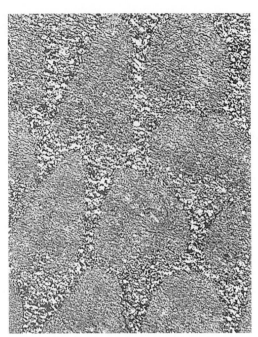

Fig. 7.16 Transmission electron micrograph of a cross section of enamel rods that shows differences in rod sheath and rod core crystal orientation. (Avery JK. *Oral development and histology.* 3rd ed. Stuttgart: Thieme Medical; 2002.)

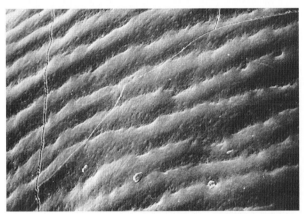

Fig. 7.15 Scanning electron micrograph of perikymata in Fig. 7.14 at a much higher magnification, which shows alternating ridges and valleys. (Avery JK. *Oral development and histology.* 3rd ed. Stuttgart: Thieme Medical; 2002.)

of ameloblasts before the next group of rods contact the enamel surface (Fig. 7.15). This manifestation is more prominent on the facial surface of the tooth near the cervical region (see Fig. 7.14). Another feature of outer enamel near its surface is the zone of prismless enamel, which is 20 to 40 μm thick. Throughout this zone, no Schreger band effect is noted. This zone is not accentuated except near the cervical region and in deciduous teeth. The prismless zone of enamel is important because it appears as a structureless microcrystalline environment of enamel rods oriented nearly perpendicular to the enamel surface. This enhances the integrity of the enamel surface and should be recognized when a bevel for restorations is prepared.

PERMEABILITY

Enamel permeability is a feature of clinical importance. The passage of fluid, bacteria, and bacterial products through enamel is an important consideration in clinical therapy. Permeability of enamel is caused by several factors, some of which are evident as they relate to leakage around faulty restorations and decomposition of the tooth by dental caries. These latter examples need no further explanation, but fluid and fine particles can also pass through unbroken enamel by way of pathways described previously in this chapter, such as lamellae, cracks, tufts, and spindles. These all contribute to the microporosity of enamel. The minute spaces between or around enamel rods and through crystal spaces within rods are also important and are called microlamellae. Differences in crystal orientation can cause enamel to have minute spaces that can be seen at high magnification (Fig. 7.16). Also, surface irregularities, such as those found in central fissures and near the cervical region, are important in influencing permeability.

Enamel and dentin are both composed of hydroxyapatite crystals, although the crystals in enamel are about 30 times larger than those in dentin (Fig. 7.17). Crystal size is a factor in the extreme hardness of enamel in contrast to dentin.

CLINICAL COMMENT

When caries has spread from the tooth's surface to near the dentinoenamel junction, the hypocalcified tufts allow a lateral spread along this junction. Other hypocalcified structures in enamel, such as lamellae and incremental lines, can also modify the spread of caries.

CLINICAL COMMENT

Decalcifying agents such as lemon juice and sodas can remove mineral from the surface of the enamel crystals. However, the various constituents of saliva, including calcium and phosphate, help to maintain the integrity of the enamel surface.

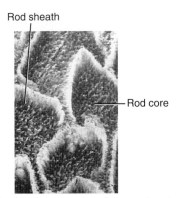

Fig. 7.18 Acid-etched enamel rod core dissolved to greater extent than rod sheath, which provides for attachment of sealant.

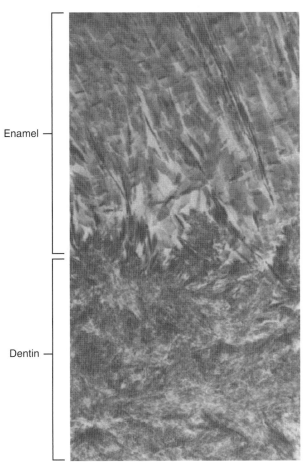

Fig. 7.17 Dentinoenamel junction. Enamel is above and dentin below. Crystallites of enamel and dentin are different in size and orientation. Whereas crystals of human enamel may be 90 nm (900 Å) in width and 0.5 μm in length, those of dentin are only 3 nm (30 Å) in width and 100 nm (1000 Å) in length. Crystals of dentin are similar in size to bone. (Electron micrograph × 35,000.)

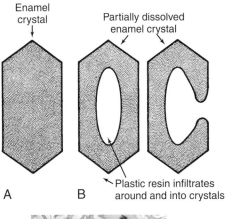

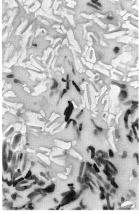

Fig. 7.19 A, Intact enamel crystal. B, Loss of crystal core in acid-etched enamel. C, Demineralized enamel crystals. Medium-toned areas show plastic replacing enamel, lightest areas are dissolved crystals, and the darkest areas are intact enamel crystals.

CLINICAL COMMENT

Some etched areas of enamel can be remineralized by solutions of sodium fluoride or stannous fluoride. Tests show that the fluoride ion penetrates the porous, etched surface enamel. Low levels of fluoride stimulate remineralization.

ETCHING

Etching with dilute acids, such as citric acid, may alter the surface of enamel. This dilute acid selectively etches the ends of the enamel rods and provides adherence of a plastic sealant to the surface of enamel rods (Fig. 7.18). The rod sheath resists demineralization to a greater extent than the rod core. The core of the crystal is rich in coronated apatite and is more sensitive to demineralization than is the peripheral hydroxyapatite (Fig. 7.19). The purpose of this procedure is to produce an intact surface and thus prevent caries.

CLINICAL COMMENT

The use of sealants, especially in children, can help prevent caries in susceptible areas of the teeth. In order for the sealant to be effective and retained, the surface enamel must be etched to improve adhesion.

CONSIDER THE PATIENT

A radiograph would reveal a lengthened root with excessive cemental deposition that is the result of hypereruption of the tooth. Because of the hypereruption, space is provided for compensating cemental deposition.

QUANDARIES IN SCIENCE

Enamel is a unique tissue that does not have the ability to heal after it matures. Although it is the most mineralized tissue in the body, it is still subject to challenges by bacteria and wear by occlusal attrition. The dental practitioner has a complete armamentarium of techniques and materials to treat caries and occlusal attrition, and restore function. Whereas the mechanical issues of enamel are easily fixed, the genetic issues are not well understood, and therefore the resultant treatments are technical and not usually related to the genetic basis of the specific dental problem. Many scientists are actively researching the genetic basis of various enamel disorders, such as amelogenesis imperfecta, with the hopes of treating this genetic disorder in utero or informing the patient of what to expect when their children inherit the genes. Active researchers have a much clearer understanding of the biology of enamel formation and the proteins involved in enamel growth and maturation. The precise mechanisms involved in the synthesis, secretion, and maturation of enamel crystals are beginning to be elucidated, and perhaps in the future, the practicing dentist will be able to use natural enamel as a restorative agent.

SELF-EVALUATION QUESTIONS

1. Describe the shape and size of the enamel rods.
2. Define Hunter-Schreger bands.
3. Define striae of Retzius. What is a synonym?
4. Describe gnarled enamel. Where is it located?
5. What are perikymata and imbrication lines?
6. What are the location and importance of tufts?
7. Define and give the cause of neonatal lines.
8. What is prismless enamel?
9. What is the inorganic component of enamel, dentin, and bone?
10. What is the organic component of enamel?

CLINICAL CASE

A 20-year-old man presents at the local dental clinic with shallow, noncavitated enamel erosions on many interproximal tooth surfaces and some occlusal surfaces, mostly on the mandibular molars. He explains to his primary care dentist that he brushes inconsistently, doesn't floss, and drinks lemonade and liters of soft drinks containing sugar daily. The dentist explains to him that both drinks can cause dissolution of the enamel surface, allowing cariogenic bacteria to begin to colonize the eroded area. The dentist reinforces the need to brush consistently, floss, and minimize intake of acidic soft drinks containing sugar. After a thorough cleaning and oral examination and not finding any cavitated lesions, the dentist decides to use a sealant to help prevent future issues and asks the patient to return in 6 months.

Although mature enamel is highly mineralized, the exposed surfaces of the teeth in the oral cavity are subject to many types of insults, including demineralization by acidic liquids. Enamel is dense but does contain developmental defects such as enamel spindles, tufts, and enamel lamellae. Also, enamel contains microspaces around the enamel rods that allow acid-containing substances to penetrate the enamel once the prismless layer is dissolved.

Protective mechanisms of the enamel include remineralization by salivary components such as calcium and phosphate, which can precipitate out of solution and participate in the remineralization process. When etched, the enamel will dissolve in a very specific and standardized manner. The dentist will use this characteristic to etch the enamel surface and then apply a sealant or a composite resin to prevent a carious attack in noncompliant patients or patients who are susceptible to caries. The use of sealant is highly effective in suppressing or preventing caries in children but a little less so in adult patients, who have a much greater bite force and therefore can wear off the sealant in a shorter amount of time.

SUGGESTED READING

Amizuka N, Uchida T, Fukae M, et al. Ultrastructural and immunocytochemical studies of enamel tufts in human permanent teeth. *Arch Histol Cytol.* 1992;55(2):179–190.

Bhaskar SN, ed. *Orban's oral histology and embryology.* 13th ed. St. Louis: Mosby; 2011.

Boyde A, Lester KS, Martin LB, et al. Basis of the structure and development of mammalian enamel as seen by scanning electron microscopy. *Scanning Microsc.* 1988;2:1479–1490.

Condò R, Cioffi A, Riccio A, et al. Sealants in dentistry: a systematic review of the literature. *Oral Implantol (Rome).* 2013;6(3):67–74.

Diekwisch TG, Berman BJ, Anderton X, et al. Membranes, minerals, and proteins of developing vertebrae enamel. *Microsc Res Tech.* 2002;59(5):373–395.

Fearnhead RW, ed. *Tooth enamel V.* Yokohama: Florence Publishers; 1989.

Horning D, Gomes GM, Bittencourt BF, et al. Evaluation of human enamel permeability exposed to bleaching agents. *Braz J Oral Sci.* 2013;12(2):114–118.

Kodaka T, Nakajima F, Higashi S. Structure of the so-called "prismless" enamel in human deciduous teeth. *Caries Res.* 1989;23:290–296.

Satchell PG, Anderton X, Ryu OH, et al. Conservation and variation in enamel protein distribution during vertebrate tooth development. *J Exp Zool.* 2002;294(2):91–106.

Simmer JP, Hu JC. Dental enamel formation and its impact on clinical dentistry. *J Dent Educ.* 2001;65(9):896–905.

Weintraub JA, Stearns SC, Rozier RG, et al. Treatment outcomes and costs of dental sealants among children enrolled in Medicaid. *Am J Public Health.* 2001;91(11):1877–1881.

Xu HH, Smith DT, Jahanmir S, et al. Indentation damage and mechanical properties of human enamel and dentin. *J Dent Res.* 1998;77(3):472–480.

Zeichner-David M, Diekwisch T, Fincham A, et al. Control of ameloblast differentiation. In: Ruch JV, ed. Odontogenesis: embryonic dentition as a tool for developmental biology. Int J Dev Biol. 1995;39:69-92.

Zeichner-David M, Vo H, Tan H, et al. Timing of the expression of enamel gene products during mouse tooth development. *Int J Dev Biol.* 1997;41:27–38.

8

Dentin

LEARNING OBJECTIVES

- Describe the various types of dentin and the structures they contain.
- Describe the dental process that lies in the dental tubules.
- Discuss the relationship of the enamel to the dentin at their junction.

OVERVIEW

This chapter focuses on **dentin**, the hard tissue that constitutes the body of the tooth. Dentin is a living, sensitive tissue not normally exposed to the oral environment. Root dentin is covered by cementum, and crown dentin is covered by enamel. Dentin, like bone, is composed primarily of an organic matrix of collagen fibers and the mineral hydroxyapatite. It is classified as **primary, secondary**, or **tertiary** on the basis of the time of its development and the histologic characteristics of the tissue. Primary dentin is the major component of the crown and root and consists of **mantle** dentin, globular dentin, and **circumpulpal** dentin. Mantle dentin is deposited first, along the dentinoenamel junction in a band about 150 μm wide, and is mineralized by matrix vesicles and not a mineralization front. Mantle dentin does not contain dentin sialoprotein or dentin phosphoprotein in the mineralizing extracellular matrix. It is thought that mantle dentin is secreted by immature odontoblasts. The collagen fibers of this dentin are larger than those of the circumpulpal dentin, which forms later. Mantle dentin is separated from the circumpulpal dentin by a zone of disturbed dentin formation called **globular** dentin, which is notable because of the spaces between the globules, termed **interglobular spaces**. Globular dentin is believed to be a result of deficient mineralization caused during the final maturation of the odontoblast.

Dentin continues to form, although the collagen fibers are smaller, until the teeth erupt and reach occlusion. As the teeth begin to function, the dentin is termed *secondary dentin* and is normal circumpulpal dentin. Dentin is responsive to the environment. When caries or mechanical trauma affect the pulp, dentin is deposited underlying that area and is termed **reactionary/response, reparative**, or *tertiary dentin*. This dentin is deposited to protect the pulp. Bordering the pulp is **predentin**, which is newly formed dentin before calcification and maturation. Predentin is composed of 90% type I collagen fibers and 10% noncollagenous proteins, which calcify within 24 hours as the odontoblasts deposit a new band of collagen fibers (Box 8.1).

Fig. 8.1 demonstrates uptake of 3H-proline 30 minutes after an exogenous injection. Much of the injected proline is hydroxylated to hydroxyproline, which is specific for collagen. The silver halide grains over the ameloblasts, which do not have a collagenous extracellular matrix, are a result of the enamel proteins containing the amino acid proline.

In addition to classifying dentin, this chapter describes properties and characteristics of dentin. Like osteoblasts that form bone, the odontoblasts that form dentin lie on the surface of the forming hard tissue. Unlike bone, the odontoblastic processes exist in tubules and penetrate the dentin from the pulp toward the dentinoenamel junction. Dentin, like bone, is deposited by appositional growth and produces incremental lines, but unlike bone, dentin does not remodel. In addition, a **granular** dentin anomaly appears along the root surface. This developmental defect is likely caused by incomplete molecular information transferred by the inner root sheath cells to the underlying neural crest cells on the pulp side of the developing root, resulting in the young odontoblast moving in an incorrect direction and then reversing itself to move pulpward. The odontoblasts may die because of trauma or old age, and **dead tracts** then develop in dentin. The tubules may later calcify as they fill with mineral. When this occurs, the dentin is termed **sclerotic** or **transparent** dentin.

PHYSICAL PROPERTIES

Dentin, which forms the bulk of the tooth, is yellowish in contrast to the whiter enamel. It appears darker if a root canal procedure has been performed. Dentin is composed of 70% inorganic hydroxyapatite crystals, 20% organic collagen fibers with small amounts of other proteins, and 10% water by weight. With 20% less mineral than enamel, dentin is softer, although it is slightly harder than bone or cementum. Therefore it is more radiolucent than enamel but much more dense or radiopaque than pulp. Dentin is resilient or slightly elastic, and this allows the impact of mastication to occur without fracturing the brittle overlying enamel. This resilience is partly the result of the presence throughout the matrix of tubules, which extend from the dentinoenamel junction to the pulp.

CLINICAL COMMENT

Metallic restorations, such as gold inlay, crown, or silver amalgam, are excellent thermal conductors. Therefore it is appropriate to place a cement base under these restorations to protect the pulp by minimizing pain conduction.

BOX 8.1   Components of the Extracellular Matrix of Dentin

Collagens
- Type I
- Type I trimer
- Type V
- Type III
- Type VI, IX, X, XI, XII

Proteoglycans
- Decorin (PG II)
- Biglycan (PG I)
- Chondroitin, 4- and 6-sulfate–containing
- Dermatan sulfate
- Keratan sulfate
- Perlecan (heparan sulfate)

Lipids
- Phospholipids (phosphatidylcholine, phosphatidylethanolamine)
- Cholesterol
- Cholesterol ester
- Triacylglycerols

Proteolytic enzymes, etc.
- Enamelysin
- Matrix metalloproteinases (MMPs)
- Tissue inhibitors of matrix metalloproteinases (TIMPs)
- Gelatinases

Glycoproteins/sialoproteins
- Osteonectin
- Dentine sialoproteins (DSPs)
- Dentine phosphoproteins (DPPs)
- Bone sialoprotein
- Osteopontin
- Bone acidic glycoprotein 75
- Syndecan 2
- α-2-HS-glycoprotein (AHSG)
- Laminin

Serum-derived proteins
- Albumin
- Fibronectin
- Immunoglobulins

Phosphoproteins
- Dentine matrix protein 1, 2
- γ-carboxyglutamate A
- Osteocalcin
- Matrix Gla protein

Growth factors
- Transforming growth factors (TGFs)
- Chondrogenic-inducing factor
- Bone morphogenic proteins (BMPs 2, 4, 7)
- Fibroblast growth factors (FGFs)
- Insulin-like growth factors (IGFs)
- Amelin-1 transient expression

DENTIN CLASSIFICATION

Dentin includes primary, secondary, and tertiary dentin. Based on structure, primary dentin is composed of mantle and circumpulpal dentin. Examples of these classifications are given in Fig. 8.2A. Fig. 8.1B shows the **S curve** of the dentinal tubules through primary and secondary dentin. Primary dentin forms the body of the tooth; secondary dentin forms only after tooth eruption and is a narrow band that borders the pulp. Tertiary or reparative dentin is formed only in response to trauma to the pulp (Box 8.2).

Primary Dentin

Mantle dentin is the first primary dentin formed. It is deposited first at the dentinoenamel junction (Fig. 8.3) and extends approximately 150 μm from the junction pulpward to the zone of **interglobular** or globular dentin. Mantle dentin is so named because it serves as a covering or mantle over the rest of the dentin. Normal circumpulpal dentin directly underlies mantle and globular dentin and comprises the bulk of the tooth's primary dentin. Circumpulpal dentin may be 6 to 8 mm thick in the crown and a little thinner in the roots.

Zones of dentin have structural differences. Mantle dentin is composed of large collagen fibers, some of which are 0.1 to 0.2 μm in diameter, in contrast to the circumpulpal dentinal matrix, which is 50 to 200 nm. Thus the fibers in circumpulpal dentin are 10 times smaller than those in mantle dentin. Mantle dentin is also slightly less mineralized and contains fewer defects than circumpulpal dentin. Mantle dentin is nearly free of developmental defects. It interdigitates with enamel at the scalloped dentinoenamel junction peripherally and in the zone of globular dentin centrally. The area of globular dentin usually exists only in the crown but may extend into the root. Such a zone of dentinal matrix is not completely mineralized, and the area of globular calcospherites has not fused correctly (see Fig. 8.3 and Fig. 8.4C).

Globular dentin contains hypomineralized areas between the globules, termed *interglobular spaces*. Fig. 8.4 shows examples of various structures in dentin. Interglobular spaces are not true spaces but are less mineralized areas between the calcified globules. The dentinal tubules run without interruption through this zone, indicating a defect in mineralization, not a defect in matrix formation (see Fig. 8.3). Interglobular dentin is especially noticeable with vitamin D deficiency, which affects mineralization of teeth and bones. Primary dentin constitutes the bulk of dentin in crowns and roots of teeth. It is characterized by the continuity of tubules from pulp to dentinoenamel junction and by incremental lines that indicate a daily rhythmic deposition pattern of approximately 4 μm of dentin.

CLINICAL COMMENT

The sensitivity of dentin is an important clinical consideration after placement of a restoration that conducts heat or cold. Dentin responds to such stimuli by deposition of reactionary dentin and by changes in the dentin tubules underlying the restoration. The sensitivity of the tooth will diminish after a few weeks because of these changes.

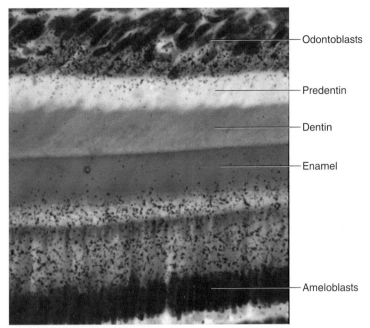

Fig. 8.1 This autoradiograph shows the distribution of silver halide grains over the odontoblasts, predentin, dentin, enamel, and ameloblasts 30 minutes after an injection of 3H-proline in a rat incisor. In the predentin, the 3H-proline is hydroxylated to hydroxyproline, which is a precursor to collagen. In the enamel, the 3H-proline is incorporated into the enamel proteins.

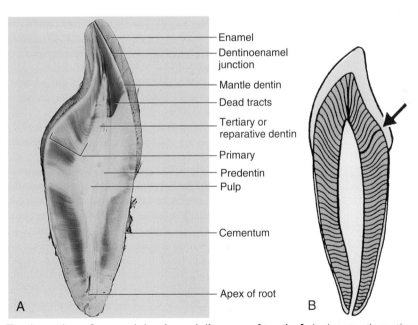

Fig. 8.2 Tooth section of enamel dentin and diagram of tooth. **A**, Incisor tooth section illustrating structures in enamel, dentin, and cementum. **B**, Diagram of dentin showing S curvature of the dentinal tubules, especially at the arrow. (Avery JK. *Oral development and histology.* 3rd ed. Stuttgart: Thieme Medical; 2002, with modification.)

Secondary Dentin

Secondary dentin forms internally to primary dentin of the crown and root. It develops after the crown has come into clinical occlusal function and the roots are nearly completed (Fig. 8.5). This dentin is deposited more slowly than primary dentin, and its incremental lines are only about 1.0 to 1.5 μm apart. Dental scientists theorize that after the crown begins clinical function, the brain signals the dentin to slow the rate of production. This keeps the pulp from being obliterated by the previous rapid rate of dentin formation. The tubules of primary and secondary dentin are generally continuous unless the deposition of

BOX 8.2   Types of Dentin

Primary dentin (prior to eruption)
- Mantle dentin
- Interglobular dentin
- Circumpulpal dentin
- Peritubular dentin
- Intertubular dentin

Secondary dentin
- Normal circumpulpal dentin (after eruption)

Tertiary dentin
- Reactionary/response
- Reparative
- Osteodentin
- Sclerotic dentin

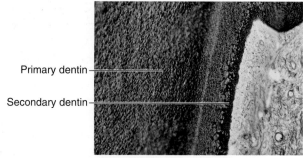

Fig. 8.5 Primary dentin *(left)* and secondary dentin *(right)*. Note the demarcation between the two. (Bhaskar SN, ed. *Orban's oral histology and embryology*. 11th ed. St. Louis: Mosby; 1991.)

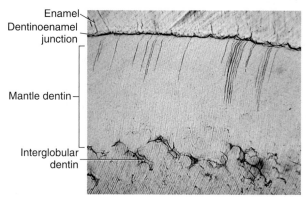

Fig. 8.3 Histologic section of mantle dentin. Area bounded by dentinoenamel junction above and interglobular dentin below.

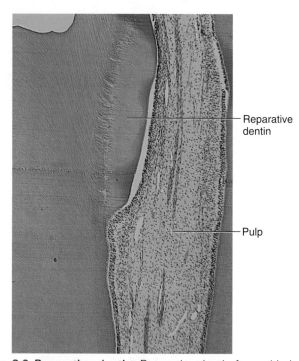

Fig. 8.6 Reparative dentin. Reparative dentin formed in localized area under cavity preparation. Open tubules underlying the cavity floor caused the response of reparative dentin.

secondary dentin is uneven. In molar teeth, for example, more secondary dentin is deposited on the roof and floor of the coronal pulp chamber than on the lateral walls. This leads to protection of the pulpal horns as occlusal function occurs.

Tertiary Dentin: Reactionary/Response and Reparative

Reparative or tertiary dentin results from pulpal stimulation and forms only at the site of odontoblastic activation. Whether the formation is the result of attrition, abrasion, caries, or restorative procedures, this dentin is deposited underlying only those stimulated areas (Figs. 8.6 and 8.7). It may be deposited rapidly, in which case the resulting dentin appears irregular, with sparse and twisted tubules and possible cell inclusions (see Fig. 8.6B–E). Odontoblasts, fibroblasts, and blood cells have been found in this type of dentin. In contrast, if it is formed

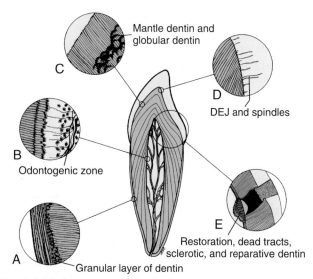

Fig. 8.4 Various structures in dentin. **A**, Granular layer of dentin and adjacent cementum. **B**, Odontogenic zone and predentin. **C**, Mantle dentin and interglobular or globular dentin. **D**, Dentinoenamel junction and spindles. **E**, Restoration, dead tracts, sclerotic dentin, and reparative dentin.

slowly because of fewer stimuli, the dentin appears more regular, much like primary or secondary dentin (see Figs. 8.6 and 8.7A). Reparative dentin at times resembles bone more than dentin and is then termed **osteodentin** (see Fig. 8.7C); it is the type of dentin that is formed under an exposure that has a hardset calcium hydroxide as the pulp-capping medicament. It can also appear as a combination of several types (see Fig. 8.7E). Recent terminology suggests that the term *reactionary/response dentin* be used when the original odontoblasts function in deposition and that *reparative dentin* be used when newly recruited (replacement) odontoblasts begin depositing dentin. The latter case occurs with a more severe injury to the tooth, such as a pulp exposure, which necessitates recruitment of progenitor cells that then differentiate into new odontoblasts. It is interesting to speculate why the newly recruited odontoblasts do not recapitulate development and produce mantle dentin but instead produce various other types of dentin, including osteodentin initially and tubular dentin at a much later time

during the pulpal healing sequence. Perhaps this is because of the urgency of protecting the pulp from further damage and thereby forming a "scar," which then seals the pulp during dentin bridge formation.

CONSIDER THE PATIENT

Case 1: A patient complains of pain in a tooth after placement of a large gold crown. The tooth is very sensitive to hot or cold fluids or foods. Why?

PREDENTIN

Predentin is a band of newly formed, unmineralized matrix of dentin at the pulpal border of the dentin (Fig. 8.8). Predentin is evidence that dentin forms in two stages: first, the organic matrix is deposited, and second, an inorganic mineral substance is added. Mineralization occurs at the predentin–dentin junction at the mineralization front where predentin becomes a new

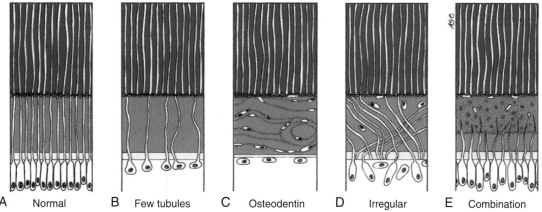

A Normal   B Few tubules   C Osteodentin   D Irregular   E Combination

Fig. 8.7 Normal and reparative dentin. A, Normal dentin. **B** to **E,** Reparative dentin. **B,** Decrease in number of tubules. **C,** Cell inclusions. **D,** Irregular and twisted tubules. **E,** Combination of types.

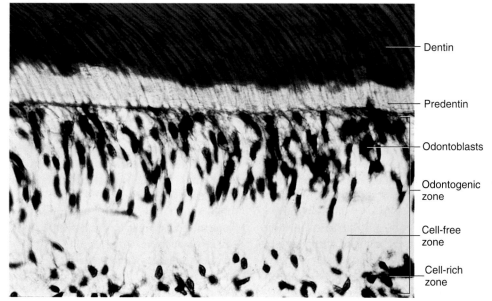

Dentin
Predentin
Odontoblasts
Odontogenic zone
Cell-free zone
Cell-rich zone

Fig. 8.8 Photomicrograph of predentin zone that borders pulp with mature dentin above. Odontogenic zone is below predentin and comprises odontoblasts and cell-free and cell-rich zones.

layer of dentin. During primary dentin formation, 4 µm of pre-dentin is deposited and calcified each day. After occlusion and function, this activity decreases to 1.0 to 1.5 µm per day.

TUBULAR AND INTERTUBULAR RELATIONS

Primary and Secondary Tubules

As dentin is formed by odontoblasts, space is provided for the lengthening process of the odontoblast that moves pulpward from the dentinoenamel junction. The tubules normally begin at this junction but may extend into the forming enamel matrix. The process begins forming before either enamel or dentin matrix begins forming. Thus the spindles that are extensions of the odontoblastic process extend a short distance into enamel. The odontoblastic process then forms an S curve, which extends to the pulp. The odontoblasts initially have multiple processes when they first differentiate and are synthesizing and secreting mantle dentin but withdraw them at the junction of the globular/circum-pulpal interface when the cell undergoes the final differentiation process. As the process elongates, it branches, and its second-ary processes appear at nearly right angles to the main process (Fig. 8.9) and are contained within **canaliculi** located perpen-dicular to the dentinal tubule. These cells and their processes give the dentin vitality. The surface area ratio of the dentinoenamel junction to the pulpal surface is about 1:5. Therefore the tubules are farther apart at the dentinoenamel junction than at the pulpal surface (see Figs. 8.2 and 8.9). In addition, the tubules are smaller in diameter in the outer dentin (1 µm) than at the pulpal border (3 to 4 µm). The ratio of the number of tubules at the dentinoe-namel junction to the number at the pulpal border is about 4:1. This relates to the odontoblast's gradual increase in size as its pro-cess grows in length. Also, more tubules are in the crown than in the root. Approximately 30,000 to 50,000 tubules per square mil-limeter exist in the dentin near the pulp. The lateral branches of the odontoblastic processes are seen throughout dentin, crown, and root. These lateral branches are termed *canaliculi, secondary branches*, or *microtubules* (see Fig. 8.9), and are less than 1 µm in diameter. Some of these lateral branches lead to an adjacent dentinal tubule, and some appear to terminate in the intertubu-lar matrix. Each of these secondary tubules contains branches of the odontoblastic process that contact the adjacent odontoblasts, allowing intercellular communication through gap junctions.

Intratubular or Peritubular Dentin and Sclerotic Dentin

The dentinal matrix that immediately surrounds the den-tinal tubule is termed **intratubular** or **peritubular** dentin (Fig. 8.10). Peritubular dentin is present in tubules throughout dentin except near the pulp. It is called *peritubular* because it is a hypermineralized collar surrounding the tubules. However, because it is formed within and at the expense of the tubules, *intratubular dentin* is a more accurate term. Intratubular den-tin is missing from the dentinal tubules in interglobular dentin. This is an area of deficient mineralization like the area of pre-dentin, which is also not calcified. In some areas, the hypermin-eralized intratubular dentin completely fills the tubules, as in the area near the dentinoenamel junction overlying the pulp horns.

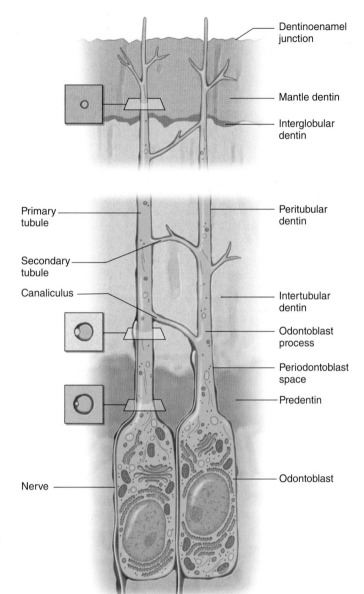

Fig. 8.9 Odontoblast process in the dentinal tubule and extending from the dentinoenamel junction above to the pulp below. Side branches of odontoblast processes in tubules are in inner dentin called secondary tubules and in outer dentin termed canaliculi.

This condition is also found in the peripheral tubules of the root near the cementum. These are areas of very small tubules and areas where external stimulation may play a role. *Sclerotic den-tin* or *transparent dentin* (Fig. 8.11) is the term for dentin with tubules that are completely obliterated. The name is derived from the transparent nature of dentin in its appearance under a light microscope, which manifests itself when the tubules are no longer present. Sclerotic dentin increases in amount with age and is believed to be another mechanism to protect the pulp, like reactionary/response and reparative dentin. Permeability to the pulp is eliminated in these areas, and sclerotic dentin is found in areas of attrition, abrasion, fracture, and caries of the enamel. Sclerotic dentin is not formed by odontoblasts but is a sequela due to the death of the odontoblasts. The odontoblast is responsible for deriving the dentinal fluid from the blood plasma and maintains the dentinal fluid by pumping ions, especially calcium and phosphorus, among others, to maintain the fluid consistency. When the odontoblast dies, this fluid spontaneously crystallizes because it is supersaturated with calcium and phosphate, occluding the dentinal tubules at the pulp–predentin/dentin interface.

Intertubular Dentin

The main body of dentin is located between or around the dentinal tubules. Intertubular dentin is the body of dentin, which comprises the crown and root. This dentin consists of the same type of organic matrix fibers (type I collagen fibers and inorganic crystals of hydroxyapatite) as that of intratubular dentin. Intertubular dentin, however, is less highly calcified and changes little throughout life. The collagen fibers of the matrix form a meshwork oriented nearly perpendicular to the intratubular dentin. They exhibit a typical 640-Angstrom (Å) cross banding similar to those of bone or cementum.

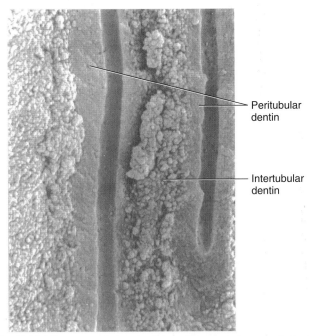

Fig. 8.10 Diagram of dentinal tubules showing peritubular and intertubular dentin. Note that side branches of dentinal tubules are in the intertubular dentin. (Berkovitz BKB, Holland GR, Moxham BJ. *Oral anatomy, histology, and embryology.* 4th ed. St. Louis: Elsevier; 2009.)

Peritubular dentin

Intertubular dentin

> ### CLINICAL COMMENT
> Dentinal tubules increase in size by the loss of intratubular or peritubular dentin. This dentin is subject to decalcification by caries or acid cleansing of the cavity, which also removes the smear layer. This dentin is about 40% more highly calcified than the remainder of the dentin.

> ### CLINICAL COMMENT
> Dentin is a permeable hard tissue with tubules leading from the dentinoenamel junction to the pulp. Therefore, in cavity preparation, sealing of dentinal tubules is a requisite for effective restorative dentistry.

INCREMENTAL LINES

All dentin is deposited incrementally, which means that as a certain amount of matrix is deposited daily, a hesitation in activity follows. This hesitation in formation results in an alteration of the matrix known as **incremental lines, imbrication lines,** or

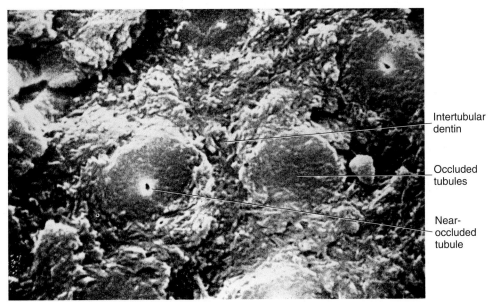

Intertubular dentin

Occluded tubules

Near-occluded tubule

Fig. 8.11 Scanning electron micrograph of sclerotic dentinal tubules. The micrograph shows the minute size of nearly occluded dentinal tubules and some completely occluded tubules. Tubule occlusion is a mechanism to protect the pulp. (Avery JK. *Oral development and histology.* 3rd ed. Stuttgart: Thieme Medical; 2002.)

lines of von Ebner. Although daily lines are difficult to distinguish, lines formed by increments over several days (possibly every 5 days), resulting in 20-μm lines, are believed to be the ones von Ebner described (Fig. 8.12). Analysis of soft x-ray films has shown these lines to represent hypocalcified bands, at least in the primary teeth and the permanent first molars, indicating that dentin is formed before birth. Prenatal dentin and postnatal dentin are separated by an accentuated contour line known as the **neonatal line** (Fig. 8.13). This line reflects the abrupt change in environment, including hormonal and nutritional changes, that occurs at or near birth.

GRANULAR LAYER

When a thin, calcified section of root is studied under transmitted light, a granular-appearing layer of dentin is seen underlying the cementum that covers the root. This layer is known as the **granular layer** or **granular layer of Tomes** (Fig. 8.14). This zone increases slightly in width, proceeding from the cementoenamel junction to the root apex. The zone is believed to be the result of a coalescing and looping of the terminal portions of the dentinal tubules. It is possible that the odontoblast is initially disoriented as it begins dentin formation. The odontoblast turns at right angles to the root surface and proceeds pulpward, causing the dentinal matrix in this area to be defective (Fig. 8.15). This disorientation of the odontoblasts could be the result of the initial incomplete information transmitted by the inner root sheath cells resulting in the granular layer. In the crown, ameloblasts direct this process more efficiently, although on occasion, odontoblasts cross the dentinoenamel junction and come back, leaving enamel spindles on the enamel side of the dentinoenamel junction.

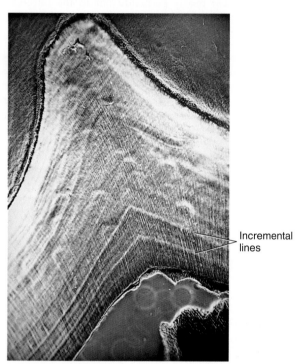

Fig. 8.12 Microradiograph of 20-μm incremental lines (lines of von Ebner) in dentin. Fine daily incremental lines can be seen microscopically between the 20-μm lines.

Incremental lines

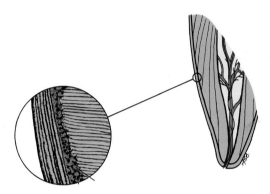

Fig. 8.14 Diagram of the appearance and location of the granular layer of dentin along the cementodentinal junction of the root.

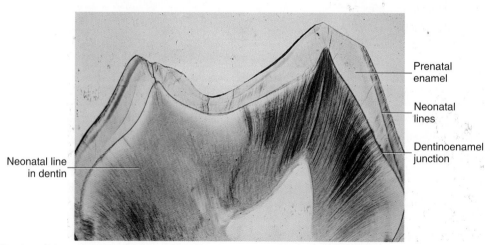

Neonatal line in dentin

Prenatal enamel

Neonatal lines

Dentinoenamel junction

Fig. 8.13 Neonatal line is seen at birth in both enamel and dentin, because prenatal enamel has fewer defects than postnatal enamel. The neonatal line is more easily seen in enamel because of the color change between pre- and postnatal enamel. Dentin has a neonatal line that is difficult to see at this magnification but is located midway through dentin.

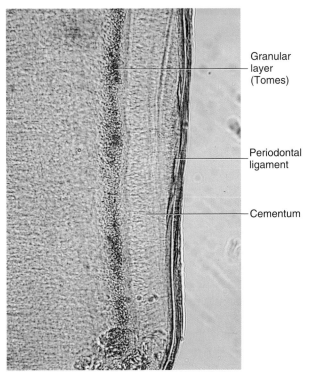

Fig. 8.15 Histologic appearance of the granular layer of dentin *(center)* and cementum *(right)*, with periodontal ligament remnants *(far right)*.

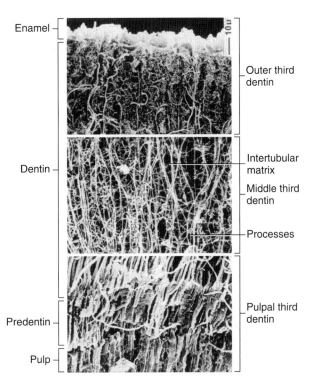

Fig. 8.16 Photomicrograph of odontoblasts (bottom) with their processes intact and extending upward to dentinoenamel junction (top). Peritubular and intertubular dentinal matrix has been removed, exposing odontoblastic processes.

ODONTOBLASTIC CELL PROCESSES

Odontoblastic cell processes are cytoplasmic extensions of the cell body that are positioned at the pulp–dentin border. Opinions vary about whether these processes extend through the entire thickness of dentin. This difference in opinion is caused in part by the difficulty in preserving and visualizing these processes. Recently, improved techniques of immunofluorescence labeling, freeze fracture, and polymer replacement have revealed that these processes extend to the dentinoenamel junction (Fig. 8.16). In some instances, they also extend into the enamel for a short distance as enamel spindles (Fig. 8.17). The odontoblastic processes are largest in diameter near the pulp (3 to 4 μm) and taper to 1 μm near the dentinoenamel junction. During development, these processes were divided near the dentinoenamel junction into branched processes (Fig. 8.18), but as the odontoblast matured, the processes were retracted and formed a single main process.

Periodically, along the odontoblastic process, lateral branches arise at nearly right angles to the main odontoblastic process, extend into the intertubular dentin and, where they contact adjacent odontoblast processes, form gap junctions (Fig. 8.19). Within the odontoblastic process are microtubules, small filaments, occasional mitochondria, and microvesicles that can be visualized using the transmission electron microscope. Organelles (e.g., mitochondria) are not normally found in the odontoblast process but are found within the cell body. All these structures are indicative of the protein-synthesizing character of the odontoblast. Collagen is deposited along the predentinal

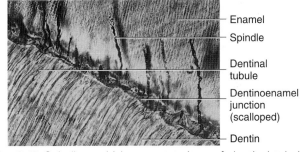

Fig. 8.17 Spindles, which are extensions of dentinal tubules, pass across the dentinoenamel junction into inner enamel.

border and to a lesser extent along the tubule wall. Nerve terminals can be seen close to the odontoblastic cell body and within the dentinal tubule in the region of the predentin. These are described in Chapter 9. Loss of the odontoblastic process usually results in the appearance of dead tracts in dentin. In the dentin underlying an area of attrition or a carious lesion, odontoblasts may die and processes disintegrate, producing a group of open tubules that contain debris and spaces. If these tubules are open to overlying caries, bacteria may enter them and migrate to the pulp, causing inflammation. The areas of dead tracts may appear black when the teeth are sectioned and viewed by transmitted light because of the additive properties of light rays and because air may penetrate these tubules and create this appearance (Fig. 8.20).

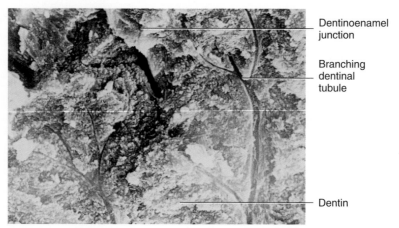

Dentinoenamel junction

Branching dentinal tubule

Dentin

Fig. 8.18 Scanning electron micrograph of dentinal tubules branching near the dentinoenamel junction.

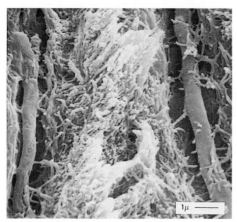

Fig. 8.19 Scanning electron micrograph of dentin near the dentinoenamel junction, illustrating the odontoblastic processes. Side branches of the odontoblastic process extend into intertubular dentin.

CONSIDER THE PATIENT

Case 2: A patient asks why carious dentin does not elicit pain during its removal.

CLINICAL COMMENT

A carious attack can sometimes result in the death of the odontoblast underlying the surface lesion. The dentinal tubules normally contain a living odontoblast process, dentinal fluid, and sometimes a nerve terminal. After the odontoblast dies, the dentinal fluid will crystallize and fill the dentinal tubule with sclerotic dentin (transparent dentin), thus preventing further insult to the pulp.

DENTINOENAMEL JUNCTION

The junction between dentin and enamel, termed the *dentinoenamel junction*, is scalloped, which enhances contact and adherence of the two structurally different tissues. This can be seen microscopically in Figs. 8.14 and 8.17. Scalloping has been found to be accentuated in the cusps where the incisal or occlusal contact is greatest. Features in addition to scalloping that characterize the

dentinoenamel junction are enamel spindles and fine branching of the terminal dentinal tubules in the mantle dentin (see Figs. 8.17 and 8.18). The odontoblastic processes extend to the dentinoenamel junction unless stimulation has caused a change in the tubule and its contents. Fig. 8.19 shows the processes with their side branches, and Fig. 8.20 gives an example of changes in dentin underlying a restoration. Loss of tubular contents results in dead tracts *(black streaks)* that indicate air in the tubules. Below the dead tract area in Fig. 8.20 is sclerosed dentin, which protects the pulp from bacteria or bacterial products in the tubules underlying the restoration.

PERMEABILITY

The outer surface of dentin is approximately five times larger in surface area than the inner surface. Because the tubule diameter is only 1 µm near the dentinoenamel junction, the tubules are farthest apart at this junction. They are, however, much closer together at the pulpal surface because the tubules are larger (3 to 4 µm) and the dentinal surface is five times smaller (Fig. 8.21). The tubules are consequently cone-shaped and permit increased permeability from the cavity wall or floor to the pulp. The system of branching tubules increases the permeability. Also, because the peritubular dentin is more highly calcified than the intertubular dentin, the etching of a cavity causes an increase in the diameter of the tubule. The only feature that protects the pulp is that it has higher osmotic pressure than the area of the dentinoenamel junction. Fluid is constantly being forced outward by this increased pressure of the pulp. Therefore, when some dentinal tubules are cut, a small droplet of fluid appears on the cut surface of the cavity preparation. Against the direction of this flow, minute particles such as bacteria or bacterial products percolate down the dentinal tubules to the pulp. Again, loss of the odontoblastic process, which produces a dead tract, results in increased permeability. For these reasons, the permeability factor is a major consideration in cleansing of the cavity preparation and the placement of a cavity liner to prevent microleakage. In Fig. 8.21, the shaded area indicating caries signifies that bacteria find the shortest distance to the pulp along the dentinal tubules. The figure also shows the deposition of reparative or reactionary/response dentin to the cavity preparation.

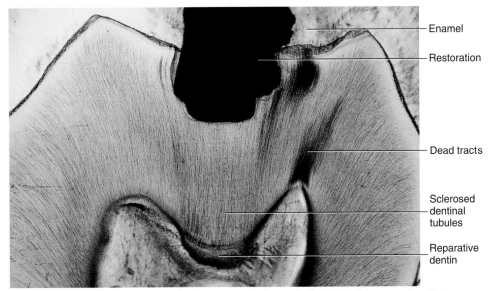

Fig. 8.20 Black dead tracts (open tubules) underlie a black (dense) restoration that appears associated with sclerosed dentinal tubules. Tubules lie adjacent to the reparative dentin, which is seen on the roof of the pulp chamber. Each of these tubules probably resulted from stimulation from the overlying restoration.

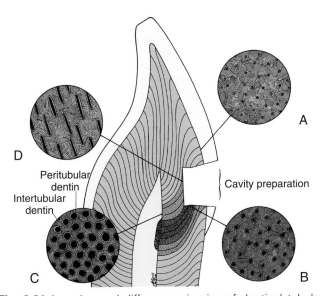

Fig. 8.21 Location and differences in size of dentinal tubules at the dentinoenamel junction **(A)** and at pulp **(C)** and relationship between tubules in cavity floor **(B** and **D)** and the pathway of caries through dentin. Size of tubules at the pulp border **(C)** can be compared with those in the floor of the cavity **(B** and **D)** and at the dentinoenamel junction **(A)**. Deposition of reparative dentin underlies invading caries. (Avery JK. *Oral development and histology*. 3rd ed. Stuttgart: Thieme Medical; 2002, with modifications.)

CLINICAL COMMENT

Dentin is a vital tissue that contains living cell processes. Because these branching processes permeate the dentin so completely, it is not possible to touch a cavity preparation in dentin with an explorer without inflicting pain.

The tubules of dentin are effectively blocked by the production of a smear layer on the floor or walls of the cavity during preparation. The **smear layer** is composed of the fine particles of cut dentinal debris that are produced by cavity preparation. These particles enter the tubules as smear plugs at the cut surface of the cavity preparation. The effectiveness of the plug is dependent on the size of the tubules and the size of the cut particles of dentin.

REPAIR PROCESS

Dentin is laid down throughout life. Pathologic effects of dental caries, attrition, abrasion, and cavity preparation cause changes in dentin. The changes are described as odontoblastic degeneration, formation of dead tracts, calcification of tubules leading to sclerosis, and tertiary or reparative dentin formation. Stimulation of the odontoblasts leads to increased dentinogenesis underlying an area of pathologic change. If the stimulation is mild enough for the odontoblast to survive, reactionary/ response dentin will be formed. This is believed to be a protective mechanism of the pulp to maintain its vitality. A second situation arises after death and degeneration of the odontoblast. When dead tracts appear, sclerosis of the dentin may occur, and further reparative dentin secreted by replacement odontoblast in the pulp forms. In this instance, the pulp is again protected by this walling-off action, which blocks the tubules underlying the area of trauma (see Figs. 8.20 and 8.21). With appropriate coverage, pulps can maintain their vitality. Dead tracts and sclerosis of dentin do not occur if leakage is prevented. An example of this is shown in Figs. 8.22 and 8.23, in which the pulp is vital in the first molar under a full crown. The pulp in the second molar is not visible because the crown was not cut through its center. This unusual section shows teeth dend the surrounding supporting bone.

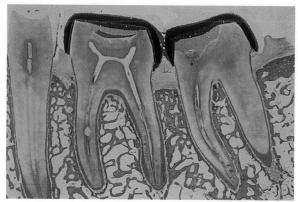

Fig. 8.22 Thin section of two human mandibular molar teeth in situ with gold crowns. The pulp of the first molar appears normal with no sign of sclerotic dentin or dead tracts.

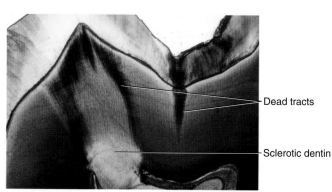

Dead tracts

Sclerotic dentin

Fig. 8.23 Dead tracts and sclerotic dentin. Dead tracts and sclerotic (transparent) dentin can be seen in this photomicrograph of a ground section of a molar tooth. Caries at the surface (not seen in this picture) has caused the odontoblasts to die, causing the dentinal tubules to fill with air and appear black. The sclerotic dentin close to the pulp is due to odontoblasts dying and the consequent crystallization of the dentinal fluid within the dentinal tubules. This is due to the fluid being supersaturated with calcium and phosphate, which spontaneously crystallize when not being maintained by the odontoblast.

CLINICAL COMMENT

The pulp is covered by a smear layer of dentinal particles, which block the tubules and aid in walling off the pulp, and by the formation of reparative dentin.

CONSIDER THE PATIENT

Discussion 1: Metals are good conductors of heat and cold. (Similar complaints may result after placement of an amalgam or an inlay.) However, the clinician can offer the patient assurance that the tooth will respond to the pain with internal healing. The clinician knows that reactionary/response dentin forms slowly and eventually will insulate the pulp nerves from the metal restoration. Within 6 months or a year following such a restoration, the patient may note that the pain no longer exists. This indicates that the reactionary/response dentin has formed.

Discussion 2: The odontoblastic process is believed to function in pain conduction in dentin and is nonliving in carious dentin. During cavity preparation, pain arises only from the adjacent living dentin.

SELF-EVALUATION QUESTIONS

1. Name the type of dentin that comprises the greater part of the crown and root.
2. Name the newly formed area of collagen matrix that borders the pulp.
3. Describe the location and composition of the granular layer of dentin.
4. Name several factors that affect the permeability of the dentin.
5. What are the location and composition of mantle dentin?
6. What is the smear layer and what is its importance to permeability of dentin?
7. Why is dentin considered a vital tissue?
8. What is sclerotic dentin and where is it most likely to be seen?
9. What is secondary dentin and when does it form?
10. What is interglobular dentin and how does it form?

QUANDARIES IN SCIENCE

The extracellular matrix (ECM) of predentin and dentin is highly evolved and contains many substances that potentially function during development, wound healing, and repair/regeneration. On stimulation, soluble molecules can be released from the ECM that have the ability to recruit cells necessary for repair/regeneration and induce progenitor cells to differentiate into replacement odontoblasts. How these molecules participate in the maintenance of dentin and how it is maintained by the odontoblast are still the subjects of many dental scientists who are studying this interesting tissue. Whether the dentist of the future will use natural substances to effect repair of the dentin and maintain pulp vitality is a question that only science and time will answer.

CLINICAL CASE

A 40-year-old female patient with a nondiagnostic medical and dental history goes to the dentist for a routine checkup after a 2-year lapse. After a thorough intraoral examination, she is discovered to have a carious lesion on the occlusal surface of her right first mandibular molar. When asked if she ever felt pain from this tooth during her 2-year absence from the dentist, the patient replies no. Radiographs show that the lesion is through the enamel, past the dentinoenamel junction, and into approximately one-third of the dentin. Following mandibular block anesthesia, caries removal was accomplished, and the cavity preparation was restored to the surface with an etched and bonded composite resin. There were no complications, and the patient left the dental office. The dentist followed up the next day, and the patient reported no negative issues.

In some circumstances, caries can progress slowly enough that the odontoblasts at the pulp interface are able to synthesize and secrete reactionary dentin in response to the carious insult, thus protecting the patient from pain. On other occasions, the caries progresses rapidly, terminally insults the odontoblast, and causes cell death. Many times, after the odontoblast dies, the dentinal fluid will crystallize in a type of tertiary dentin called sclerotic dentin, which occludes the dentinal tubules at the pulp interface and effectively prevents bacteria or other antigenic substances from entering the pulp and potentiating further pulpal inflammation. In the case of this patient, it is possible that after the initial carious attack, sclerotic dentin formed, protecting the pulp and preventing pain by preventing fluid flow within the dentinal tubules (hydrodynamic theory of pain transmission through dentin). People who suffer from severe bruxism can also induce sclerotic dentin formation, but the mechanisms are unknown.

SUGGESTED READING

Anderson DG, Chiego DJ, Glickman GN, et al. A clinical assessment of the effects of 10% carbamide peroxide gel on human pulp tissue. *J Endod*. 1999;25(4):247–250.

Bleicher F, Couble ML, Buchaille R, et al. New genes involved in odontoblast differentiation. *Adv Dent Res*. 2001;15:30–33.

Boskey AL. The role of extracellular matrix components in dentin mineralization. *Crit Rev Oral Biol Med*. 1991;2:369–387.

Dechichi P, Biffi JC, Moura CC, et al. A model of the early mineralization process of mantle dentin. *Micron*. 2007;38:486–491.

Goldberg M, Kulkarni AB, Young M, et al. Dentin: structure, composition and mineralization: the role of dentin ECM in dentin formation and mineralization. *Front Biosci (Elite Ed)*. 2012;3: 711–735.

Holland GR. The odontoblast process: form and function. *J Dent Res*. 1985;64:499–514.

Linde A. Structure and calcification of dentin. In: Bonucci E, ed. *Calcification in biological systems*. Boca Raton, FL: CRC Press; 1992.

Pashley DH. Dentin permeability and dentin sensitivity. *Proc Finn Dent Soc*. 1992;88(suppl 1):31–37.

Pashley DH. Smear layer: overview of structure and function. *Proc Finn Dent Soc*. 1992;88(suppl 1):215–224.

Priam F, Ronco V, Locker M, et al. New cellular models for tracking the odontoblast phenotype. *Arch Oral Biol*. 2005;50(2):271–277.

Stratmann U, Schaarschmidt K, Wiesmann HP, et al. The mineralization of mantle dentine and of circumpulpal dentine in the rat: an ultrastructural and element-analytical study. *Anat Embryol (Berl)*. 1997;195(3):289–297.

Szabó J, Trombitás K, Szabó I. The odontoblast process and its branches in human teeth observed by scanning electron microscopy. *Arch Oral Biol*. 1984;29(4):331–333.

Trowbridge HO, Franks M, Korostoff E, et al. Sensory response to thermal stimulation in human teeth. *J Endod*. 1980;6(1):405–412.

Yamamoto T, Domon T, Takahashi S, et al. The structure of the cemento–dentinal junction in rat molars. *Ann Anat*. 2000;182(2):185–190.

9

Dental Pulp

LEARNING OBJECTIVES

- Describe the anatomy of the pulp and the histology of the odontoblasts; fibroblasts; Schwann cells; the endothelial cells of the arteries, veins, and capillaries; pericytes and perivascular cells; and undifferentiated cells within the pulp proper and macrophages.

- Describe the structure and distribution of the blood vessels.
- Discuss the extracellular matrix of the pulp, predentin and dentin, pulp stones, and diffuse calcifications and changes that take place during the aging process.

OVERVIEW

Dental pulp is the soft, loose connective tissue located in the central portion of each tooth. It has a crown (coronal part) and a root (radicular part). Pulp is a delicate, specialized connective tissue containing thin-walled blood vessels, nerves, and nerve endings enclosed within dentin. Each pulp opens into the tissue surrounding the tooth, the periodontium, through the apex of the root canal. Accessory canals may be present at the apex of the tooth.

Pulp has a central zone and a peripheral zone, which are observed in both the coronal and radicular pulp. The central zone contains arterioles, veins, and nerve trunks that enter the pulp from the apical canal and proceed to the coronal pulp chamber. Fibroblasts are the preponderant cell, existing in an extracellular matrix (ECM) of glycosaminoglycans and collagen fibers. Odontoblasts are the second most prevalent cell. The odontogenic zone in the periphery consists of odontoblasts and cell-free and cell-rich zones. Adjacent to the cell-rich zone is a parietal layer of nerves.

Odontoblasts form dentin throughout life, which causes the pulp to grow smaller with time. The terminal blood cells in the periphery are in thin-walled continuous and fenestrated capillaries situated among the odontoblasts and are under local humoral control. Larger vessels with smooth muscle cell support in their walls exist centrally and are under postganglionic sympathetic control. Several theories exist concerning pain conduction through dentin. The hydrodynamic theory is the most popular. It defines the movement of the odontoblast into contact with pulpal and intratubular nerve endings. Recent findings indicate, however, that odontoblasts are capable of receiving, conducting, and transmitting impulses to nerve endings in close proximity.

Pulp has several functions, such as initiative, formative, protective, nutritive, and reparative activities. All these clinical features are important to the production and maintenance of teeth.

Pulp may regress after trauma or with age and may contain diffuse areas of collagen fiber bundles and pulp stones. These pulp stones may be attached, embedded, or free in the pulp tissue. Pulp may also contain diffuse calcifications.

ANATOMY OF THE PULP

Human beings have 52 pulps in their teeth, 20 in the primary dentition and 32 in the permanent dentition (Fig. 9.1). All pulps have similar morphologic characteristics, such as a soft, gelatinous consistency in a chamber surrounded by dentin, which contains the peripheral extensions of the pulpal odontoblasts. The total volume of the pulps of the permanent dentition is approximately 0.38 mL, and the mean volume of a single human tooth is 0.2 mL. The pulps of molar teeth are approximately four times larger than those of the incisors (see Fig. 9.1).

Coronal Pulp

The two forms of pulpal tissue are coronal and radicular (Figs. 9.2 and 9.3). **Coronal pulp** occupies the crown of the tooth. It is much larger than root pulp and has a structure different from the root tissue. In general, the coronal pulp follows the contour of the outer surface of the crown. Coronal pulp has six surfaces: mesial, distal, buccal, lingual, occlusal, and the floor. Coronal pulp has pulp horns, which are protrusions of pulp that extend into the cusps of the teeth. The number of pulp horns depends on the number of cusps (see Fig. 9.1). At the cervical region, the coronal pulp joins the root pulp. With age, the coronal pulp decreases in size because of continued dentin formation (see Fig. 9.2).

Radicular Pulp

Pulpal root canals extend from the cervical region to the apex of the root. **Radicular pulp** of the anterior teeth is singular, whereas the posterior teeth have multiple root pulps. Radicular pulp is tapered or conical and, like coronal pulp, becomes smaller with age because of continued dentinogenesis (see Figs. 9.2 and 9.3). The apical foramen may become narrowed by cementum deposition.

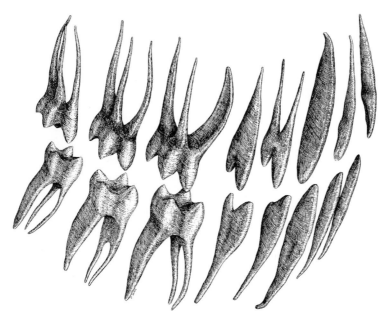

Fig. 9.1 Three-dimensional diagram of pulp organs of permanent human teeth. *Upper row,* maxillary arch, left central incisor through third molar; *lower row,* mandibular arch, left central incisor through third molar.

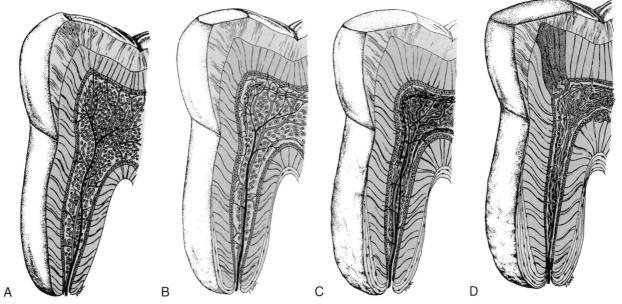

A   B   C   D

Fig. 9.2 Diagram of series of pulps during the life cycle. **A**, Young stage. **B**, After some attrition. **C**, At middle age. **D**, In old age. Pulp size and number of cells decrease, and fibrous tissue increases. Attrition also affects pulp horn, with appearance of dead tracts and sclerotic dentin. (Bhaskar SN, ed. *Orban's oral histology and embryology.* 11th ed. St. Louis: Mosby; 1991, with modification.)

Apical Foramina and Accessory Canals

The **apical foramen** is the opening of root pulp into the periodontium. This opening varies from 0.3 to 0.6 mm, being slightly larger in the maxillary teeth than in the mandibular teeth. The apical foramen generally is centrally located in the newly formed root apex but becomes more eccentrically located with age (see Fig. 9.3; Fig. 9.4). If several apical canals exist, the larger is designated the *apical foramen* and the more lateral ones are called the *accessory canals* (see Fig. 9.4). Accessory canals may result from the presence of blood vessels obstructing dentin formation or from a break in the epithelial root sheath that induces initial root formation. The incidence of accessory canals is about 33% in permanent teeth. Accessory canals are located on the lateral sides of the apical region and may be found in the bifurcation area of multirooted teeth. Clinically, accessory canals are important because they represent contact of the pulp with the periodontal tissues and can contain bacteria and bacterial endotoxins that induce inflammation. If inflammation of the pulp is present, it can spread to the periodontium or vice versa.

HISTOLOGY OF PULP

The pulp consists of coronal and root pulp. Coronal pulp is larger and contains many more elements than root pulp. Root pulp acts as a conducting tube to carry blood to and from the coronal area to the apical canal. Both pulp areas contain the same elements, although the cells, fibers, blood vessels, and nerves are more numerous in coronal pulp. Centrally, the pulp is composed of large veins, arteries, and nerve trunks surrounded by fibroblasts and collagen fibers embedded in an ECM (Fig. 9.5A). Peripherally along the dentin in both coronal and radicular pulp are the formative cells of dentin, odontoblasts. The **odontogenic zone** includes these odontoblasts, the **cell-free zone**, the **cell-rich zone**, and the **parietal plexus of nerves** (Raschkow) (see Fig. 9.5B). The cell-free zone is known as the **zone of Weil** or the **Weil basal layer**. Adjacent to this zone is a zone of high cell density called the *cell-rich zone*, and pulpal to this zone is the **parietal layer of nerves** (see Fig. 9.5B). Thus the peripheral area of pulp is highly organized. The odontogenic zone appears most notably in coronal pulp and relates to the process of dentin

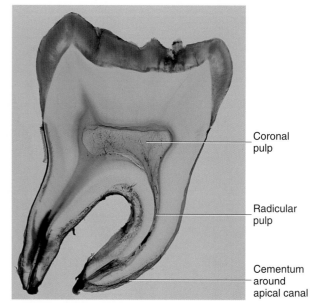

Fig. 9.3 Calcified section of older tooth showing decreased size of coronal and root pulp.

Coronal pulp

Radicular pulp

Cementum around apical canal

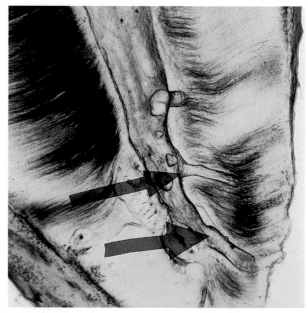

Fig. 9.4 Section of tooth apex illustrating an accessory canal *(upper arrow)* and main apical canal *(lower arrow)*.

formation, although the function of the cell-rich and cell-free zones in this process is still uncertain. In addition to the regions of the central and peripheral pulp is the area of the pulp horns. Here, the odontoblasts are crowded and appear palisaded (pseudostratified) in contrast to their appearance in the remainder of the coronal area (Fig. 9.6). In the middle area, root pulp odontoblasts are short and cuboidal.

Odontoblasts

The major function of odontoblasts is to produce and maintain the dentin ECM. This matrix contains a complex ECM consisting of 90% type I collagen matrix and a 10% noncollagenous matrix (see Box 9.2).

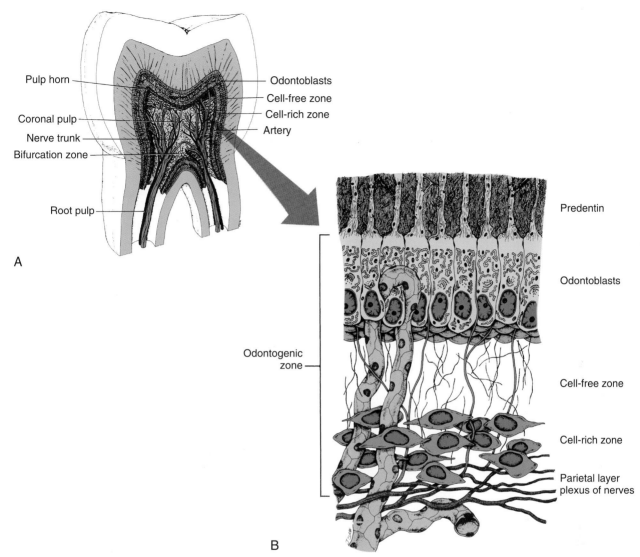

Fig. 9.5 Diagram of pulp organ illustrating pulpal architecture. **A,** There appears high organization of the peripheral pulp and the appearance of centrally located nerve trunks *(dark)* and blood vessels *(light).* **B,** Odontogenic zone of pulp. *Top to bottom:* predentin, odontoblasts, cell-free and cell-rich zones, and parietal layer of nerves. (Bhaskar SN, ed. *Orban's oral histology and embryology.* 11th ed. St. Louis: Mosby; 1991.)

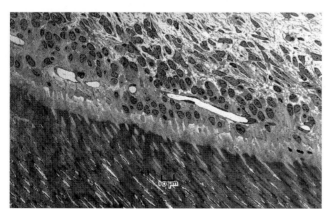

Fig. 9.6 Photomicrograph of odontoblasts in the coronal area of the pulp organ. Pulpal capillaries are shown among these cells. (Copyright Daniel Chiego Jr., PhD.)

The ECM of predentin is secreted unmineralized and then mineralizes to dentin. All the substances synthesized and secreted by the odontoblast become entrapped in the ECM of predentin and then dentin. Currently, it is thought that the soluble substances included in the ECM of predentin and dentin are chemotactic for stem cells, and certain substances induce the stem cells to differentiate into replacement odontoblasts. Scientists are avidly working on finding the critical substance(s) that allows pulpal regeneration. Odontoblasts line the perimeter of the pulp from the time they begin organizing to form dentin to the time they are quiescent and no longer producing dentin at a rapid rate. Odontoblasts are small and oval when they first differentiate but soon become columnar (Figs. 9.7–9.9).

These cells then develop processes or extensions around which dentin forms. As the process lengthens, the amount of dentin thickens. Then the odontoblastic process develops many

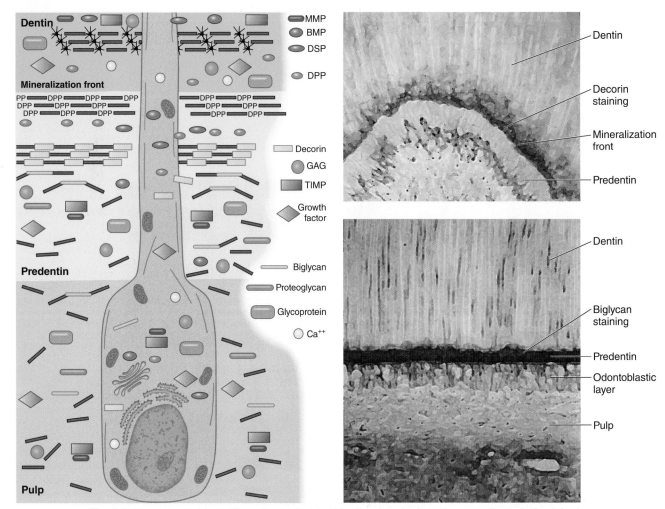

Fig. 9.7 The odontoblast. The odontoblast in this drawing depicts the complicated physiologic capabilities of this cell. The odontoblast not only synthesizes, secretes, and maintains the extracellular matrix (ECM) of predentin and dentin but also adds many different molecules paramount to the integrity of this tissue. The complex nature of the odontoblast and the included ECM of predentin and dentin have also been implicated in repair and regeneration of the pulp after compromise, as many of the included molecules are solubilized and are able to be recognized by stem cells located in various niches of the pulp.

side branches that are contained within canaliculi. When these branches develop, space is provided in the dentin for them (Fig. 9.10). Odontoblasts are larger in coronal pulp than in the root and appear columnar in pulp horns (see Fig. 9.6)

These tall, columnar cells are about 35 μm long in the pulp horns, whereas in radicular pulp, they are more cuboidal, and cells of the apical region appear flat. The process of the odontoblast is the largest part of the cell, extending from the pulp to the dentinoenamel junction. In the crown, the process could be several millimeters long, but it is shorter in the root.

The active cell has a large nucleus in its basal part and a Golgi apparatus in its apical part. Abundant rough-surface endoplasmic reticulum and numerous mitochondria are scattered through the cell body (Fig. 9.11). The process arises from the odontoblast at the predentil border, where the cell constricts as the process enters the dentinal tubule (see Fig. 9.10). The process passes through the predentin, where a few mitochondria are located. As it continues into the mineralized dentin, the process is devoid of major organelles but contains filaments,

membrane-bound vesicles, and microtubules throughout its length to the dentinoenamel junction. How far the process extends into the dentin has been the subject of much discussion. Recent evidence indicates that it extends all the way to, and in some instances through, the dentinoenamel junction and into the enamel as spindles (see Fig. 9.10).

The fluorescent photomicrograph in Fig. 9.12 demonstrates an iontophoretic injection of Lucifer yellow (800D MW) into one human odontoblast in a tooth slice preparation. The Lucifer yellow has labeled multiple odontoblasts and their processes since it is able to flow through gap junctions. The dilations and constrictions in the dentinal tubules are caused by nerve terminals coiling around the odontoblast process and constricting it.

Each junction has a different function. Adhering junctions or desmosomes are beltlike areas around these cells that possibly function in maintaining positional relationship between cells. This also prevents substances in the pulp from passing into the dentin. Gap junctions are openings between odontoblasts for communication of cell electrical impulses and the passage

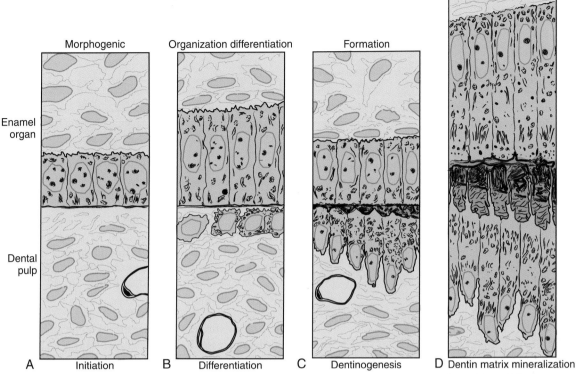

Apposition

Morphogenic   Organization differentiation   Formation

Enamel organ

Dental pulp

A Initiation   B Differentiation   C Dentinogenesis   D Dentin matrix mineralization

Fig. 9.8 Changes in an odontoblast during its differentiation from a preodontoblast (A) to beginning function (D). In the enamel organ, an ameloblast differentiates first and an odontoblast second, but an odontoblast then forms dentin before an ameloblast forms enamel.

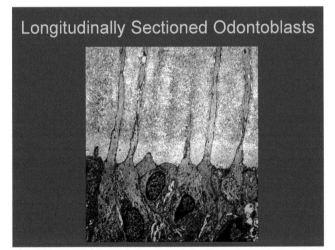

Longitudinally Sectioned Odontoblasts

Fig. 9.9 Longitudinally sectioned odontoblasts. (Copyright Daniel Chiego Jr., PhD.)

of small molecules (see Fig. 9.12; Fig. 9.13). In this manner, the odontoblasts can have synchronous activity. If stimuli reach the odontoblasts, this information spreads throughout the cell layer by gap junctions, which allow molecules less than a kilo kilodalton (kD) to pass from one cell to another (paracrine; such as calcium, cyclic adenosine monophosphate, which are important intercellular signaling molecules). Although odontoblasts are generally believed to live as long as the tooth is viable, inactivity and aging of the odontoblasts result in loss of organelles and a reduction of cell size.

CLINICAL COMMENT

The pulp horns recede with age. This is a protective measure performed by the pulp cells. Also, reparative dentin forms under cavity preparations or other areas of trauma. Cells in the pulp can be called on to become new odontoblasts and to form dentin at required sites.

Fibroblasts

Fibroblasts are the most numerous cells in pulp because they are located throughout pulp. These cells are characterized by their functional state. In young pulp, fibroblasts produce collagen fibers and ground substance. At that time, they have a large oval nucleus that is centrally located and has multiple processes (Fig. 9.14). Higher magnification of a fibroblast illustrates a Golgi apparatus, adjacent abundant rough-surface endoplasmic reticulum, and mitochondria (Fig. 9.15). This fibroblast is a protein-producing cell. In aging, these cells appear smaller and are shaped like spindles, with few organelles. Although many cells in the pulp proper resemble fibroblasts, it is difficult to determine what their exact role is in pulpal homeostasis, maintenance, turnover, and repair/regeneration. This remains an active area of scientific investigation.

Other Pulpal Cells

Nerve cells in the pulp include **Schwann cells** (Fig. 9.16). These cells form the myelin sheath of nerves and are associated with all pulp nerves. In addition, **endothelial cells** lining the capillaries,

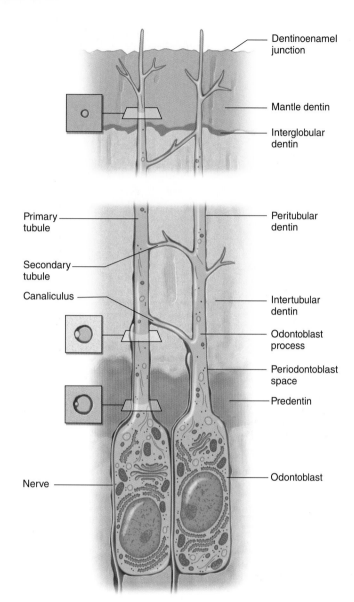

Fig. 9.10 Odontoblast and process extend through the entire thickness of dentin into the inner enamel, as noted at the top of the picture. Side branches of the odontoblastic process are shown, and cross section of tubules is at the *left*.

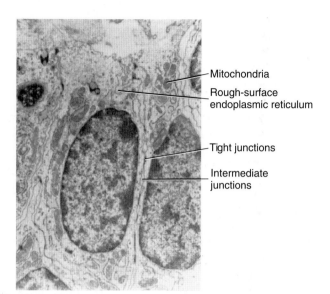

Fig. 9.11 Electron micrograph of tight, intermediate, and gap junctions, which are located between odontoblasts. Cell organelles may also be seen above the region of nuclei. (Avery JK. *Oral development and histology.* 3rd ed. Stuttgart: Thieme Medical; 2002.)

veins, and arteries of the pulp can be visualized (Fig. 9.17). Accompanying most blood vessels are **pericytes** and perivascular cells and numerous **undifferentiated cells** found in normal pulp. They function as a cell pool and are recruited when new odontoblasts or fibroblasts are needed. For example, this may happen when reparative dentin is needed for pulp exposure. **Macrophages**, normal constituents of the pulp, function in pulp maintenance because of the turnover of cells in pulp (Fig. 9.18). **Lymphocytes**, both T and B, are also found in pulp-free spaces and function in an immune capacity. Type II dendritic cells are also normal residents of the intact dental pulp; however, when the pulp is injured, the cells will diapedesis from the vascular system and migrate to the site of infection/injury. The brown stained cells in this photomicrograph demonstrate type II dendritic cells at the pulp predentin interface as well as

migrating through the odontogenic zone and having their dendritic processes in the dental tubules (Fig. 9.19). **Erythrocytes, leukocytes, eosinophils,** and **basophils** are found in pulp blood vessels.

Fibers and Ground Substance

Collagen fibers exist in the ECM, which surrounds the cells. Collagen originates from the pulpal fibroblasts throughout pulp. Both type I and type III collagen have been found in pulp. Type I is produced by odontoblasts, because this is the type of collagen found in dentin, the tissue that the odontoblasts produce. Type III is produced by pulp fibroblasts in the maintenance of the pulp proper. In young pulp, fibers are relatively sparse, and the tissue appears delicate (see Fig. 9.14). Around the fibers is the ground substance of pulp. This substance is the environment that provides life for cells in pulp and throughout the body. If pulp is irritated, fibers may accumulate rapidly. However, older pulp contains more collagen of both bundle and diffuse types (Fig. 9.20). Type IV collagen is found associated with the basement membrane surrounding blood vessels in the pulp. Other types of collagen are also found in the pulp proper but are in small amounts and not well characterized.

Pulpal Stem Cells

The ability of the dental pulp to respond to wounding is well documented. To accomplish this, there must be a reserve of cells that can be recruited to participate in the pulpal response to compromise. These undifferentiated, or stem, cells are located in several areas of both mature and immature pulp. Dental pulp stem cells are located throughout the pulp but can especially be found in the cell-rich layer of the odontogenic zone. Stem cells from the apical papilla are located around the epithelial diaphragm of the developing root in the pulp proliferative zone. Stem cells from the pulp of human exfoliated deciduous teeth

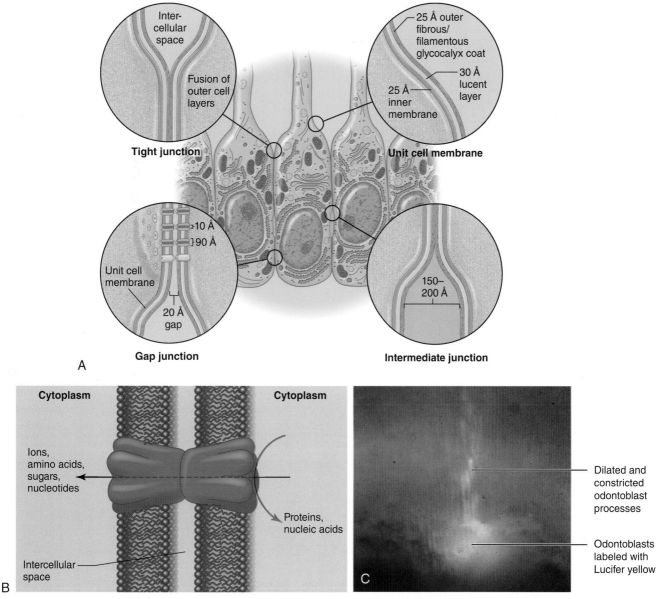

Fig. 9.12 A, Diagram of the three types of junctional complexes found between adjacent odontoblasts. Their locations can be noted in central diagram, and an illustration of a unit membrane is at *upper right.* **B,** Desmosomes. **C,** This fluorescent micrograph shows Lucifer yellow fluorescent dye (800D mw) 15 minutes after electrophoresis into one human odontoblast in a living tooth slice preparation. Because the odontoblasts are connected to one another by gap junctions, the Lucifer yellow was able to pass through the gap junctions, which allow molecules less than 1 kD through the openings and into adjacent odontoblasts and also into the odontoblast processes.

can be harvested from exfoliated teeth. Periodontal ligament stem cells are found in the periodontal ligament, and dental follicle stem cells of developing teeth are found in the dental follicle. All of these cell types have been used to regenerate the pulp with varying degrees of success, but all have potential for success. When one considers the complexity of a mature dental pulp and all the elements that work together so well, it is astounding that pulp biologists have achieved so many successes. In the future, dentists may transplant tooth pulp just as other doctors transplant other organs such as the heart, pancreas, kidneys, and liver. The future holds much hope for regenerating the pulp and

therefore hope for maintaining a vital pulp and tooth with the periodontal attachment intact (Table 9.1 and Box 9.1).

Vascularity

The pulp organ is highly vascularized, with vessels arising from the external carotid arteries to the superior and inferior alveolar arteries. It drains by the same veins. Although the periodontal and pulpal vessels both originate from these vessels, their walls are different. The walls of the periodontal and pulpal vessels become quite thin as they enter the pulp because the pulp is protected within a hard, unyielding container of dentin.

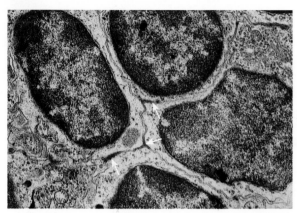

Fig. 9.13 Electron micrograph of junctions between four odontoblasts in the region of cell nuclei. Cell membranes meet at thickened, dense-staining zones where junctions are formed, as indicated by *arrows*. These dark zones are gap junctions that allow passage of small molecules between odontoblasts.

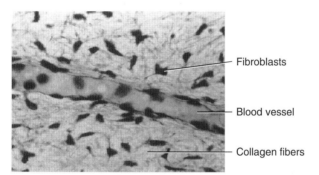

Fig. 9.14 Pulp fibroblasts, collagen fibers, and blood vessels in young pulp. (Avery JK. *Oral development and histology.* 3rd ed. Stuttgart: Thieme Medical; 2002.)

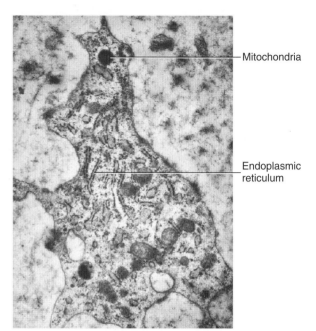

Fig. 9.15 Electron micrograph of pulp fibroblasts showing rough-surface endoplasmic reticulum and mitochondria. (Bhaskar SN, ed. *Orban's oral histology and embryology.* 11th ed. St. Louis: Mosby; 1991.)

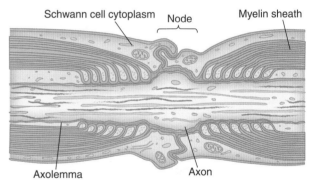

Fig. 9.16 Pulpal nerve axon surrounded by Schwann cell cytoplasm.

These thin-walled arteries and arterioles enter the apical canal and pursue a direct route up the root pulp to the coronal area (Fig. 9.21). Along the way, vessels produce branches that pass peripherally to a plexus that lies in and adjacent to the odontogenic zone of the root (Fig. 9.22). Blood flow is more rapid in the pulp than in most areas of the body, and the blood pressure is quite high. The diameter of the arteries varies from 50 to 100 µm, which equals the size of arterioles in other areas of the body. These vessels have three layers: the inner lining, or **intima**, which consists of oval or squamous-shaped endothelial cells surrounded by a closely associated fibrillar basal lamina; a middle layer, or **media**, which consists of muscle cells from one to three cell layers thick (Fig. 9.23); and an outer layer, or **adventitia**, which consists of a sparse layer of collagen fibers forming a loose network around the larger arteries. Smaller arterioles with a single layer of muscle cells range from 20 to 30 µm, and **terminal arterioles** of 10 to 15 µm are also present. **Precapillaries** measuring 8 to 12 µm and **capillaries** measuring 8 to 10 µm in diameter are present in the peripheral pulp. Capillaries are endothelial cell–lined tubes that form a network among the odontoblasts (see Fig. 9.22). Numerous investigators have shown that lymphatic vessels are present in pulp. These vessels are thin walled, irregularly shaped, and larger than

capillaries, and they have an incomplete lamina supporting the intima and media.

CLINICAL COMMENT

The vitality of pulp results in part from the apical canal's ability to remain open. This opening can become blocked, however, as the tooth ages and cementum becomes deposited around the apical canal. Thin walls of veins are the first structure affected by cemental constriction of the apices; vascular congestion can occur, leading to pulpal necrosis.

Nerves

Several large nerves enter the apical canal of each molar and premolar, and single nerves enter the anterior teeth. These nerve trunks traverse the radicular pulp, proceed to the coronal area, and branch as they extend peripherally (Fig. 9.24). Nonmyelinated axons also enter with the myelinated axons, but

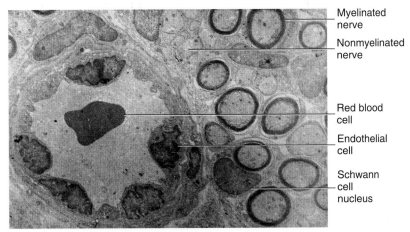

Fig. 9.17 Electron micrograph of an arteriole in the central pulp. The lumen is surrounded by endothelial cells forming the intimal layer and of muscle cells forming the media. At *right* are myelinated nerves; large nuclei belong to accompanying Schwann cells. (Avery JK. *Oral development and histology.* 3rd ed. Stuttgart: Thieme Medical; 2002.)

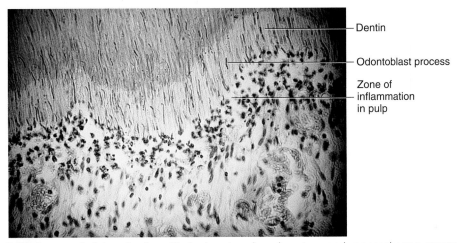

Fig. 9.18 Area underlying dentin with leukocytes, lymphocytes, and macrophages apparently responding to an irritant that resulted in inflammation. The odontoblastic processes in dentinal tubules are degenerating.

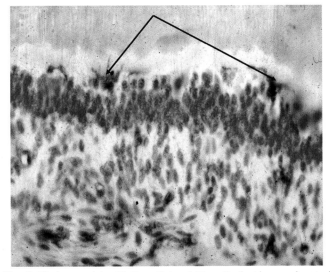

Fig. 9.19 Arrows identify Type II dendritic cells that have migrated through the odontogenic zone to reach the opening of the dentinal tubules where bacterial endotoxins have infiltrated the odontoblast layer. They were recruited from the vascular system and migrated to the source of the stimulus.

they are smaller. A young molar may have as many as 350 to 700 myelinated axons and 1000 to 2000 nonmyelinated axons entering the apex.

The large nerve trunks are invested with Schwann cells (see Figs. 9.16 and 9.17). Later, as the pulp organ matures, the subodontoblastic plexus is apparent in the roof and lateral walls of the coronal pulp and, to a lesser extent, the root canals. This network, comprising both myelinated and nonmyelinated axons, is known as the *parietal layer of nerves* or nerve **plexus of Raschkow** (see Fig. 9.24; Fig. 9.25). From the parietal layer, the nerves lose their myelin sheath, pass into the odontogenic zone, and then terminate among the odontoblasts or extend into the dentinal tubules with the odontoblastic process.

Nerve Endings

Most pulpal nerve endings are in the odontogenic region of the pulp horns. Some terminate on or in association with the odontoblasts (Figs. 9.26 and 9.27). Others are found in the predentinal tubules, usually in the region of pulp horns or roof of the coronal area (see Fig. 9.27). These nerve endings are

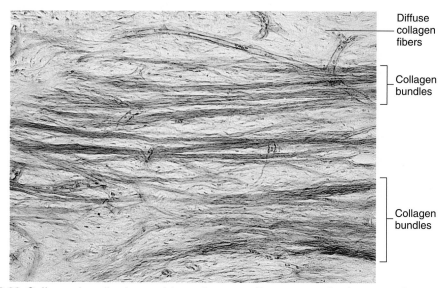

Fig. 9.20 Collagen bundles in an older pulp organ. Trauma may also have contributed to collagen in this pulp.

TABLE 9.1   Stem Cell Types in Dental Pulps (6, 7, 10–15, 17, 18, 20).

Properties	DPSC	SCAP	SHED	PDLSC	DFPC
Location	Permanent tooth pulp	Apical papilla of developing root	Exfoliated deciduous tooth pulp	Periodontal ligament	Dental follicle of developing tooth
Proliferation rate	Moderate	High	High	High	High
Heterogeneity	Yes	Yes	Yes	Yes	Yes
Multipotentiality	Odontoblast, osteoblast, chondrocyte, myocyte, neurocyte, adipocyte, corneal epithelial cell, melanoma cell, iPSC	Odontoblast, osteoblast, neurocyte, adipocyte, iPSC	Odontoblast, osteoblast, chondrocyte, myocyte, neurocyte, adipocyte, iPSC	Odontoblast, osteoblast, chondrocyte, cementoblast, neurocyte	Odontoblast, osteoblast, neurocyte
Tissue repair	Bone regeneration, neuroregeneration, myogenic regeneration, dentin–pulp regeneration	Bone regeneration, neuroregeneration, dentin–pulp regeneration, root formation	Bone regeneration, neuroregeneration, tubular dentin	Bone regeneration, root formation, periodontal regeneration	Bone regeneration, periodontal regeneration

DFPC, Dental follicle precursor cells; *DPSC*, dental pulp stem cells; *iPSC*, inducible periodontal stem cell; *SCAP*, stem cells from the apical papilla; *SHED*, stem cells from the pulp of human exfoliated deciduous teeth; *PDLSC*, periodontal ligament stem cells.
Estrela C, Alencar A, Kitten G, et al. Mesenchymal stem cells in the dental tissues: perspectives for tissue regeneration. *Braz Dent J.* 2011;22(2):91–98.

BOX 9.1   What Do Stem Cells Need to Differentiate Into Replacement Odontoblasts After Pulp Exposure?

Stimulus: Injury
Chemotactic factor: released from nervous system, vascular system, cells, dentin extracellular matrix (ECM), or preprogrammed
Cytoskeletal reorganization
Motility: cilia
Induction factor
Attachment substrate: consisting of basement membrane components? Type IV collagen, fibronectin, laminin, etc.

Vascular response: neovascularization
Neural response: secretion of vasoactive neuropeptides and trophic factors and neural regeneration
Activation of specific ion channels: Na^+, Ca^{++}, K^+, etc.
Intercellular communication: formation of gap junctions
Upregulated secretion of ECM components

presumed to function in pain reception, although recently, a small proportion of these endings have been reported to have transient receptor potential receptors for cold and, in fact, can discriminate the cold modality. Few nerve endings are located along the larger muscular blood vessels in the central pulp. All these nerve endings have a similar appearance and are highly vascular. They are believed to function in regulation of blood flow, constriction, or dilation of large blood vessels of the pulp.

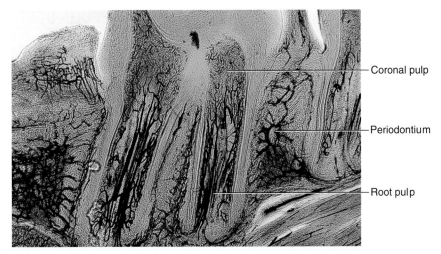

Fig. 9.21 Vascular injection to illustrate blood vessel organization in pulp and periodontium. Larger vessels conduct blood in the central pulp, and smaller capillaries are in the peripheral pulp.

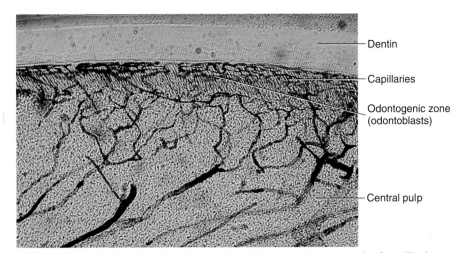

Fig. 9.22 Vascular injection into blood vessels to illustrate the network of capillaries among odontoblasts in the odontogenic zone. Dentin, which protects pulp, is seen at the top of the picture. The central pulp is in the lower part of the micrograph. (Avery JK. *Oral development and histology.* 3rd ed. Stuttgart: Thieme Medical; 2002.)

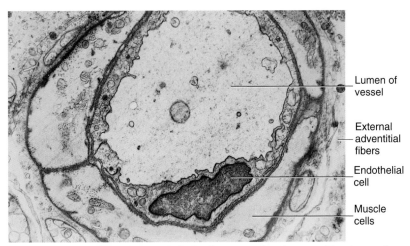

Fig. 9.23 Ultrastructure of a pulp arteriole in the central pulp area. The lumen is surrounded by endothelial cells; a nucleus is seen below. These cells compose the intima layer. Surrounding the intima is a layer of muscle cells that form the media. External adventitial fibers are also present. (Avery JK. *Oral development and histology.* 3rd ed. Stuttgart: Thieme Medical; 2002.)

These nerve endings are postganglionic sympathetic nerves, with cell bodies located in the Superior Cervical Ganglion. There are no other synapses in pulp. Nerve terminals closely associated with odontoblast processes are demonstrated in dentinal tubules in the pulp horn of a rat molar in the transmission electron micrograph in Fig. 9.28.

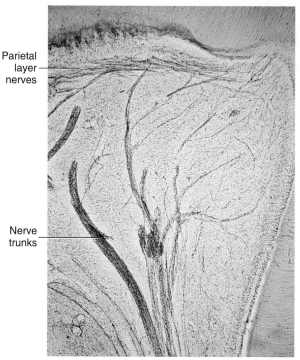

Fig. 9.24 Nerve trunks pass from the radicular pulp into the coronal area. These nerves extend to the periphery, where they form a plexus of nerves adjacent to the odontogenic zone above. (Bhaskar SN, ed. *Orban's oral histology and embryology.* 11th ed. St. Louis: Mosby; 1991.)

PAIN AND THE PULP–DENTIN COMPLEX

Pain is a function of the high concentration of nerve endings within the tooth. Pulp is highly sensitive to temperature changes, electrical and chemical stimuli, and pressure as applied to the inner enamel, dentin, or pulp. Until recently, teeth were considered one of the few body structures that perceive only the modality of pain, but recent research suggests that specific nerves in the pulp also transmit the modality of cold. The close relationship between nerve endings and the odontoblasts and their processes is significant. Moreover, the nerve endings in the dentinal tubules and the pulp may be some distance from where the pain is perceived, at the dentinoenamel junction and the inner enamel. Several theories attempt to explain this phenomenon.

The first theory is called the **direct innervation theory**, which is based on the belief that the nerves extend to the dentinoenamel junction. However, studies have not shown nerves present at this junction. In a second theory, other scientists believe the odontoblastic process is the receptor and that it conducts the pain to nerve endings in the peripheral pulp and in the dentinal tubules. This theory has been termed the **transduction theory** (Fig. 9.29).

A third theory, the **hydrodynamic theory**, was developed to explain the transmission of pain through the thickness of dentin (see Fig. 9.29). This theory is based on the premise that when dentin is stimulated, fluid and the odontoblastic process move within the tubules, making contact with the nerve endings in the inner dentin and adjacent pulp. When these nerve endings are contacted, they deform and act as mechanoreceptors to produce an impulse. Several factors support this theory. For example, when a stimulus such as cold is applied to the dentin, the odontoblastic process moves outward, but when heat is applied, the odontoblastic process moves inward. Other evidence is seen in the close relationship of the nerve endings and the odontoblastic process.

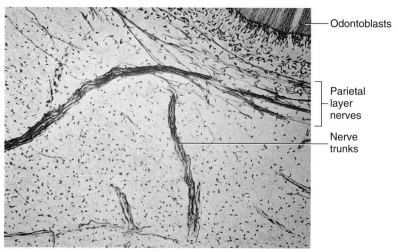

Fig. 9.25 Myelinated nerves extending into the parietal nerve plexus in the peripheral pulp. From this area, they extend between odontoblasts to terminate among them or in dentinal tubules. (Avery JK. *Oral development and histology.* 3rd ed. Stuttgart: Thieme Medical; 2002.)

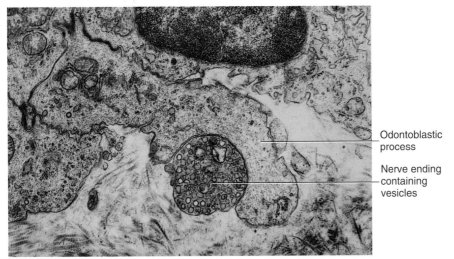

Fig. 9.26 Ultrastructure of a nerve ending in close contact with the odontoblastic process in predentin. The nerve contains small vesicles believed to contain a neurotransmitter substance. The nerve terminal interdigitates with the odontoblastic process. (Bhaskar SN, ed. *Orban's oral histology and embryology.* 11th ed. St. Louis: Mosby; 1991.)

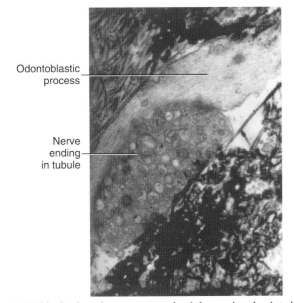

Fig. 9.27 Vesiculated nerve terminal in a dentinal tubule closely approximating an odontoblastic process. The nerve and process are close to each other. Dark-stained mineral of dentin is shown above and below the tubule.

The odontoblast is a unique cell that forms dentin throughout life. It forms reactionary or response dentin, for example, in response to various stimuli. In addition, it plays a role in conducting stimuli through dentin and in affecting nerve endings in the peripheral pulp.

FUNCTIONS OF THE PULP

Pulp has several functions, none of which is more important than providing vitality to the teeth with its cells, blood vessels, and nerves. The loss of pulp after a root canal does not mean the tooth will be lost; on the contrary, the tooth will function without pain. The tooth, however, has lost the protective mechanism that the pulpal nerves provided.

Pulp has several other functions. It is **inductive**, because in early development the pulp (papilla) interacts with the oral epithelium and initiates tooth formation. Pulp organs are **formative**, because odontoblasts of the pulp form the dentin that surrounds and protects pulp. Pulp is **protective** in its response to stimuli, such as heat, cold, pressure, and operative cutting procedures. The formation of sclerotic dentin, the process of mineral deposition in the tubules, originates in pulp and protects pulp from invasion of bacteria and bacterial products. Pulp is **nutritive**, because it carries oxygen and nutrition to the developing and functioning tooth. Finally, pulp has the ability to be **reparative** (Fig. 9.30) through its response to operative cutting or dental caries by the formation of reactionary and reparative dentin.

CLINICAL COMMENT

A cracked tooth may result from masticatory impact on a hard object. It can cause a fracture of a restoration margin. As a result, bacterial organisms or their toxins may penetrate the tooth and cause inflammation of the pulp, pain, and eventually pulpal pathosis.

REGRESSIVE CHANGES

Numerous regressive changes in the pulp and surrounding dentin are related to environmental stimuli and to aging. It is often difficult to determine which factor has caused the specific change seen. As the tooth ages, pulp decreases in size because of the continued deposition of dentin. This decrease in size usually occurs because of uniform deposition around the entire perimeter of the pulpal border (Fig. 9.31). In addition, changes occur in the dentin with both aging and injury. Areas of dentinal changes, such as dead tracts and mineral deposits, appear in zones of trauma. Reparative dentin usually forms under traumatized areas (see

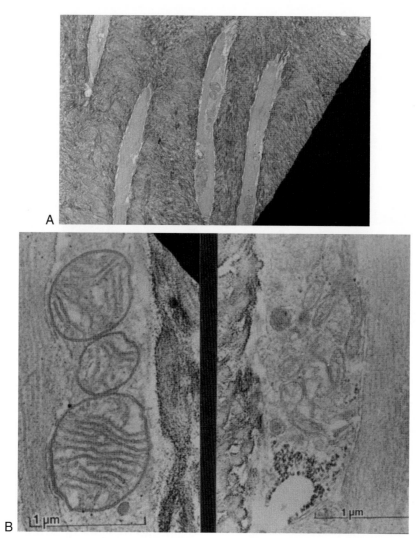

Fig. 9.28 A, This low magnification transmission electron micrograph demonstrates innervated dentinal tubules in the coronal pulp horns of the first mouse molar. Each tubule is innervated. **B,** This transmission electron micrograph demonstrates a series of dentinal tubules above the pulp horns of a rat molar. Within each dentinal tubule, an odontoblast process can be observed closely approximating a nerve terminal. The nerve terminals have mitochondria and secretory vesicles within the cytoplasm of the terminal. There are no synaptic junctions of membrane specializations in the pulp or between odontoblast processes and nerve terminals except between the smooth muscle cells of an arteriole and a postganglionic sympathetic terminal.

Fig. 9.31). In addition, as a result of both aging and trauma, pulpal cells decrease in general, as do cellular perinuclear cytoplasm and organelles in the cytoplasm, such as mitochondria and endoplasmic reticulum. This indicates that cell activity has decreased. Therefore aging decreases the ability of the pulp to respond to injury and to repair itself. With injury, however, deposition of dentin appears in a specific location (see Fig. 9.31).

Fibrous Changes

Fibrosis, which is seen in some pulps more than others, is believed to be caused more by injury than by aging. In some cases, diffuse fibrosis with collagen fibers appears throughout the pulp. Occasionally, the fibers nearly obliterate the pulp. What mechanism causes this condition is not certain, although it is believed to result from pulpal injury, at least in part. Scarring caused by injury is an important factor. One characteristic of aging is an increase in collagen fibers, which become more evident with the decreasing size of the pulp (see Fig. 9.20). Some pulps contain diffuse areas of collagen, and others have bundles of collagen fibers, probably because of injury or unknown systemic factors.

Pulp Stones

Pulp stones or **denticles** are round to oval calcified masses appearing in either the canal or coronal portions of the pulp organ (Fig. 9.32). They appear in teeth that have suffered injury, such as microtrauma, and in otherwise normal pulps. Pulp stones also occur in unerupted as well as erupted teeth. These denticles are noted in most pulps of permanent teeth, especially in individuals older than 50 years. They are classified according to their structure as true or false. **True denticles** have dental tubules like dentin. Odontoblasts may be on the surface of these denticles, and their processes are evident in their tubules. **False denticles**

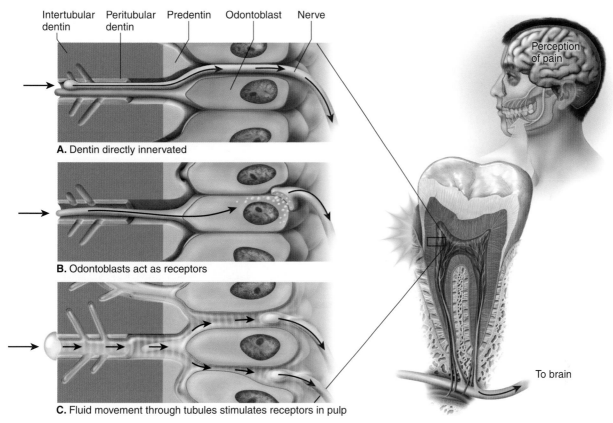

A. Dentin directly innervated

B. Odontoblasts act as receptors

C. Fluid movement through tubules stimulates receptors in pulp

Intertubular dentin Peritubular dentin Predentin Odontoblast Nerve

Perception of pain

To brain

Fig. 9.29 Summary of theories on the passage of nerve impulses through dentin. At the top **(A)**, impulses are shown stimulating nerves in dentin; this is termed the *direct stimulation theory*. In the center **(B)**, an odontoblast is depicted as a receptor passing impulses to nerves in the peripheral pulp and hence on to the brain; this is the transduction theory. At the bottom **(C)**, the diagram displays the concept of fluid and odontoblast movement. This movement causes pressure on the nerve endings, which stimulates them. The odontoblast thus acts as a mechanoreceptor to nerve endings which, in turn, conduct impulses to the brain. This is termed the *hydrodynamic theory*. (Nanci A. *Ten Cate's oral histology.* 8th ed. St. Louis: Mosby; 2013.)

are concentric layers of calcified tissue (Fig. 9.33). In the center of these false stones may be a group of cells that appear necrotic. One theory of denticle formation is that these cells are believed to serve as the nidus of denticle formation. Another theory is that pulp stones are the result of microtrauma within the pulp and form mineralized structures in response to the injury.

All denticles begin small and grow, sometimes nearly obliterating the pulp. Denticles may appear free in pulp, attached to dentin, or embedded in dentin. Therefore they are classified as **free, attached**, or **embedded denticles**. One pulp may have all three types (see Fig. 9.33 and Box 9.2). Investigators believe that a free denticle may become attached and later embedded as dentin is deposited around the denticle. Most denticles are false pulp stones that are free in the pulp.

Recently, researchers have been correlating pulp stones with cardiovascular disease. Several original manuscripts have suggested a strong correlation between the presence of pulp stones and arteriosclerosis.

Diffuse Calcifications

Diffuse calcifications appear as irregular calcified deposits along collagen fiber bundles or blood vessels in the pulp. This is considered a pathologic condition and usually appears as a sprinkling of small or occasionally large masses of mineral. These calcifications appear more often in the root canal than in the coronal area of the pulp.

PULPAL WOUND HEALING

Fig. 9.34A is an example of an experimental pulp exposure 2 days after surgery on a previously intact Rhesus monkey tooth showing a clot. Four days after exposure (see Fig. 9.34B) demonstrates clot retraction and streaming of progenitor cells toward the walls of the cut dentin, which has soluble chemotactic substances attracting the progenitor cells. At 6 days (see Fig. 9.34C), the progenitor cells have migrated to the exposure site, becoming a continuous sheet of cells across the exposure and forming gap junctions. Cells deep to the exposure also are in contact with the cells lining the exposure site and exhibit morphologic characteristics of cells becoming terminally differentiated, including dark-staining nuclei and enhanced cytoplasmic-to-nuclear ratios. Nine days after exposure (see Fig. 9.34D), differentiating replacement odontoblasts can be seen at the pulp medicament interface, around dentin chips

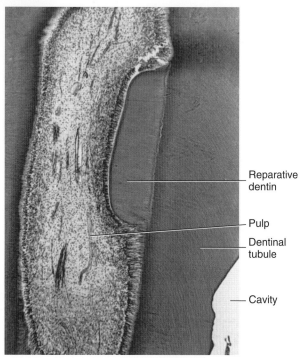

Fig. 9.30 Reparative dentin is deposited underlying areas
of stimulation by caries, abrasion, cavity preparation, and
restorations. It is limited to the area underlying dental tubules
leading from the cavity floor. (Avery JK. *Oral development and
histology.* 3rd ed. Stuttgart: Thieme Medical; 2002.)

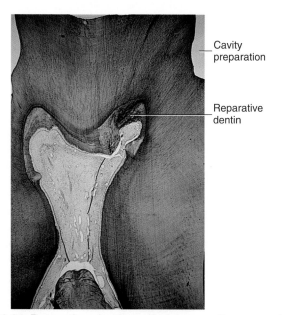

Fig. 9.31 Reparative dentin underlying cavity preparation
on the mesial-occlusal-distal aspects of a crown. Reparative
dentin on roof and sides of coronal pulp chamber underlie cut
dentinal tubules that lead from cavity preparation. (Avery JK.
Oral development and histology. 3rd ed. Stuttgart: Thieme
Medical; 2002.)

that have been pushed into the pulp during the surgical procedures, and along the walls of the cut dentin. At 12 days after
exposure (see Fig. 9.34E), disoriented odontoblasts can be seen
mineralizing the newly secreted predentin ECM. The replacement odontoblasts are dissimilar to the original odontoblasts

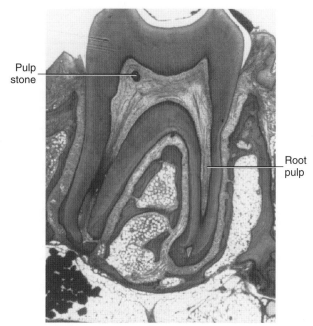

Fig. 9.32 Fibrous changes and pulp stone in coronal pulp. A
pulp stone appears in the coronal area of a molar tooth.

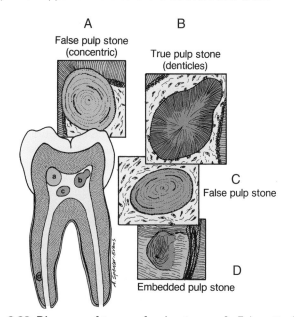

Fig. 9.33 Diagram of types of pulp stones. **A**, False attached
denticle. **B**, True denticle with tubules. **C**, False free denticle.
D, Embedded denticle.

BOX 9.2   Classification of Dental Pulp Calcification

Pulp stones were classified according to the most prevalent types occurring
in the population.
   Type I: single pulp stone present in pulp chamber
   Type IA: multiple pulp stones present in pulp chamber
   Type II: single pulp stone present in root canal
   Type IIA: multiple pulp stones present in root canal
   Type IIB: multiple pulp stones present in pulp chamber and root canal
   Type III: continuous type extending from pulp chamber to root canal

Satheeshkumar P, Mohan M, Saji S, et al. Idiopathic dental pulp
calcifications in a tertiary care setting in South India. *J Conserv Dent.*
2013;16(1):50–55.

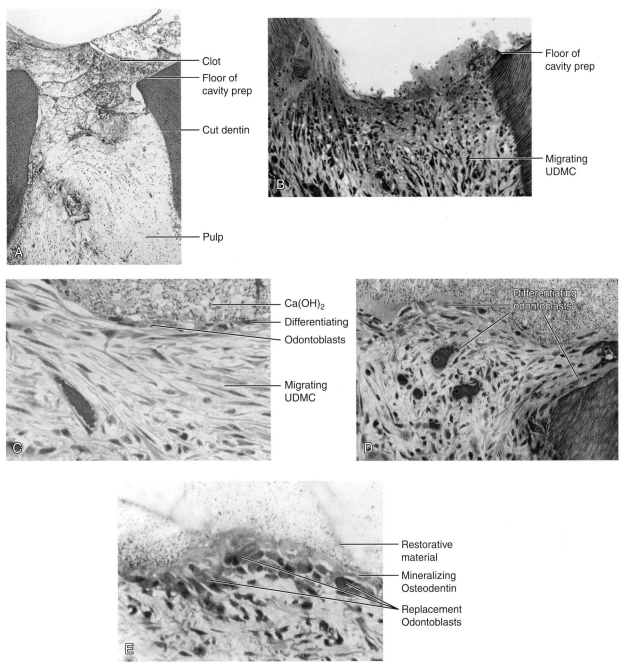

Fig. 9.34 A, Pulp exposure and blood clot 2 days after surgery. Cellular debris and fibrin strands can be seen across the exposure site. **B,** Pulp exposure 4 days after surgery. Cells can be seen migrating from the pulp proper toward the cut dentin walls and toward the periphery of the exposure site. **C,** Pulp exposure 7 days after surgery. Precursor replacement odontoblasts can be seen parallel to the medicament (calcium hydroxide; Ca[OH]$_2$) interface. The replacement odontoblasts have dark staining nuclei and are in contact with adjacent cells and also cells in the pulp proper. Other, less-differentiated cells can be seen migrating toward the periphery of the exposure site. **D,** Healing of pulp exposure 9 days after surgery. Cells at the pulp interface are contiguous with one another and have an enlarged diameter composed mostly of cytoplasm with dark-staining nuclei. Newly formed reparative dentin and replacement odontoblasts can be seen lining the cut dentin walls and around the dentin chips pushed into the pulp by the surgical procedure. **E,** A newly formed mineralized dentinal bridge can be seen at the pulp medicament interface. Newly differentiated replacement odontoblasts can be seen deep to the newly formed dentin extracellular matrix and randomly oriented, rather than the pseudostratified layer of polarized odontoblasts seen during normal embryologic tooth development.

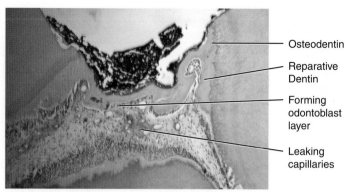

Fig. 9.35 **Three months postexposure.** This photomicrograph depicts a healing Rhesus monkey pulp 3 months after an exposure and capping with hard-set calcium hydroxide (Ca[OH]$_2$). A dentinal bridge can be seen across the exposure site with osteodentin closest to the medicament. Along the walls of the exposure, reparative dentin can be observed. The floor of the pulp demonstrates a significant accumulation of reactionary dentin.

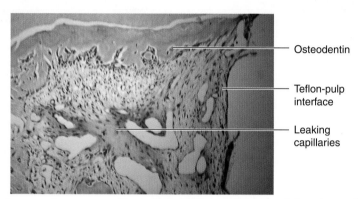

Fig. 9.36 **30 days post exposure.** Reparative dentin can be seen lining the walls of this pulp exposure. Osteodentin is also included as a component of this repair process 30 days after injury. Replacement odontoblasts can be seen lining the newly formed reparative dentin. The pulp exposure has been capped with Teflon. Teflon is a material that does not allow substances to adhere to the surface; therefore some of the necessary substances for regulated pulpal healing are missing. Primarily a substrate that is advantageous for the progenitor cells to adhere to, including fibronectin and laminin. These molecules are derived from the blood plasma and are two components of the basement membrane that the original odontoblasts attached to during embryologic development. Therefore there was no development of a dentinal bridge. (Heys DR, Fitzgerald M, Heys RJ, et al. Healing of primate dental pulps capped with Teflon. *Oral Surg Oral Med Oral Pathol.* 1990;69:227-237.)

that were derived from neural crest cells after induction by the ameloblasts. They are not well polarized, they are secreting the ECM in a 360-degree direction, and they do not produce tubular dentin. After exposure and capping with calcium hydroxide (Ca[OH]$_2$), osteodentin is normally secreted as the initial dentinal bridge that functions to protect the vital pulp and prevent further trauma. After osteodentin, tubular dentin will be formed, although when this occurs varies both with time and the extent of the injury. Fig. 9.35 demonstrates healing at

the exposure site 3 months after exposure. Reactionary dentin, reparative dentin, and osteodentin can all be seen in the photomicrograph in Fig. 9.35.

A study using Teflon as a pulp-capping agent was designed to better understand pulpal wound healing (Fig. 9.36). Because attachment proteins from the extravasated plasma, including laminin and fibronectin, could not adhere to the "wet" surface of the Teflon, cells could not form an attachment and therefore could not differentiate (Fig. 9.37A).

CLINICAL CASE

During excavation of a deep cavity, a pulp exposure is probable. When this occurs, there are usually bacteria present, and the prep will need to be cleaned, any hemorrhage controlled, and $Ca(OH)_2$ placed. When first placed, $Ca(OH)_2$ has a pH of around 11, which is bactericidal; over time, it becomes neutral. Because the $Ca(OH)_2$ approximates the edges of the cut dentin, it also functions to seal off the outside environment from the pulp and therefore is protective. Under the scanning electron microscope, hard-set $Ca(OH)_2$ exhibits a porous nature and therefore allows adhesion of attachment molecules that have been released from the injured vascular system, including laminin and fibronectin, which the undifferentiated mesenchymal cells (stem cells, progenitor cells, etc.) need to attach to in order to terminally differentiate into replacement odontoblasts.

Finally, the placement of glass ionomer over the $Ca(OH)_2$ ensures that it will not fracture during intrusive occlusal forces and allows the final restorative material to be innocuously placed.

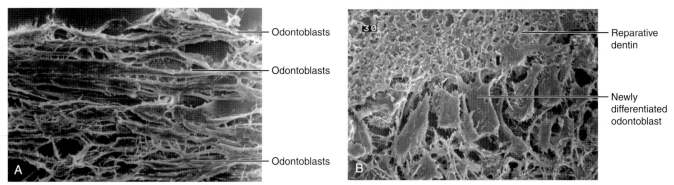

Fig. 9.37 A, The cells in this scanning electron micrograph are at the interface between the Teflon pulp-capping material and the pulp deep to a pulp exposure occurring 30 days earlier. The cells morphologically resemble fibroblasts. Multiple connections can be observed between the cells, but there is no differentiation into replacement odontoblasts. Because plasma proteins such as laminin and fibronectin were released from cut blood vessels after pulp exposure but could not adhere to the Teflon, the progenitor cells could not differentiate and remain morphologically and phenotypically fibroblasts. **B,** This scanning electron micrograph shows newly differentiated replacement odontoblasts at the interface between calcium hydroxide ($Ca[OH]_2$) and the newly formed dentinal bridge 30 days after surgery. No tubules can be seen in the newly formed reparative dentin. Odontoblasts are of varied morphology and are not coupled to adjacent odontoblasts.

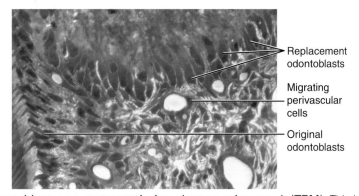

Fig. 9.38 Odontoblast zone on transmission electron micrograph (TEM). This low-magnification TEM shows the dentin pulp complex in a rat incisor. Odontoblasts and their processes can be seen entering the predentin–dentin interface. Capillaries and included endothelial cells can be seen parallel with the predentin and dentin. The loose connective tissue of the pulp proper can be seen deep to the odontoblasts.

However, when $Ca(OH)_2$ was used as a capping agent, replacement odontoblasts did differentiate and formed a dentinal bridge. Again, the newly differentiated odontoblasts did not resemble the original odontoblasts but still functioned in the wound healing cascade, ending with a functional dentin bridge (see Fig. 9.37B).

Fig. 9.38 demonstrates healing after an exposure in a rat pulp. Large replacement odontoblasts can be seen lining the exposure site, while the original odontoblasts can be seen on the opposite pulpal wall. Large perivascular cells appear to be migrating from the vasculature close to the exposure site (see Boxes 9.3–9.6).

BOX 9.3   Does Wound Healing After Exposure Recapitulate Development?

No interaction with ameloblasts or inner root sheath cells: no epithelial interaction

No mantle dentin formed

Due to the injury, no nerves and no blood vessels in the immediate proximity

Differences in the reparative dentin extracellular matrix: nontubular osteodentin and irregular dentin formed

Distinctly different cellular arrangement at medicament/odontoblast interface

Replacement odontoblasts morphologically different from original odontoblasts, but are they biochemically different?

BOX 9.4   Selected Biological Sequelae to Deep Cavity Preparation/Pulp Exposure

Initial odontoblastic response including cell death, breakdown of junctional attachment and communication, upregulation of substances for secretion of reparative extracellular matrix

Neural response:
1. Efferent: release of neuropeptides/transmitters/neurotrophic factors
2. Afferent: nociception
3. Neurogenic inflammation/response

Vascular response with increased capillary permeability releasing bloodborne factors

Inflammatory cascade and release of cellular mediators

Release of soluble factors from predentin/dentin

Cell signaling resulting in mitogenesis, chemotaxis, recruitment, and differentiation of cells necessary for repair/regeneration of injured pulp tissue

Reestablishment of an intact odontoblast layer and coordinated reparative dentinogenesis

BOX 9.5   Clinical Case Scenario

Operative Dentistry for Deep Caries/Pulp Exposure

When excavating a deep cavity, there is probability of a pulp exposure. When this occurs, there are usually bacteria present, and the prep will need to be cleaned, hemorrhage controlled, and hard-set pulp-capping material such as calcium hydroxide, white mineral trioxide, or Biodentine must be placed. When first placed, these materials have a pH of around 11, which is bactericidal and becomes neutral over time. Because these pulp-capping materials approximate the edges of the cut dentin, they also function to seal the outside environment from the pulp and therefore are protective. Under the scanning electron microscope, hard-set pulp-capping materials, including calcium hydroxide, exhibit a porous morphology and therefore allow adhesion of attachment molecules that have been released from the injured vascular system, including laminin and fibronectin. These attachment factors allow undifferentiated mesenchymal cells (stem cells, progenitor cells, etc.) to attach to the material surface in order to terminally differentiate into replacement odontoblasts.

Finally, the placement of a type of glass ionomer over these pulp-capping materials ensures that the calcium hydroxide will not fracture during intrusive occlusal forces and allows the final restorative material to be innocuously placed.

▌ SELF-EVALUATION QUESTIONS

1. Describe the characteristics of the odontogenic zone.
2. Compare the odontoblast in coronal pulp with the odontoblast in root pulp.
3. What are the most prominent cells of pulp, and what are their functions?
4. What are five other cell types found in normal pulp?

BOX 9.6   Clinical Case Study with Translational Basic Science

A 26-year-old male patient presents with acute, sharp pain in the second molar in the upper right quadrant of the maxilla. After appropriate diagnostic procedures and a thorough health history, you determine that the second maxillary molar could have pulpal involvement. Radiographs that were taken demonstrate a large periapical radiolucency surrounding the root apices.

What are the mechanisms associated with the formation of the periapical radiolucency?

Induction of bone resorption initiated by necrotic pulp tissue and bacterial endotoxins (e.g., lipopolysaccharides & lipoteichoic) leaking into the periodontal ligament space and binding to toll-like receptors 4 and 2 on fibroblasts, lymphocytes, and/or macrophages and subsequently mediated by inflammatory and proinflammatory cytokines and regulated by osteoblasts physiologically coupled to osteoclasts.

5. Describe the various blood vessels of pulp and how they differ from blood vessels of the periodontium.
6. Give descriptions and locations of nerve endings in pulp.
7. Name five functions of pulp.
8. Name and describe various types of denticles (pulp stones).
9. What are the types of junctional complexes found between odontoblasts?
10. Name and describe the types of reparative dentin.

CLINICAL COMMENT

Pulp stones begin to develop as early as functional occlusion. They normally are asymptomatic unless they impinge on blood vessels or nerves and usually do not present a problem to the dentist. Pulp stones are thought to be a result of microtrauma to the pulp resulting in ectopic calcifications.

CONSIDER THE PATIENT

This condition can be caused by internal resorption of the root and crown dentin. The crown appears pink because the transparent enamel reveals the blood vessels in the pulp.

QUANDARIES IN SCIENCE

The dental pulp contains a heterogeneous population of cells that maintain the pulp proper and the dentin protecting this sensitive organ. The dense innervation of the pulp belies the importance of this tissue in maintaining the overall health of the body, as does the number of reserve cells (various types of stem cells) contained within the stroma of the matrix. Because scientists do not fully understand the biology of the pulp, it is interesting to speculate on why it is so densely innervated with sensory nerves that contain many different types of neurotransmitters that are usually colocalized with other neurotransmitters within discrete nerve terminals located in the dentinal tubules, around the odontoblasts, and within the pulp proper. Do the different conformations of nerve terminals and different neurotransmitters function only during the transmission or modulation of nociception, or do they have other roles, such as modifying the responsiveness of the odontoblasts to iatrogenic or environmental insult or in the recruitment of replacement odontoblasts? The varieties of nerves, nerve terminals, and putative neurotransmitters that have been reported in the mature dental pulp have raised many questions relative to their functional significance. Evidence suggests that pulpal neurons have a significant role in modulating wound healing by releasing substances that can upregulate protein synthesis and modulate inflammation. Could changes in odontoblastic activity be mediated by neuropeptides, neuromodulators, and/or neurotransmitters released by sensory nerves that maintain the homeostatic balance of the pulp–dentin complex and affect how this balance is restored after injury?

CLINICAL CASE

A 12-year-old boy presents at the dentist's office and complains that his right first mandibular premolar is painful. After taking a thorough patient history and radiographs and performing an oral exam, the dentist diagnoses deep caries with a possible pulp exposure. Because the tooth has an open apex, the dentist refers the patient to an endodontist to do a regenerative endodontic procedure that involves stimulating stem cells at the apical papilla to differentiate into odontoblasts and pulp tissue to preserve pulpal integrity.

Regenerative endodontic therapy is a promising new therapy that tries to preserve teeth that are not fully formed in young patients. It is based on tissue engineering and stem cell evidence that suggests that the cells in the apical papilla and in the surrounding periodontal structures have the potential to be induced to differentiate into cells capable of achieving apexification. The procedure requires nonaggressive endodontic instrumentation to remove any infected pulp tissue within the coronal and root canal pulp; expose the ECM of the predentin and dentin; induce bleeding that will bring stem cells, growth factors, and nutrients to the apical environment and allow the root to finish growing; close the apical foramen; and form a dentinal bridge. A medicament such as mineral trioxide or a hard-set Ca(OH)$_2$ is placed in the root and allowed to harden, and the surface is tightly sealed. The process of forming a mineralized tissue, sometimes described as cementum-like, usually takes between 3 and 24 months.

SUGGESTED READING

American Association of Endodontists (AAE). Regenerative endodontics. Available at: http://www.aae.org/regeneration/.

Avery JK. *Oral development and histology*. 3rd ed. Stuttgart: Thieme Medical; 2002.

Avery JK. Pulp. In: Bhaskar SN, ed. *Orban's oral histology and embryology*. 11th ed. St. Louis: Mosby; 1991.

Avery JK, Chiego Jr DJ. Cholinergic system and the dental pulp. In: Inoki R, Kudo T, Olgart L, eds. *Dynamic aspects of dental pulp: molecular biology, pharmacology and pathophysiology*. New York: Chapman & Hall; 1990.

Baume LJ. The biology of pulp and dentine. In: Myers HM, editor. *Monographs in oral science*. Vol 8. New York: S. Karger; 1980.

Berdal A, Lézot F, Néfussi JR, et al. Mineralized dental tissues: a unique example of skeletal biodiversity derived from cephalic neural crest. *Morphologie*. 2000;84(265):5–10.

Boabaid F, Gibson CW, Kuehl MA, et al. Leucine-rich amelogenin peptide: a candidate signaling molecule during cementogenesis. *J Periodontol*. 2004;75(8):1126–1136.

Chan E, Darendeliler MA. Physical properties of root cementum. Part V. Volumetric analysis of root resorption craters after application of light and heavy orthodontic forces. *Am J Orthod Dentofacial Orthop*. 2005;127(2):186–195.

Chiego Jr DJ. An ultrastructural and autoradiographic analysis of primary and replacement odontoblasts following cavity preparation and wound healing in the rat molar. *Proc Finn Dent Soc*. 1992;88(suppl 1):243–256.

Goga R, Chandler NP, Oginni AO. Pulp stones: a review. *Int Endod J*. 2008;41(6):457–468.

Goldberg M, Six N, Chaussain C, et al. Dentin extracellular matrix molecules implanted into exposed pulps generate reparative dentin: a novel strategy in regenerative dentistry. *J Dent Res*. 2009;88(5):396–399.

Gronthos S, Mankani M, Brahim J, et al. Postnatal human dental pulp stem cells (DPSCs) in vitro and in vivo. *Proc Natl Acad Sci U S A*. 2000;97:13625–13630.

Hargreaves KM, Giesler T, Henry M, et al. Regeneration potential of the young permanent tooth: what does the future hold? *J Endod*. 2008;34(suppl 7):S51–S56.

Heys DR, Fitzgerald M, Heys RJ, et al. Healing of primate dental pulps capped with Teflon. *Oral Surg Oral Med Oral Pathol*. 1990;69:227–237.

Jin QM, Zhao M, Webb SA, et al. Cementum engineering with three-dimensional polymer scaffolds. *J Biomed Mater Res A*. 2003;67(1):54–60.

Koike T, Polan MA, Izumikawa M, et al. Induction of reparative dentin formation on exposed dental pulp by dentin phosphophoryn/collagen composite. *Biomed Res Int*. 2014;2014:745139.

Murray PE, Garcia-Godoy F, Hargreaves KM. Regenerative endodontics: a review of current status and a call for action. *J Endod*. 2007;33:377–390.

Nanci A. *Ten Cate's oral histology*. 8th ed. St. Louis: Mosby; 2012.

Ostby BN. The role of the blood clot in endodontic therapy. *An experimental histologic study. Acta Odontol Scand*. 1961;19:324–353.

Rex T, Kharbanda OP, Petocz P, et al. Physical properties of root cementum. Part IV. Quantitative analysis of the mineral composition of human premolar cementum. *Am J Orthod Dentofacial Orthop*. 2005;127(2):177–185.

Sedgley CM, Botero TM. Dental stem cells and their sources. *Dent Clin North Am*. 2012;56:549–561.

Smith AJ, Tobias RS, Cassidy N, et al. Influence of substrate nature and immobilization of implanted dentin matrix components during induction of reparative dentinogenesis. *Connect Tissue Res*. 1995;32(1-4):291–296.

Sotelo-Hitschfeld P, Bernal L, Zimmermann K. Odontoblasts are cold sensory cells in teeth. *Temperature*. 2023;10(1):9–12. https://doi.org/10.1080/23328940.2021.1933365.

Srivastava KC, Shrivastava D, Nagarajappa AK, et al. Assessing the prevalence and association of pulp stones with cardiovascular diseases and diabetes mellitus in the Saudi Arabian population—a CBCT based study. *Int J Environ Res. Public Health*. 2020;17:9293. https://doi.org/10.3390/ijerph17249293.

Teti G, Salvatore V, Ruggeri A, et al. In vitro reparative dentin: a biochemical and morphological study. *Eur J Histochem*. 2013;57(3):e23.

Turkal M, Tan E, Uzgur R, et al. Incidence and distribution of pulp stones found in radiographic dental examination of adult Turkish dental patients. *Ann Med Health Sci Res*. 2013;3(4):572–576.

Yamamoto T, Domon T, Takahashi S, et al. The structure of the cemento-dentinal junction in rat molars. *Ann Anat*. 2000;182(2):185–190.

Zou SJ, D'Souza RN, Ahlberg T, et al. Tooth eruption and cementum formation in the Runx2/Cbfa1 heterozygous mouse. *Arch Oral Biol*. 2003;48(9):673–677.

10

Cementum

LEARNING OBJECTIVES

- Describe the development of cementum and its function on the surface of the root.
- Describe the nature and the physical properties of intermediate cementum, cellular cementum, and acellular cementum.

- Discuss the aging of cementum, the formation of cementicles, and the repair of cementum.

OVERVIEW

Cementum has two major functions. It seals the tubules of root dentin and serves as an attachment for periodontal fibers to keep the tooth in its socket. Cementum has the ability to reverse root resorption by means of deposition as it forms a smooth patch on the cemental surface.

Two types of hard tissue cover tooth roots. The first, called **intermediate cementum**, is a homogenous epithelial derivative originating from inner epithelial root sheath cells. The second, called **cellular–acellular cementum**, is a thicker deposit of a bonelike substance produced by cementoblasts that differentiate from the undifferentiated cells in the dental follicle. The latter is laid down in increments, usually an acellular layer followed by a cellular layer. Cementum simulates bone by displaying cells within lacunae and cell processes within canaliculi. Cementum also exhibits incremental lines but does not have a vascular and neural supply that is characteristic of bone. As a result, the cementum has unique characteristics, such as lack of neural sensitivity and a greater ability than bone to resist resorption. Both are important clinical features. Aging cementum exhibits a rough and irregular surface caused by resorption of the cemental surface. This cementum also is associated with free, attached, or embedded cementicles. These oval to round ectopic calcifications are similar to the denticles in pulp. They are calcified bodies that may be embedded, attached to cementum, or free in the periodontal ligament.

ROLE OF CEMENTUM ON THE ROOT SURFACE

The hard tissue that covers the entire root surface is very thin but manages to carry out two important functions. First, it seals the surface of the root dentin and covers the ends of the open dental tubules, preventing dentinal fluid flow and subsequent pain associated with the hydrodynamic theory of pain transmission through dentin. Second, perforating fibers (Sharpey

fibers) of the periodontal ligament become embedded in the cementum. These fibers function as an attachment for the periodontal ligament fibers to the tooth root and aid in maintaining the tooth in its socket. This chapter discusses sealing of the root surface (Fig. 10.1).

CLINICAL COMMENT

Cementum can aid in maintaining the teeth in functional occlusion if it is deposited at the apical aspect of the root, especially in patients with chronic bruxism. Because cementum is the slowest growing tissue compared with the other periodontal tissues, it will be the last tissue to be involved in maintenance of functional occlusion in cases of loss of occlusal height.

DEVELOPMENT OF CEMENTUM

The first cementum deposited on the root's surface is called *intermediate cementum* and is formed by the inner epithelial root sheath cells that formed during root dentin formation and is an epithelially derived keratin-like protein. This deposition occurs before the root sheath cell layer disintegrates (Fig. 10.2). Intermediate cementum is situated between the granular dentin layer of Tomes and the secondary cementum that is formed by the cementoblasts. These cementoblasts arise from the dental follicle (sac). The thin layer of intermediate cementum is approximately 10 μm thick. After being deposited, this layer mineralizes to a greater extent than the adjacent dentin or the cellular–acellular cementum. Under proper magnification, a thin line of radiopacity is seen covering the root.

The cellular–acellular cementum is a specialized hard tissue covering the root surfaces of teeth (see Figs. 10.2 and 10.3). The initial thin layer of this cementum is acellular and is deposited on intermediate cementum. Subsequent layers alternate between cellular and acellular. Thus cementum is deposited incrementally. Both grossly and histologically, this cementum resembles bone because it is a hard tissue with cells contained in lacunae

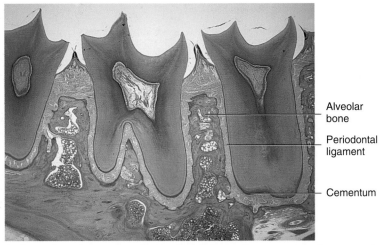

Fig. 10.1 Relation of tooth roots to the periodontium. Cementum is shown on the root apex. It covers the entire root surface overlying dentin. (Avery JK. *Oral development and histology.* 3rd ed. Stuttgart: Thieme Medical; 2002.)

Labels on figure: Alveolar bone; Periodontal ligament; Cementum

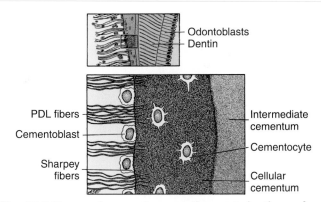

Fig. 10.2 Types of cementum on the root dentin surface. Intermediate cementum on the right overlying dentin cellular cementum in the center of the field and periodontal attachment fibers *(PDL)* on the left. (Avery JK. *Oral development and histology.* 3rd ed. Stuttgart: Thieme Medical; 2002.)

Labels on figure: Odontoblasts; Dentin; PDL fibers; Cementoblast; Sharpey fibers; Intermediate cementum; Cementocyte; Cellular cementum

that exhibit canaliculi (see Fig. 10.2). However, unlike bone, cementum does not contain blood vessels, nerves, or Haversian systems or Volkmann canals, which are the nutrient canals containing blood vessels and nerves in bone (see Fig. 10.3).

Cementum is limited to the roots of teeth. In 60% of cases, cementum is formed on the cervical enamel for a short distance; in 30%, it stops at the cervical line just meeting the enamel; and in 10%, a small gap exists between them. This order of frequency is known as **overlap, meet, and gap (OMG)** (Fig. 10.4 and Table 10.1).

INTERMEDIATE CEMENTUM

Intermediate cementum is a thin, noncellular, amorphous layer of hard tissue approximately 10 μm thick. It is deposited by the inner layer of the epithelial cells of the root sheath. Deposition occurs immediately before the epithelial root cells disintegrate

as a sheet and migrate away from the root into the periodontal tissue (see Fig. 10.2).

Intermediate cementum is the first layer of hard tissue deposited, and it seals the tubules of dentin. Because of its epithelial origin, intermediate cementum is composed of an enamelin-like protein rather than collagen, which is the protein typical of cellular or secondary cementum. Intermediate cementum is completely formed before deposition of the secondary cementum begins. As an amorphous, noncellular layer, it is similar to the aprismatic enamel layer on the crown surface of teeth. This cementum calcifies to a greater extent than either the adjacent cellular cementum or the dentin and therefore has a harder consistency (see Fig. 10.2).

CLINICAL COMMENT

Cementum functions as a protective covering for the root surface, a seal for the open dentinal tubules, and an attachment for the periodontal fibers that hold the tooth in its socket.

CELLULAR AND ACELLULAR CEMENTUM

Cementum is deposited directly on the surface of the intermediate cementum at a thickness of about 30 to 60 μm at the cervical region of the crown (see Fig. 10.3; Fig. 10.5). It increases gradually to a thickness of 150 to 200 μm at the root apex (Fig. 10.6).

The cementum appears to be more cellular as the thickness increases to maintain its viability (Fig. 10.7). The thin layer near the cervical region requires no cells to maintain vitality because fluids bathe its surface.

Cementum forms more slowly than the adjacent dentin (see Fig. 10.5). After the inner epithelial root sheath cells induce odontoblasts on the pulp side of the developing root, they begin to secrete predentin and stimulate the formation of the root dentin. Then they deposit intermediate cementum on the surface of the dentin. These cells then begin to degenerate and migrate from the root surface into the periodontal ligament. Then the

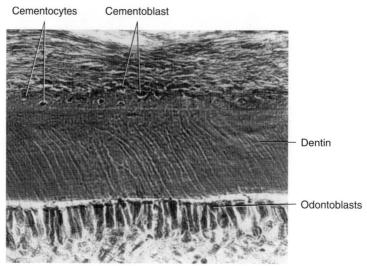

Fig. 10.3 Young cementum deposition on root dentin. Some cementoblasts become enmeshed in cementum matrix and develop into cementocytes living in lacunae. (Avery JK. *Oral development and histology.* 3rd ed. Stuttgart: Thieme Medical; 2002.)

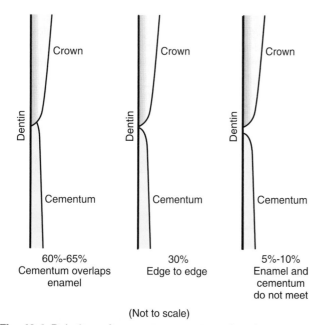

(Not to scale)

Fig. 10.4 Relation of cementum to enamel at the cemento-enamel junction. Overlap, meet, and gap (OMG) describe the order of frequency of these conditions. (Daniel SJ, Harfst SA. *Mosby's dental hygiene: concepts, cases, and competencies.* 2nd ed. St. Louis: Mosby; 2008.)

TABLE 10.1 **Relationship of Cementum to Enamel at the Cementoenamel Junction**	
Relationship of How Enamel and Cementum Meet During Development	**Percentage of Cases**
Cementum overlaps enamel	60
Cementum meets enamel	30
Small gap exists between cementum and enamel	10

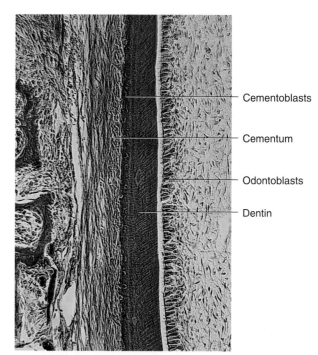

Fig. 10.5 Development of cellular cementum. Epithelial root sheath cells have moved from the root surface of dentin to a position peripheral to the cementum in the periodontal ligament. Cementoblasts are forming cementum along left side of band of dentin and cementum. (Avery JK. *Oral development and histology.* 3rd ed. Stuttgart: Thieme Medical; 2002.)

cementoblasts, which originate from the dental follicle, begin to form increments of cementum along the root surface.

Cementum is always thickest at the apex of the root (see Fig. 10.6). Cementum forms through the deposit in increments of a collagenous matrix that then becomes secondarily mineralized. The young unmineralized extracellular matrix (ECM) is called

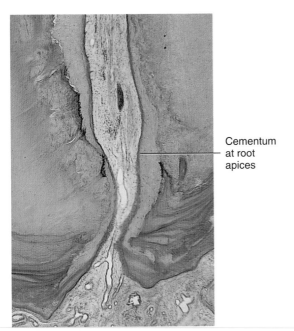

Cementum at root apices

Fig. 10.6 Thick cementum on root apices of an older tooth. Cementum is deposited around apical foramen and is lining the pulpal wall near the apex, constricting the foramen. (Avery JK. *Oral development and histology.* 3rd ed. Stuttgart: Thieme Medical; 2002.)

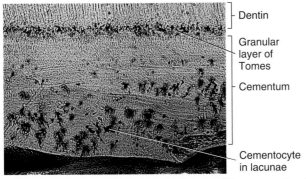

Dentin

Granular layer of Tomes

Cementum

Cementocyte in lacunae

Fig. 10.7 Histology of the granular layer of Tomes and cells in the lacunae in cementum. Cementum near the apex has the greatest number of lacunae. (Avery JK. *Oral development and histology.* 3rd ed. Stuttgart: Thieme Medical; 2002.)

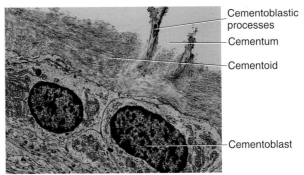

Cementoblastic processes

Cementum

Cementoid

Cementoblast

Fig. 10.8 Ultrastructure of cementoblasts on the surface of young cementum. Cementoblasts become cementocytes as their processes (and later their cell bodies) become incorporated in the matrix. (Avery JK. *Oral development and histology.* 3rd ed. Stuttgart: Thieme Medical; 2002.)

Lacuna   Cell process

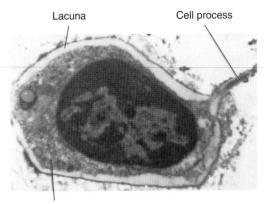

Viable cementocyte

Fig. 10.9 Ultrastructure of cementocyte near the surface of cementum. Cementocytes in this region appear viable and communicate with adjacent cementocytes by gap junctions on their processes. (Avery JK. *Oral development and histology.* 3rd ed. Stuttgart: Thieme Medical; 2002.)

cementoid, and its formation is similar to that of bone from osteoid and dentin from predentin.

Some cementoblasts become incorporated in the forming cementum along the developing front as cementum continues to form around the cementoblasts (see Fig. 10.7; Figs. 10.8–10.11). These cells are then termed *cementocytes* because they reside in lacunae, have cytoplasmic processes included in canaliculi that contact adjacent cementocytes, and form gap junctions. Cementocytes appear most notably in the thick apical cementum (see Fig. 10.7). The cementocytes found deep in the cementum are polygonal and have fewer organelles (see Fig. 10.9). Part of the reason for this appearance, especially in thicker cellular cementum, is that since the blood supply to cementum is through diffusion from the vasculature located in the periodontal ligament, the deeper cells are less likely to get enough oxygen and nutrients to maintain a healthy morphology and physiology.

Although many blood vessels are near the surface, none actually enter the cementum. In laboratory tests, cementum is slightly more permeable to dyes than bone or dentin. However, the permeability of viable cementum is unknown. Cementum is deposited in increments, resulting in incremental lines similar to those of bone, dentin, and enamel (Fig. 10.12). Cementum has many characteristics of hard tissue, although some elements are absent. Therefore cementum is not exactly like any other tissue in the human body. A thin layer of acellular cementum covers the cervical half of the root surface to a distance of approximately 20 μm. A deposit of cellular cementum then covers the acellular layer on the cervical root to a total thickness of 50 μm. Cellular cementum is then deposited on the apical root dentin to a thickness of 150 to 200 μm.

Without the presence of nerves, cellular cementum is insensitive to pain, which is an important clinical feature. Cementum is also more resistant to resorption than bone, and the lack of cementum vascularity may be part of the reason.

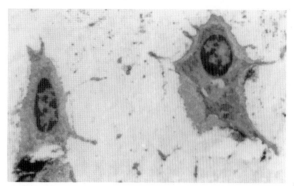

Fig. 10.10 Ultrastructure of two cementocytes lying deep in cementum. These cells contain few organelles and appear to be inactive. (Avery JK. *Oral development and histology.* 3rd ed. Stuttgart: Thieme Medical; 2002.)

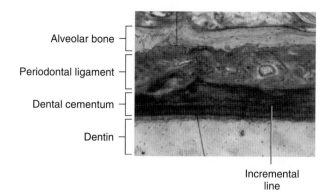

Fig. 10.12 Histology of cementum on the root surface. Horizontal incremental lines in cementum appear similar to those of bone, dentin, or enamel.

Alveolar bone

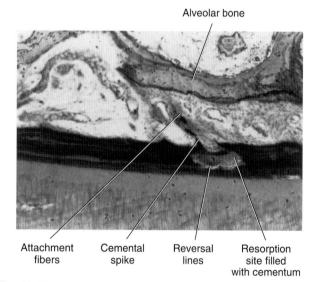

Attachment fibers | Cemental spike | Reversal lines | Resorption site filled with cementum

Fig. 10.11 Aging cementum showing projection of cemental spikes into ligament. A reversal line indicates root resorption and anatomic repair. Cementum builds up around bundles of periodontal ligament attachment fibers. (Avery JK. *Oral development and histology.* 3rd ed. Stuttgart: Thieme Medical; 2002.)

Deep within cementum, many lacunae appear empty, implying that these cells gradually die. Some of these cells have long processes that lie in canaliculi and are in contact with adjacent cementocytes (see Figs. 10.7–10.10). Near the surface of cementum, the cells appear active with organelles such as the Golgi apparatus, rough-surface endoplasmic reticulum, and mitochondria, which are all associated with protein secretion (see Fig. 10.10). Layers of cellular cementum may alternate with noncellular layers in their formation, although the reason is unknown. Deeper in the cementum, the cells may be less active (see Fig. 10.9).

The collagen fibers formed within the cementum are associated with the cementum's function on the root's surface. More superficially, cementum has bundles of noncalcified fibers that are associated with the function of attachment of periodontal fibers. These perforating fibers (Sharpey fibers) are called *extrinsic fiber bundles of cementum,* whereas the intrinsic fibers

TABLE 10.2 Organic and Mineral Composition of Cementum, Dentin, and Bone

Substance	Percentage of Organic Material (Collagen)	Percentage of Mineral (Calcium, Phosphorus)
Cementum	50–55	45–50
Dentin	30	68–70
Bone	30–35	60–65

of cementum ECM are formed from cementoblasts and maintained by cementocytes.

PHYSICAL PROPERTIES

As one group of hard connective tissues, cementum contains slightly less mineral than dentin or bone (Table 10.2). It is yellow and can be distinguished from enamel because cementum, unlike enamel, has no luster. Cementum is slightly lighter in color than dentin, which makes it difficult to distinguish between the two. It is softer than dentin, however, which aids in its identification.

AGING OF CEMENTUM

With aging, the relatively smooth surface of cementum becomes more irregular (see Fig. 10.11). This is caused by the calcification of some ligament fiber bundles where they were attached to the cementum. Such occurrences appear on most surfaces of cementum, but to no greater degree than near the apical zone. In aging, a continuing increase of cementum in the apical zone may obstruct the apical canal (see Fig. 10.6).

Microscopically, only the lacunae near the surface may have cells that appear viable, whereas deeper lacunae appear empty. Cementum resorption is one characteristic of aging cementum (see Fig. 10.11). Resorption becomes active for a period and then may stop. Deposition of cementum occurs in that period, creating reversal lines. Resorption can also occur in root dentin, and cemental repair can cover this defect (Fig. 10.13). As the tooth ages, occlusal height is reduced. Since the tooth

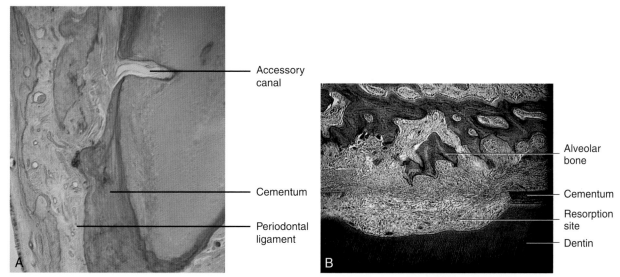

Fig. 10.13 A, Multiple layers of cementum can be seen in the photomicrograph at the apex of an older human tooth. The cementum has been laid down in an irregular fashion, causing a constriction in the periodontal ligament. An accessory (lateral) canal can also be seen passing through the cementum into the dentin. One of the possibilities for accumulations of cementum at the apex is loss of occlusal height and is a consequence of the tooth trying to maintain functional occlusion. **B**, Cemental and dentin resorption with periodontal soft tissue occupying the area. Alveolar bone develops in this space to compensate for root loss. The length of the periodontal fibers is thus maintained. (B, Avery JK. *Oral development and histology.* 3rd ed. Stuttgart: Thieme Medical; 2002.)

needs to be in functional occlusion, this reduction is compensated for by changes in the periodontal ligament first, then the alveolar bone proper, and finally the cementum, as Fig. 10.13A demonstrates.

CEMENTICLES

A cementicle is a calcified ovoid or round nodule found in the periodontal ligament. Cementicles may be found singly or in groups near the surface of the cementum (Figs. 10.14 and 10.15). The origin of a cementicle may be a nidus of epithelial cells. Cementicles are composed of calcium phosphate and collagen in the same amount as cementum (45% to 50% inorganic and 50% to 55% organic). Cementicles may be free in the ligament, attached, or embedded in the cementum (see Figs. 10.14 and 10.15). They are more prevalent along the

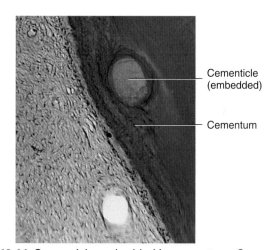

Fig. 10.14 Cementicle embedded in cementum. Cementicles may be found as free, attached, or embedded cementicles. They may begin free but gradually become attached and then become deeply embedded in the cementum. (Avery JK. *Oral development and histology.* 3rd ed. Stuttgart: Thieme Medical; 2002.)

root in an aging person, although they may also be found at a site of trauma.

CEMENTAL REPAIR: FUNCTIONAL AND ANATOMIC

Cemental repair is a protective function of the cementoblasts after resorption of root dentin or cementum. These cells are

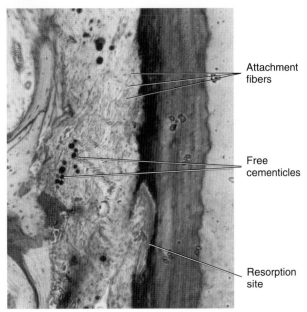

Fig. 10.15 Two groups of free cementicles in the periodontal ligament. A resorption area in the cementum is at the right. (Avery JK. *Oral development and histology*. 3rd ed. Stuttgart: Thieme Medical; 2002.)

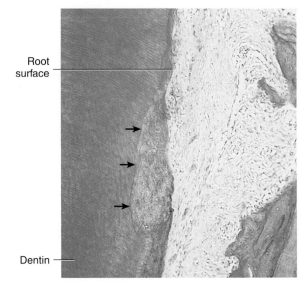

Fig. 10.16 Reversal line in cementum *(arrows)*. The root surface is again smooth as a result of cementum deposit in the resorption area (anatomic repair). (Avery JK. *Oral development and histology*. 3rd ed. Stuttgart: Thieme Medical; 2002.)

programmed to maintain a smooth surface of the root. Defects arise because of trauma of various kinds, such as traumatic occlusion, tooth movement, and hypereruption caused by the loss of functional occlusion from an opposing tooth. Loss of cementum is accompanied by a loss of attachment fibers to the root surface. When this occurs, repair cementum may be deposited by cementoblasts in the defect. If the repair fills in the defect to conform to the original morphology of the root surface, it is known as *anatomic repair*. However, this does not happen consistently; thus when a defect in the cementum contains a thin layer of new cementum and reattached perforating fibers, it is a *functional repair*. After this happens, the attachment fibers readily appear and are found embedded in the repair cementum (see Fig. 10.11). A cemental deposit means the development of a reversal line. This is seen at the point where resorption stops and deposition begins (Fig. 10.16). In an older individual, the surface cementum no longer exhibits a smooth surface (see Fig. 10.15).

More often, because of the lack of vascularity and innervation, cementum has a difficult time with repair, and the normal result of injury is ankylosis, where the surrounding alveolar bone proper will fuse with the cementum with no intervening periodontal ligament (Figs. 10.17 and 10.18).

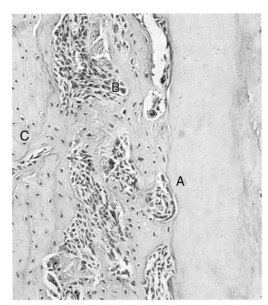

Fig. 10.17 Ankylosis. This photomicrograph demonstrates ankylosis between the cementum on the root surface **(A)**, the alveolar bone proper **(C)**, and the area that was the periodontal ligament **(B)**, which is now filled in with bone and connective tissue and fused with the cementum and the alveolar bone proper.

CLINICAL COMMENT

Cementum is resistant to resorption in younger tissues. This is the reason that orthodontic tooth movement results in alveolar bone resorption rather than tooth root loss. Cemental repair is an important root protective mechanism. In the case of orthodontic tooth movement, the first tissue to remodel is the periodontal ligament, then the alveolar bone proper lining the alveolus, and, finally, if necessary, the cementum.

CONSIDER THE PATIENT

Root exposure is common in both aging and periodontal disease. In these conditions, when there is an apical migration of the epithelial attachment, exposure of cementum and dentin occurs. Pain is associated with exposed dentin and cementum because dentinal tubules open into pulp, where nerves are located. Also, cementum is thin or nonexistent on the cervical root. Patients with root exposure should be careful. Root caries is also common in root exposure. This occurs because the exposed cementum and dentin are less resistant to caries than is enamel. The pain decreases in time because pulpal odontoblasts respond to the stimuli of exposed dentinal tubules, with deposition of reparative dentin in the pulp underlying this area.

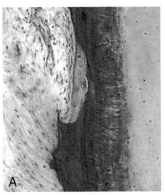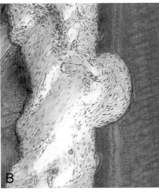

Fig. 10.18 A, Anatomic repair. The surface of the cementum has been previously resorbed by osteoclasts but has now been replaced by new cementum to the original surface of the root. **B,** Functional repair. The cementum has been resorbed by previous osteoclastic activity. The cementum has not filled in this defect, but the periodontal ligament fibers have reattached to the newly formed cementum surface and are now functional.

Alternative Nomenclature for Types of Cementum

- Cementum
- Intermediate cementum
- Primary acellular intrinsic fiber cementum
- Primary acellular extrinsic fiber cementum
- Secondary cellular intrinsic fiber cementum
- Secondary cellular mixed fiber cementum
- Acellular afibrillar cementum

CLINICAL CASE

A 15-year-old female patient complains about pain from the left mandibular central incisor after the hygienist finished scaling her teeth. The dentist was consulted and reviewed the radiographs but could not find any reason why the tooth was sensitive after ruling out an inflamed tooth pulp, caries, and periodontal disease.

After applying several endodontic tests, including an electric pulp tester and hot and cold cotton pellets, it was determined that the tooth was vital. However, when the dentist used an explorer at the cervical region of the tooth, the patient felt pain. The dentist applied a desensitizing agent to the tooth and told the patient to brush with desensitizing toothpaste and to come back if the pain remained or increased within 2 weeks.

The intermediate and the acellular primary intrinsic fiber cementum secreted at the cervical region of the tooth to seal the exposed dentinal tubules is very thin and can be scaled or abraded off the surface, reexposing the dentinal tubules and causing pain by allowing dentinal fluid flow and initiating the hydrodynamic theory of pain conduction through dentin. Also, during tooth development, the cementum sometimes does not meet or overlap the enamel, leaving exposed dentinal tubules and resulting in pain. In either case, the dentist will usually suggest brushing with a desensitizing toothpaste and will sometimes seal the cementum/dentin surface with various types of desensitizing agents that have been reported in the dental literature to be efficacious for sensitive teeth.

SELF-EVALUATION QUESTIONS

1. What is the origin of intermediate cementum?
2. Where on the root is cementum thinnest and where is it thickest?
3. Name three types of cementicles.
4. Describe the appearance of healed root surfaces.
5. Why is cementum insensitive to pain?
6. What is the function of cementum?
7. What is the origin of cementoblasts and cementocytes?
8. Name two characteristics of aging cementum.
9. What are the percentages that cementum overlaps, meets, or gaps enamel?
10. What are some reasons for cemental resorption?

QUANDARIES IN SCIENCE

Cementum does not have a nerve or blood supply and therefore does not remodel readily after injury. Cementum covers the root surface, protects the underlying dentin, and contains perforating fibers (Sharpey fibers) of the periodontal ligament. There are many questions about the biology of cementum that are still unanswered. During periodontal disease, a loss of attachment of periodontal fibers occurs and, although the periodontist can clean and treat the diseased area, it is difficult to initiate reattachment of the periodontal fibers. The ECM of cementum is mostly collagen type I with a small amount of noncollagenous proteins. Bacteria and their associated endotoxins (lipopolysaccharide and lipoteichoic acid) readily attach to the surface of cementum and are difficult to remove. There are many theories associated with whether the bacterial antigens that adsorb to the surface of cementum due to electrostatic forces are actually incorporated into the surface of the ECM of the cementum. Modern treatments sometimes use a combination of a decalcifying agent combined with mechanical debridement and, although these techniques are well established, there is still little reattachment of the periodontal fibers realized. Why reattachment is difficult to achieve is a matter under considerable investigation. The answer hopefully will result in more effective treatment in the future.

SUGGESTED READING

Bravman RJ, Everhart DL, Stahl SS. A cementum-bound antigen: its reaction with serum antibody and localization, in situ. *J Periodontol.* 1979;50(12):656–660.

Hammarström L, Alatli I, Fong CD. Origins of cementum. *Oral Dis.* 1996;2(1):63–69.

Harrison JW, Roda RS. Intermediate cementum. Development, structure, composition, and potential functions. *Oral Surg Oral Med Oral Pathol Oral Radiol Endod.* 1995;79(5):624–633.

Schroeder HE. Oral structure biology. New York: Thieme Medical; 1991.

Yamamoto T, Hasegawa T, Yamamoto T, et al. Histology of human cementum: its structure, function, and development. *Jpn Dent Sci Rev.* 2016;52(3):63–74.

Zeichner-David M. Regeneration of periodontal tissues: cementogenesis revisited. *Periodontol 2000.* 2006;41:196–217.

Periodontium: Periodontal Ligament

OVERVIEW

The periodontal ligament is a fibrous connective tissue between the alveolar bone proper and the cementum covering the root. This ligament covers the root of the tooth and connects with the tissue of the gingiva. The periodontal ligament occupies the periodontal space and is composed of fibers, cells, and intercellular substance. The latter consists of collagen fibers and ground substance, which in turn contains proteins and polysaccharides. The periodontium develops from dental follicular tissue that surrounds the tooth. The cells forming the ligament fibers, alveolar bone, and cementum develop from the follicle. The periodontium has a thickness of 0.15 to 0.38 mm, is thinnest in the midroot zone, and decreases slightly in thickness with age. The ligament is composed of collagen fiber bundles that attach the cementum to the alveolar bone proper. Interstitial areas contain the blood vessels and nerve trunks, which communicate freely with vessels and nerves at the apex of the roots and the alveolar bone. This tissue is highly cellular, containing fibroblasts and vascular, neural, bone, and cemental cells. The primary function of the periodontal ligament is support for the teeth. The ligament also transmits neural input to the masticatory apparatus and has a nutritive function essential to maintaining the ligament's health, which has important clinical implications.

ORGANIZATION OF THE PERIODONTAL LIGAMENT

Two groups of principal fibers are named according to their location with respect to the teeth. The **gingival group** is located around the necks of the teeth, and the **dentoalveolar group** surrounds the roots of the teeth (Fig. 11.1). These principal fibers are bundles of primarily type I collagen fibers strategically positioned at inclinations important to their functions along the root surface from the cervical region to the tooth's apex (see

parts *1* to *6* in Fig. 11.1). The collagen bundles are embedded in the cementum of the root and extend into the alveolar bone. Therefore they act as a suspensor ligament for the teeth.

Between each group of fibers is a space termed the **interstitial space (areas)** (Fig. 11.2), which is not actually a space. Interstitial areas contain a network of blood vessels, nerves, and lymphatics that maintain the vitality of the periodontal ligament and a network of finer fibers that interlace in the spaces and support the dense collagen fiber bundles. The function of the interstitial space relates to the constant stretching and contraction of the fiber bundles during mastication. Most supporting fibers are collagenous, but a few have been described as elastic-like and of a structure different from that of collagen. These are termed **oxytalan fibers** (Fig. 11.3). Oxytalan fibers are small in diameter and appear to interface with the collagen bundles, supporting the collagen bundles and the blood vessel walls. These fine, elastic-like fibers stain with special stains that reveal their location to be almost longitudinal within the ligament and perpendicular to the principal fibers when the fibers are viewed through a light microscope (see Fig. 11.3).

Gingival Fiber Group

The principal fibers of the periodontal ligament in the gingival area are known as the **gingival fibers**. They consist of four groups of fibers, each having a different orientation and all supporting the gingiva (Fig. 11.4). The **free gingival fibers** arise from the surface of the cementum in the cervical region and pass into the free gingiva. The **attached gingival fibers** arise from the alveolar crest and pass into the attached gingiva. The **circular** or **circumferential fibers** are continuous around the neck of the tooth and resist gingival displacement. The **alveolar crest fibers** arise from the cementum at the neck of the tooth and terminate in the alveolar crest. **Transseptal fibers** originate in the cervical region of each crown and extend to similar locations on the mesial and distal surfaces of each adjacent tooth (Figs. 11.5 and 11.6). This fiber

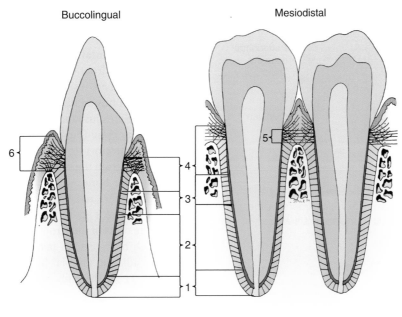

Buccolingual   Mesiodistal

1. Apical
2. Oblique
3. Horizontal
4. Alveolar crest
5. Transseptal
6. Gingival group

Fig. 11.1 Principal fiber groups of the periodontal ligament. All fibers listed in the buccolingual plane are also present in the mesiodistal plane. The transseptal fiber group number 5, however, is seen only in mesiodistal plane, as these fibers are attached tooth to tooth. All other principal fibers are attached tooth to the gingiva or alveolar bone.

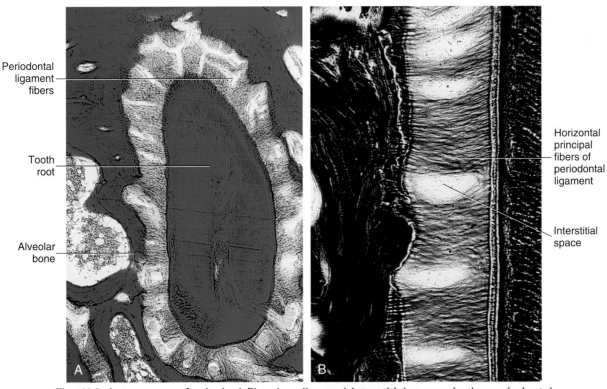

Periodontal ligament fibers

Tooth root

Alveolar bone

Horizontal principal fibers of periodontal ligament

Interstitial space

Fig. 11.2 Appearance of principal fiber bundles and interstitial spaces in the periodontal ligament. **A,** As they appear in cross-sectional plane. **B,** In plane longitudinal to tooth.

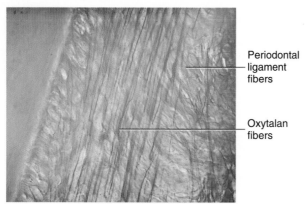

Fig. 11.3 Histologic appearance of oxytalan fibers in the periodontal ligament oriented parallel to the tooth's surface.

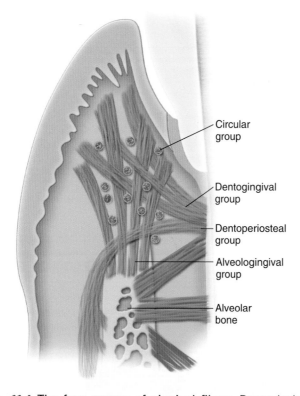

Fig. 11.4 The four groups of gingival fibers. Dentogingival fibers extend from the cervical cementum into free and attached gingiva. Alveologingival fibers extend from the alveolar crest into gingiva. Circular fibers surround the teeth, and the dentoperiosteal group extends from the cervical cementum into the alveolar crest. (*Nanci A. Ten Cate's oral histology. 8th ed. St. Louis: Mosby; 2013.*)

group functions in resistance to the separation of each tooth. Fig. 11.6 shows that transseptal fibers are found in the mesiodistal plane and are not present in the buccolingual plane. All these fiber groups are illustrated in Fig. 11.1 and listed in Table 11.1.

Dentoalveolar Fiber Group

The dentoalveolar fiber group consists of five differently oriented principal fiber groups named according to their origin and insertion in the dentoalveolar process. The **alveolar crest group**

originates at the cervical area, just below the dentinoenamel junction, and extends to the alveolar crest and into the gingival connective tissue (see Fig. 11.6). These fibers resist intrusive forces. The **horizontal fiber group** extends in a horizontal direction from the midroot cementum to the adjacent alveolar bone proper. These fibers resist tipping of the teeth, as illustrated in Fig. 11.7. The **oblique fiber group** extends in an oblique direction from the area just above the apical zone of the root upward to the alveolar bone (Fig. 11.8), and the fibers resist vertical or intrusive masticatory forces. The **apical fiber group** extends perpendicular from the surface of the root apices to the adjacent **fundic alveolar bone**, which surrounds the apex of the tooth root. Apical fibers resist vertical and extrusive forces applied to the tooth (see Fig. 11.8). Another group of fibers located between the roots of multirooted teeth is termed **interradicular fibers**. Such fibers extend perpendicular to the tooth's surface and to the adjacent alveolar bone and resist vertical and lateral forces (Fig. 11.9). These fibers are summarized in Table 11.1.

> ### CLINICAL COMMENT
>
> Healthy periodontal tissues are of significant importance to the health of dental patients. Chronic periodontal disease and dental caries can lead to infusion of bacteria into the bloodstream.

Interstitial Spaces

The principal fibers make up the structural and functional bulk of the periodontal ligament. They are positioned at regular intervals along the gingival–apical extent of the periodontal ligament. Between each bundle of ligament fibers an interstitial space appears. These spaces appear in both the cross-sectional and longitudinal planes of the ligament (see Fig. 11.2). The regularity of these spaces clearly relates to the vascular and neural needs of the functioning ligament. Interstitial spaces appear designed to carry these vascular and neural structures both by encircling the tooth at regular intervals and by connecting with the vessels that run longitudinal to the root (Figs. 11.10 and 11.11). These interstitial spaces are designed to withstand the impact of masticatory forces. The collagenous fiber bundles that surround these spaces are arranged at angles to the surfaces of the spaces, thus providing support for their maintenance. These spaces are compressed during mastication or tension, as noted in Fig. 11.12. For this reason, their position and support by fiber bundles are important. A network of fine fibers within these spaces can be seen supporting the nerves and nerve endings that occupy these spaces (Figs. 11.13 and 11.14).

Vascular System

The periodontal ligament has a rich blood supply that arises from the inferior and superior alveolar arteries and from branches of the facial artery from the external carotid. These vessels supply the alveolar bone and anastomose freely with the periodontal ligament. The vascular plexus that extends into the ligament traverses from the apical areas to the gingival areas, with loops that surround the teeth at regular intervals (see Fig. 11.10B). Fig. 11.10A shows the density and complexity of the ligament. When the alveolar bone and tooth have been sectioned and the

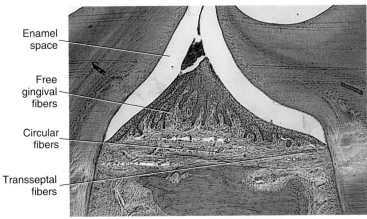

Fig. 11.5 Histology of gingival fibers in the interproximal area. The transseptal fiber group extends from mesial of one tooth to distal of an adjacent tooth. Relationship of free gingival and circular fibers to transseptal fibers is shown.

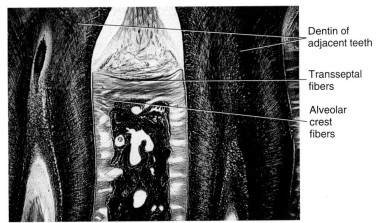

Fig. 11.6 Histology of alveolar crest fibers extending from the cementum of the cervical region to the alveolar bone. Periodontal fibers penetrate alveolar bone, and transseptal fibers extend from the tooth on the left to the right.

TABLE 11.1	**Principal Fibers**	
Fiber Group	**Location of Attachment**	**Function**
GINGIVAL FIBER GROUP		
Transseptal	Cervical tooth to tooth mesial or distal to it	Resist tooth separation mesial distal
Attached gingival	Cervical tooth to attached gingival	Resist gingival displacement
Free gingival	Cervical tooth to free gingival	Resist gingival displacement
Circumferential	Continuous around neck of tooth	Resist gingival displacement
DENTOALVEOLAR FIBER GROUP		
Apical	Apex of root of fundic alveolar bone proper	Resist vertical forces
Oblique	Apical one-third of root to adjacent alveolar bone proper	Resist vertical and intrusive forces
Horizontal	Midroot to adjacent alveolar bone proper	Resist horizontal and tipping forces
Alveolar crest	Cervical root to alveolar crest of alveolar bone proper	Resist vertical and intrusive forces
Interradicular	Between roots to alveolar bone proper	Resist vertical and lateral movement

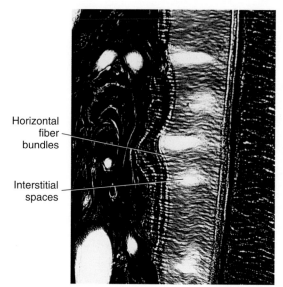

Fig. 11.7 **Histologic appearance of horizontal fiber bundles.** The bundles are perpendicular to the root and alveolar bone surface; their perforating fibers are embedded in both bone and cemental surfaces.

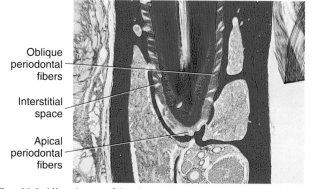

Fig. 11.8 **Histology of horizontal, oblique, and apical fiber groups of the periodontal ligament.** The angulation is shown for each of these bundle groups, which resist forces of mastication.

vascular plexus has been injected with carbon particles and then cleared, the orientation and relationship of these vessels can be demonstrated (see Fig. 11.11). Both arterioles and venules traverse these tissues, carrying blood to and away from them. Arteriovenous shunts have been demonstrated in the periodontal ligaments that provide direct connections between the arterial and venous blood supply without having to go through a capillary network. Capillaries are evident throughout the principal fiber bundles. The ligament is highly metabolically active, undergoing compaction and extension as mastication takes place. Evidence of the ligament activity is seen in cell turnover, in its ability to modify in tooth movement, and in its ability to heal. These conditions relate to the rich vascular supply of the ligament.

Neural System

The larger nerve trunks of the periodontal ligament are found in the central zone of the tooth's long axis (Fig. 11.15). Branches of these trunks pass into the ligament and alveolar bone at intervals along the path to the gingival tissues. Most nerve trunks and finer nerves are observed in the interstitial spaces, either in the tracts that traverse the ligament longitudinal to the tooth's surface or within any of the spaces between bundles along the root (see Fig. 11.13). Nerve terminals are noted throughout the ligament and especially in bundles of principal fibers. Encapsulated pressure receptors and **paciniform**, fine pain receptors, are in greatest numbers (see Fig. 11.14). These terminals are known to function during masticatory activity.

In addition to the typical sensory functions, the periodontal ligament has specialized encapsulated terminals for proprioception, with cell bodies located in the mesencephalic nucleus, which is the only central nervous system nucleus that contains first-order neuron cell bodies from sensory nerves. Knowing where the mandible is in three-dimensional space is critical for many aspects of mastication. The nerve terminals located in the

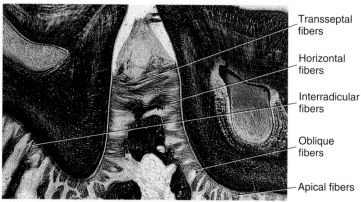

Fig. 11.9 **Histology of interradicular fiber groups of principal fibers.** These are located between the roots and alveolar bone of multirooted teeth.

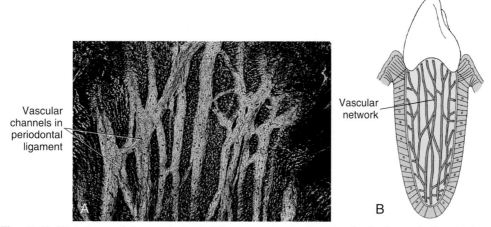

Fig. 11.10 Histology of the periodontal ligament in the longitudinal plane. A, Continuity of the interstitial system in the center of the ligament, with lateral connections throughout the interstitial spaces. **B**, Diagram of organized network of blood vessels in the ligament.

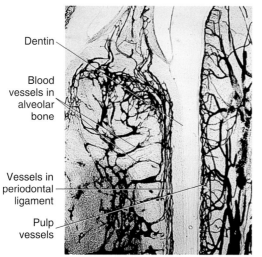

Fig. 11.11 Vascular supply of alveolar bone, periodontal ligament, and tooth pulp as seen after injection of vessels with carbon and clearing of the tissues. Bone is on the left, the periodontal ligament is in the center, dentin is to the right of center, and pulp is on the right.

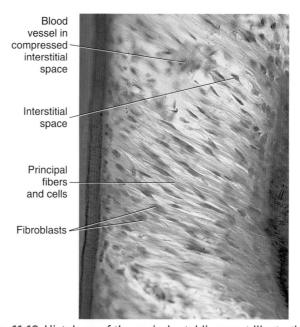

Fig. 11.12 Histology of the periodontal ligament illustrating tension. Note diminished interstitial spaces and flattening of cells when the fibers are stretched.

tendons and ligaments of the muscles of mastication and the temporomandibular joint (TMJ), as well as the periodontal ligament, allow the individual to make fine mandibular movements associated with bite force, mastication, speech, and other mouth movements when integrated with the other neural receptors in the periodontal apparatus.

CELLS OF PERIODONTAL LIGAMENT

Fibroblasts, Osteoblasts, and Cementoblasts

Several types of cells located in the ligament have formative, supportive, and resorptive functions. **Fibroblasts** are the most numerous seen in the periodontal ligament because of the high collagen density of this tissue. The abundance of fibroblasts allows rapid replacement of fibers (see Fig. 11.12). Recent investigations

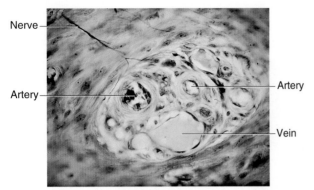

Fig. 11.13 Interstitial space viewed at high magnification. At the upper left, a nerve enters the interstitial space from the ligament. Within the interstitial space are the thick-walled artery and thin-walled veins. Beside the artery and veins are several nerve trunks.

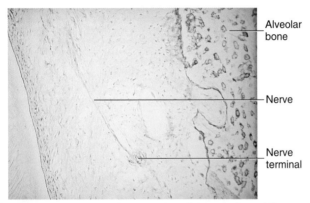

Fig. 11.14 A nerve trunk traversing the periodontal ligament along the surface of alveolar bone on the right. At the lower extremity of the trunk is an encapsulated pressure receptor (modified pacinian). These pressure-receptor endings sense the density of food during mastication.

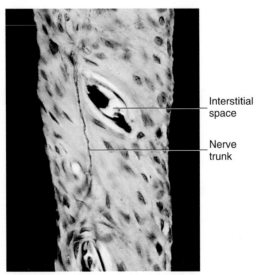

Fig. 11.15 Nerve trunk passing from the apical region toward the gingival area. Fibers of the periodontal ligament wrap around the interstitial space.

show that fibroblasts, in addition to forming new collagen fibers, function in the breakdown of worn-out fibers. Fibers are ingested and broken down into amino acids. These amino acids are taken up by other cells and are recycled into the formation of new collagen fibers. **Osteoblasts** are located along the surface of the alveolar bone. Because bone is continually turning over, the osteoblasts are busy forming new bone in the area of the alveolar bone proper. All osteoblasts differentiate locally from mesenchymal cells as the need for osteoblasts arises. **Cementoblasts** appear along the surface of the cementum. Cementum is constantly being formed as new principal fibers are embedded along the root surface. Cemental resorption may also occur for a number of reasons, such as changes in occlusal relationships or tooth movement, resulting in activity of new cementoblasts in the repair of resorbed cementum or dentin of the root and after trauma.

Macrophages and Osteoclasts

Macrophages found in the ligament are important defense cells in this location. Macrophages have mobility and phagocytic function. They phagocytose dead cells, bacteria, and foreign bodies. Some fibroblasts become macrophagic in the periodontal ligament because they have the ability to destroy collagen as well as form it (Fig. 11.16). This activity relates to the high metabolic function of the periodontal ligament. Two types of fibroblasts may exist—those that only form collagen and those that form and destroy collagen. Macrophages, lymphocytes, leukocytes, and plasma cells may also appear in the periodontium when it is stressed by disease.

Osteoclasts, in instances of both tooth movement and periodontal disease, function in bone resorption (Fig. 11.17). They appear as a normal consequence of tipping or bodily movement of a tooth (Fig. 11.18). Osteoclasts originate from monocytes within the blood vascular system and become the multinucleated cells seen in lacunae of resorption sites in hard tissue. They are recruited to an area of appositional growth or undergoing remodeling by local osteoblasts that control osteoclast activity by the mechanism of physiologic coupling.

Epithelial Rests

Epithelial rests are normal constituents of the periodontal ligament and are seen throughout life. Epithelial cells are scattered throughout the ligament, but in the early life of the tooth, they are seen along the root surface. Epithelial rests may appear as resting, proliferating, or degenerating cell masses. They also may be characterized as going through extensive periods of dormancy.

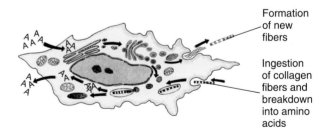

Fig. 11.16 Fibroblasts are present in the periodontal ligament in great numbers. It is probable that some of these cells function in forming and destroying collagen fibers as the need arises.

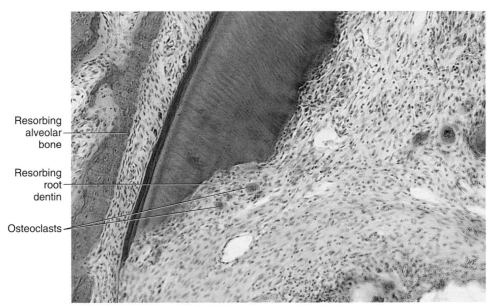

Fig. 11.17 Osteoclastic action on alveolar bone and on root dentin can be seen in this micrograph. Tooth roots *(left)* and alveolar bone *(right)* are undergoing resorption in preparation for eruption of a tooth in permanent dentition. In the lower right corner is a follicle surrounding the erupting permanent tooth crown. Osteoclasts are much larger than any other cell in the field.

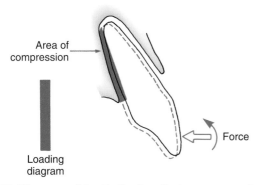

Fig. 11.18 Diagram of tooth tipping that may occur in orthodontic tooth movement or naturally as a result of malocclusion. When the tooth is tipped in the direction of the *arrow*, the resultant area of compression causes inflammation and eventually bone resorption. On the side of the force, bone formation will occur as a consequence of the inflammation caused by the stretching of the periodontal ligament fibers. (Proffit WR, Fields Jr HW. *Contemporary orthodontics.* 5th ed. St. Louis: Mosby; 2013.)

These rests are composed of a mass of epithelial cells, some four to six in number, although there may be more in cases where they are proliferating. The cells are remnants of Hertwig's epithelial root sheath. Epithelial rests can also be induced to proliferate by chronic inflammatory mediators and can form the epithelial lining of periapical cysts. Type 2 antigen-processing dendritic cells can also be found lining periapical cysts. However, epithelial rests may continue to proliferate from the epithelial cells lining the gingival sulcus. They can be observed along the root surface, as seen in Fig. 11.19. Periapical radiolucencies are caused by necrotic pulp tissue leaking into the surrounding periodontium, causing inflammation and resultant bone loss (Fig. 11.20).

Intercellular Tissue

Intercellular tissue surrounds and protects the cells of the periodontal ligament, primarily fibroblasts, and is the product of these cells. This extracellular matrix is composed of water, glycoproteins, and proteoglycans, which surround the collagen fibers. These protein and polysaccharide substances provide the cells with vital substances that arise from the blood capillaries and return unwanted waste products catabolites from these cells to the vessels.

FUNCTIONS OF THE PERIODONTAL LIGAMENT

Supportive

The most important function of the periodontal ligament is support of the teeth. Failure of this function results in tooth loss. Every time the teeth are clenched, as in mastication, the periodontal fibers are stretched and then relaxed. This system is highly efficient to compensate for the thousands of times this ligament is called into action.

Sensory

The periodontal ligament is supplied with abundant receptors and nerves that sense any movement in function. When receptors sense pressure, the nerves send signals to the brain, which informs the masticatory apparatus, including the TMJ and muscles of mastication.

Nutritive

The blood vessels of the ligament provide the essential nutrients for the ligament's vitality and for the hard tissue of cementum and alveolar bone. All cells, such as fibroblasts, osteoblasts, cementoblasts, and even the resorptive osteoclasts

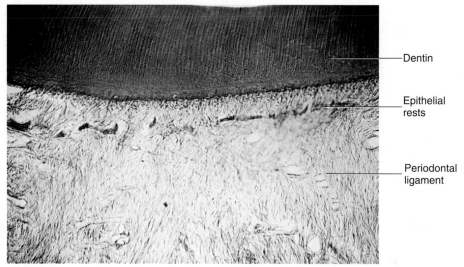

Dentin

Epithelial
rests

Periodontal
ligament

Fig. 11.19 Epithelial rests appear in the periodontal ligament near the cementum covering dentin at the top of the micrograph. This is a young specimen; thus rests are large and distinctive.

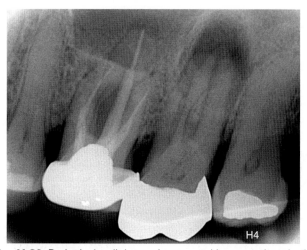

Fig. 11.20 Periapical radiolucencies caused by necrotic pulp tissue leaking into the surrounding periodontium causing inflammation and resultant bone loss.

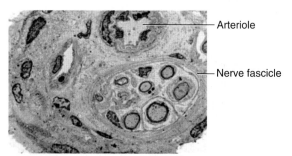

Arteriole

Nerve fascicle

Fig. 11.21 Ultrastructure of an interstitial space with a nerve bundle containing myelin and unmyelinated nerves *(lower right)* and small arterioles *(above)*.

is a continuous process. These tissues function for a lifetime if health is maintained and appropriate care is provided.

CONSIDER THE PATIENT

A patient asks about prevention of periodontal disease. What can the patient do to prevent a future problem?

CLINICAL COMMENT

Renewal capability is an important characteristic of the periodontal ligament fibers. The periodontal fibroblasts provide maintenance of the system when repair is needed.

AGING OF LIGAMENT

Aging occurs in ligamentous tissue as in all other tissues of the body. Cell number and cell activity decrease as aging takes place. In aging cementum and alveolar bone, scalloping occurs (Fig. 11.22). Some fibers are attached to the peaks of these scallops rather than over the entire surface. This is one of the more remarkable changes that occur in the aging of supporting structures of the teeth. Activity of these tissues is likely to decrease

and macrophage cells, require the nutrition that is carried by the blood vessels of the ligament (Fig. 11.21).

When an orthodontic appliance or an occlusal problem causes compaction and compression, a constriction of the blood vessels may occur. This results in a lack of vascular continuity, which leads to a diminishing of cells in the area, and the tissue becomes ischemic. The tissue then begins to appear glass-like and is described as a "hyalinized" area. Continued pressure usually leads to the appearance of osteoclasts at this site, with the loss of alveolar bone. This condition then may create space for blood vessels to grow back into this area. The periodontium therefore responds as a coordinated unit.

Maintenance

Periodontal tissues function in maintenance of the masticatory apparatus because these tissues heal readily. The interaction of the connective tissue cells with their intercellular environment

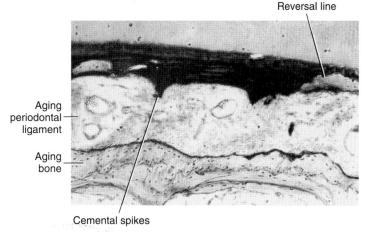

Fig. 11.22 Aging periodontal ligament, cementum, and alveolar bone. The number of fiber bundles has decreased. Cemental spikes are shown, which are caused by excessive deposition around depleted fiber bundles. Resorption sites are also noted.

during the aging process because of restricted diets, and therefore normal functional stimulation of these tissues is diminished. With aging, a healthier periodontium can result from general good health of the individual and good oral hygiene. A loss of gingival height related to gingival and periodontal disease promotes destructive changes. Unfortunately, at that time, the presence of a low-grade inflammation may be characteristic of the gingival tissue.

CLINICAL COMMENT

The four tissues comprising the periodontium are variable in their rate of regeneration, with the gingiva as the fastest and the cementum as the slowest. The periodontist is aware of these differences and uses these differences in regeneration capacity and rate in the clinical practice of periodontics.

CONSIDER THE PATIENT

The patient's role is very important. Patients assist the dental professional in the maintenance of the periodontal structures. These tissues are very susceptible to poor oral hygiene and therefore deterioration of the periodontium.

SELF-EVALUATION QUESTIONS

1. Describe the function and location of the principal fiber groups in the gingival group.
2. Describe the function and location of the principal fiber groups in the dentoalveolar group.
3. Describe the function and location of the interstitial system of the periodontal ligament.
4. Describe the vascular system of the periodontal ligament.
5. Describe the types and locations of the nerves and nerve endings in the periodontal tissues.
6. Name the cells and their functions in the periodontal ligament.
7. What are the three types of epithelial cell rests and where are they found?
8. Discuss the several functions of the periodontal ligament.
9. What are oxytalan fibers and what are their function and location?
10. Describe the characteristics of aging in the periodontal ligament.

QUANDARIES IN SCIENCE

The periodontium is a complex organ that has many functions in addition to providing attachment for the teeth. One of the functions is related to the exquisite sensory innervation of the ligament. The periodontium contains many types of sensory receptors, including proprioceptors that signal the central nervous system as to where the mandible is in three-dimensional space; these receptors affect bite force and masticatory muscle behavior. Dysfunction of the temporomandibular joint, myalgias, and muscle pain are some of the consequences of impaired neural function associated with the periodontium and are difficult to diagnose because the etiologies of the various diseases are still unknown. Periodontists can treat periodontal disease and loss of attachment with high success; however, many questions still exist about the significance of the multiple functions associated with the periodontium.

CASE STUDY

A 72-year-old male patient is referred to the periodontist for deep root planing and periodontal pocket resolution. Patient medical history is normal as are his hematologic results, with no indications of chronic or systemic diseases predisposing of his present condition. Complete intra- and extraoral exams are performed, including periodontal probing for pocket depth. Radiographs are taken and a treatment plan discussed. Several pockets will need periodontal surgery to try to preserve the tooth and its attachment apparatus. While the periodontist is scaling the root surface to remove calculus, there is profuse bleeding as she approaches the fundic bone of the socket. After cleaning the tooth surface, the periodontist places a breathable membrane in the defect to try to prevent periodontal pocket formation and tells the patient that he will need to keep the area clean and rinse with chlorhexidine to prevent a recurrence of the periodontal infection. Although the periodontium lost attachment height, the patient recovered. He is compliant but remains in a maintenance phase during his 6-month treatments with the periodontist.

Patients with periodontal disease experience inflamed and bleeding gingiva, loss of epithelial attachment, and bone loss that cannot be recovered to original height due to the deleterious effects of bacteria and bacterial byproducts (e.g, lipopolysaccharides and lipoteichoic acid, components of the plaque, and calculus). The periodontist understands the science behind the clinical practice and realizes that the disrupted tissues regenerate at different rates: first, epithelium; second, periodontal fibers; third, alveolar bone proper; and fourth, cementum. To prevent epithelial downgrowth from forming a pocket, the epithelium will have to be inhibited to allow for periodontal fiber reattachment to the new alveolar bone proper and cementum in a process known as *guided tissue regeneration*. This process requires positioning a breathable membrane, sometimes impregnated with growth factor such as platelet-derived growth factor, between the epithelium and connective tissues, thereby inhibiting downgrowth of the epithelium. Guided tissue regeneration is an excellent method for optimizing the probability of reattachment of the gingiva and periodontal ligament at the highest possible level.

SUGGESTED READING

Ahuja T, Dhakray V, Mittal M, et al. Role of collagen in the periodontal ligament: a review. *Internet J Microbiol.* 2012;10(1): 1–7.

Bonucci E. New knowledge on the origin, function and fate of osteoclasts. *Clin Orthop Relat Res.* 1981;158:252–269.

Contos JG, Corcoran Jr JF, LaTurno SA, et al. Langerhans cells in apical periodontal cysts: an immunohistochemical study. *J Endod.* 1987;13(2):52–55.

Marchi F. Secretory granules in cells producing fibrillar collagen. In: Davidovich Z, ed. *The biological mechanisms of tooth eruption and root resorption.* Birmingham, AL: EBSCO Media; 1988.

Marks Jr SC. The origin of osteoclasts: evidence, clinical applications and investigative challenges of an extraskeletal source. *J Oral Pathol.* 1983;12:226–256.

Melcher AH. Periodontal ligament. In: Bhaskar SN, ed. *Orban's oral histology and embryology.* 11th ed. St. Louis: Mosby; 1991.

Nakamura TK, Hanal H, Nakamura MT. Ultrastructure of encapsulated nerve terminals in human periodontal ligaments. *J Oral Biol.* 1982;24:126–132.

Nanci A, Somerman MJPeriodontium.. In: Nanci A, ed. *Ten Cate's oral histology: development, structure, and function.* 8th ed. St. Louis: Mosby; 2003.

Schroeder HE. *Oral structure biology.* New York: Thieme Medical; 1991.

Wong RS, Sims MR. A scanning electron-microscopic, stereo-pair study of methacrylate corrosion casts of the mouse palatal and molar periodontal microvasculature. *Arch Oral Biol.* 1987;32(8):557–566.

Periodontium: Alveolar Process and Cementum

LEARNING OBJECTIVES

- Describe the nature of alveolar bone proper and supporting bone.
- Explain how cementum participates in support of the tooth.
- Describe the condition of physiologic tooth movement and the effects of the various types of orthodontic tooth-moving devices on the hard tissues of the periodontium.

- Understand the effects of aging on the tooth-supporting structures and the condition of edentulous jaws.

OVERVIEW

This chapter discusses the hard tissues of the periodontium, which are cementum and alveolar bone. The alveolar process is the bony part of the maxilla and mandible that has the primary function of supporting the teeth. Alveolar bone is composed of alveolar bone proper, which is attached to the fibers embedded in the roots of the teeth. Supporting bone is the bone covering the mandible, and it serves as cortical plates that give support to the alveolar bone proper. This alveolar bone is in the process of continuous turnover, which enables the tissue to be responsive to manipulation, such as tooth movement resulting from normal physiologic function or orthodontic treatment. Cementum functions as the means of fiber attachment to the tooth roots and protection for the vital dentin deep to it. These fibers have the abilities to form and resorb, which are necessary for support during tooth movement. If teeth are moving in a straight line or rotating, all parts of the suspensory apparatus must change simultaneously. This phenomenon first took place during tooth eruption and continues to function for both the primary and secondary dentition. Tooth function is a prerequisite for the maintenance of the alveolar bone and cementum. Bone loss occurs during aging or periods of inactivity, resulting in possible tooth mobilization. With loss of alveolar bone, loss of periodontal fibers occurs as well. Periodontal disease can cause these conditions, with possible tooth loss that could result in an edentulous jaw (Box 12.1).

ALVEOLAR PROCESS

The alveolar process is the part of the maxilla and mandible that supports the roots of teeth and is composed of **alveolar bone proper** and **supporting bone** (Fig. 12.1). Alveolar bone proper is the bone lining the tooth socket. In clinical radiographic terms, it is defined as the **lamina dura**. Dense bone serves as the attachment bone that surrounds the roots of the teeth. Supporting bone is, as the name implies, the bone that serves as a dense cortical plate to sustain the alveolar bone proper. This cortical plate covers the surface of the maxilla and mandible and supports the alveolar bone proper. The supporting cancellous bone underlies and supports the dense cortical bone (see Fig. 12.1; Fig. 12.2). The existence of alveolar bone is entirely dependent on the presence of teeth. Alveolar bone develops initially as a protection for the soft developing primary teeth and later, as the roots develop, as a support for the teeth. Finally, as the teeth are lost, the alveolar bone resorbs. Teeth are responsible not only for the development but also for the maintenance of the alveolar process of the mandible (see Fig. 3.21). The coronal border of the alveolar process is known as the **alveolar crest** (see Fig. 12.2). This crest is normally located approximately 1.2 to 1.5 mm below the dentinoenamel junction of the teeth. It is rounded on the anterior region and nearly flat in the molar area. When teeth are viewed from the buccolingual aspect, the alveolar crest may be thin or missing. The area of bone loss where an apical root penetrates the cortical bone is known as a **fenestration**, and bone loss in the coronal area of the root is termed **dehiscence** (Fig. 12.3).

CLINICAL COMMENT

The lamina dura is an important diagnostic landmark in determining the health of the periapical tissues. Loss of density usually means infection, inflammation, and resorption of this bony socket lining.

Alveolar Bone Proper

The compact or dense bone that lines the tooth socket is of two types when viewed microscopically. This bone either contains perforating fibers from the periodontal ligament or is similar to compact bone found elsewhere in the body. Perforating fibers or **Sharpey's fibers** are bundles of collagen fibers embedded in the alveolar bone proper. These fibers are at right angles or oblique to the surface of the alveolar bone proper and along the root of the tooth (see Fig. 12.1). The fiber bundles inserting in the bone are regularly spaced and appear similar to those that insert into the root surface cementum (Figs. 12.4 and 12.5). Perforating fibers are not limited to periodontal bone. They also appear anywhere in the body where ligaments or tendons attach to cartilage or bone.

Because bone of the alveolar process is regularly penetrated by collagen fiber bundles, it can be appropriately termed *bundle bone*. Bundle bone, being synonymous with *alveolar bone proper* or *lamina dura*, appears denser radiographically than the adjacent supportive bone (Fig. 12.6). This density is probably the result of the mineral content or orientation of the mineral crystals (Ca^{++} hydroxyapatite) surrounding the fiber bundles. Blood vessels and nerves penetrate the lamina dura through small foramina. Because the mineral density is sufficient, this bone appears opaque in radiographs (see Fig. 12.6). Tension on the perforating fibers during mastication is believed to stimulate this bone and is considered important in its maintenance.

Not all alveolar bone proper appears as bundle bone because the bone lining the socket is constantly being remodeled for adaptation to the stresses of occlusal impact. Newly formed

bone does not have perforating fibers (Fig. 12.7). Teeth are constantly moving (drifting) within their sockets, resulting in loss of some fibers. Other fibers continually form and initially attach to the bone's surface and later, become embedded.

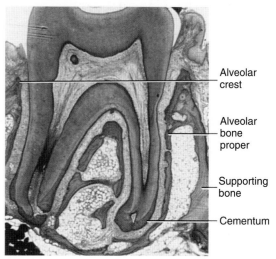

Fig. 12.2 Histology of the tooth and its supportive tissues showing relationships among alveolar bone proper, supporting bone, and cementum covering roots.

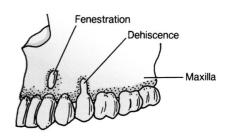

Fig. 12.3 **Loss of alveolar bone adjacent to a tooth.** Loss near the root apices is termed fenestration, whereas bone loss in the region of the cervical root is termed dehiscence.

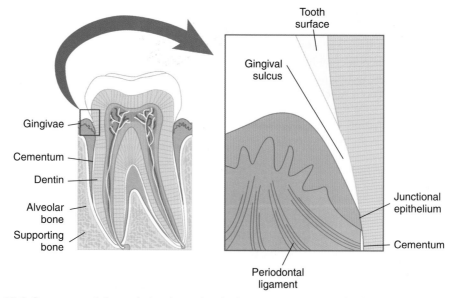

Fig. 12.1 Structures of the periodontium: alveolar bone proper, supporting bone, and cementum. (Robinson DS, Bird DL. *Essentials of dental assisting.* 6th ed. St. Louis: Saunders; 2017.)

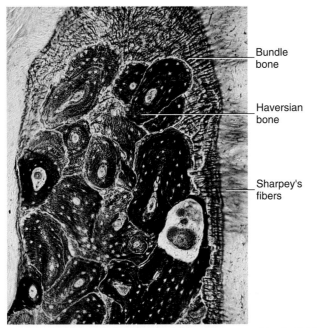

Fig. 12.4 Histology of alveolar crest area from an older individual illustrating bundle bone with penetrating (Sharpey's) fibers and Haversian-type supporting bone.

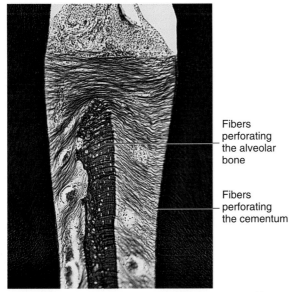

Fig. 12.5 Histology of perforating fiber bundles (Sharpey's fibers). Uniformity of position of numerous fibers in cemental and bony surfaces is shown. Fiber bundles of bone are larger and less numerous than fibers entering the cemental surface.

Supporting Compact Bone

Supporting compact bone of the alveolar process is similar to **Haversian bone** found elsewhere in the body (Fig. 12.8). Compact bone of the alveolar process extends over the lingual surface of the mandible and maxilla beside the tongue. Compact bone also covers the buccal surface of the mandible or maxilla adjacent to the lining of the cheek. Compact or cortical bone contains osteons with radiating lamellae accentuated by lacunae, which contain the osteocytes in living bone

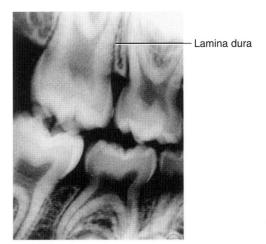

Fig. 12.6 Radiograph of alveolar bone illustrating lamina dura, the radiographically dense bone lining tooth sockets.

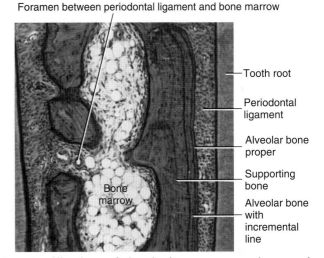

Fig. 12.7 Histology of alveolar bone proper and supporting bone. Foramina communicate between the periodontal ligament and marrow spaces in supporting bone on the left.

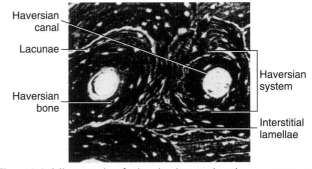

Fig. 12.8 Micrograph of alveolar bone showing a concentric Haversian system, interstitial lamellae, and lacunae.

(Fig. 12.9). Haversian and Volkmann canals form a continuous system of nutrient canals that radiate throughout the bone, which also includes a rich nerve supply. The Haversian canals extend through the long axis of the bone, and Volkmann canals enter Harversian canals at right angles. These canals form a

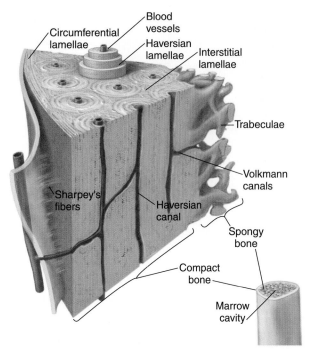

Fig. 12.9 Diagram of Haversian systems of compact bone similar to compact bone throughout body. Periosteal lamellae cover the surface of the mandible and numerous Haversian systems contain blood vessels interconnected by Volkmann canals. Lacunae containing osteocytes surround the Haversian canals. (Pollard TD, Earnshaw WC. *Cell biology.* 3rd ed. Philadelphia: Saunders; 2017.)

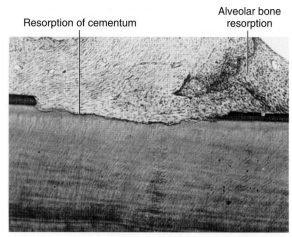

Fig. 12.10 Cemental loss by resorption, which has also destroyed adjacent alveolar bone.

nutrient network throughout bone. Bone cells or osteocytes are present in many of the lacunae and provide the maintenance and viability of the bone (see Fig. 12.9).

Supporting Cancellous Bone

The cancellous or spongy bone supporting the alveolar bone proper of the alveolar process is composed generally of heavy trabeculae or plates of bone with bone marrow spaces between them. Bone marrow contains blood-forming elements, osteogenic cells, and adipose tissues (see Fig. 12.7). The supporting bone of the maxilla in particular is filled with marrow tissue, which contains immature red blood cells and leukocytes, especially in the molar region posterior to the maxillary sinus. Bone marrow, found in bones throughout the body, is one of the largest organs in the body and represents approximately 4.5% of body weight.

CEMENTAL SUPPORT

Cementum functions as a support by attaching to perforating fibers of the periodontal ligament at the root surface. The surface of cementum functions like bundle bone because the perforating fibers cover the entire surface of the roots (see Fig. 12.5). Some areas of the cementum are inactive, with the absence of fiber bundles, or they undergo surface resorption (Fig. 12.10). The collagen fiber bundles of cementum are smaller in diameter but more numerous than the bundles of alveolar bone proper (see Fig. 12.5). The principal fiber bundle system of the

> ### BOX 12.2 Rationale for Periodontal Regeneration Therapy
>
> Regeneration of tooth support is the primary goal in periodontal therapy. Recently, proteins, including growth factors such as platelet-derived growth factor and enamel matrix proteins, are playing a role in periodontal therapeutics. Bacterial products released when periodontal disease is active can cause destruction of the alveolar bone, periodontal ligament, and cementum. When the bacterial infection is eliminated by the periodontist, regeneration can begin. Several problems exist at this time, including that different tissues regenerate at different rates, sometimes forming a periodontal pocket instead of allowing attachment to the enamel surface. To alleviate this problem, the periodontist can insert a biologic membrane that will prevent the downward growth of the epithelial attachment and allow the slower-growing alveolar bone, cementum, and periodontal ligament enough time to regenerate. Various growth factors and/or drugs can be impregnated in the membrane to facilitate growth and reattachment of the bone, periodontal ligament, and cementum.

periodontal ligament is balanced in function, although distributed differently on the two surfaces.

Characteristic of the two surfaces, bone and cementum, is their ability to resorb and later to rebuild hard tissue. Cementum is more resistant to resorption than bone, hence the ability to move teeth through bone without the loss of the tooth surface. Some investigators believe that the reduced ability of cementum to remodel due to the absence of a nerve and blood supply in cementum, unlike bone, is important to this resistance. The distribution of penetrating fibers over the surface of the cementum could also relate to resorption. Cementum will resorb, as will dentin, in cases of stress caused by traumatic occlusion or of tooth movement resulting from drift or orthodontic treatment (Box 12.2). This process of normal physiologic root and cemental resorption is one of the sequelae of primary tooth shedding during permanent tooth eruption.

TOOTH MOVEMENT

Physiologic Movement

The eruptive process involves major remodeling of the alveolar process to compensate for root growth and changes in positional relations of the primary and permanent teeth. Repositioning of teeth occurs, for example, during facial growth. Movement occurs in facial and buccal directions as the arches increase in dimension (Fig. 12.11). The height of the alveolus changes in relation to root growth as part of the facial growth process. Accommodation is made for increased dimension of the permanent teeth. In one situation, a **leeway space** (Fig. 12.12) is created in the arches by the replacement of larger primary molars by smaller permanent premolars. This important situation helps compensate for the **incisor liability factor**, which is the replacement of the smaller primary incisors with larger permanent ones (Fig. 12.13). Part of this increase is compensated by the inclination of the permanent incisors (see Fig. 12.13B). Also important is **mesial drift**, a significant occurrence during the mixed dentition period. When the teeth are clenched during normal masticatory function, an anterior force is exerted on the teeth; most cusps are inclined anteriorly, and their occlusal inclined planes therefore produce an anterior force. This is in part the result of proximal wear. Summation of these forces

defines the principle of mesial drift of the teeth. The alveolar process compensates for tooth-related factors, such as increased arch size, as well as effects of occlusal function. The effect of tooth loss or hypereruption is mesial drift, which can result in disruption of normal occlusal function.

CONSIDER THE PATIENT
A patient asks what would occur if cementum were more easily resorbed than alveolar bone.

CLINICAL COMMENT
The rate of mesial drift varies from 0.05 to 0.7 mm per year. This may be related to dietary factors and age.

Orthodontic Movement

Tooth movement by orthodontics is possible only if bone resorption takes place in the direction in which the tooth is being moved. Such movement causes pressure on the surface of the alveolar bone in the direction of tooth movement. Tooth movement also causes tension on the periodontal ligament on the opposite surface of the root. These stresses cause activation of cells and changes in the vascular and neural tissue along the bone and cemental surfaces that are mediated through the periodontal ligament (Fig. 12.14). The alveolar bone and cementum show remarkable ability to be modified. As bone resorption occurs on one surface of the lamina dura (or bone lining the socket), the tooth is allowed to move in that direction, and bone consequently forms on the opposite side of the socket. This stabilizes the tooth in a new position.

For example, if a tooth is tipped, as in Fig. 12.15A, several areas of the periodontium are compressed, and several exhibit tension. The **tipping movement** is necessary to accomplish the change in occlusion desired. Pressure applied on a specific point on the tooth causes compression in a limited area between the

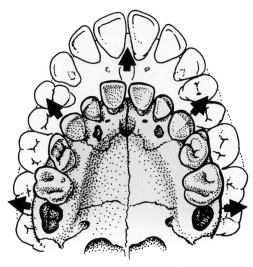

Fig. 12.11 Growth of the face results in migration of teeth laterally and anteriorly. This accompanies an increasing dimension of arch posteriorly as permanent molars develop and erupt.

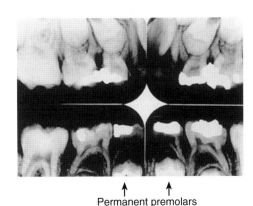

Permanent premolars

Fig. 12.12 Radiograph of permanent premolars replacing primary molars. A smaller premolar produces a leeway space in the arch.

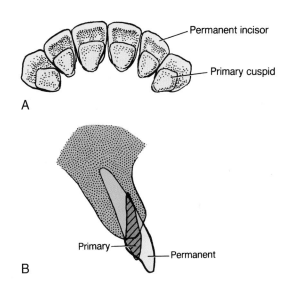

Permanent incisor

Primary cuspid

A

Primary

Permanent

B

Fig. 12.13 A, Comparison of interdental spacing of primary and permanent incisor teeth. **B,** Inclination comparison of anterior primary and permanent teeth.

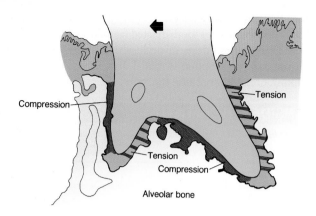

Fig. 12.14 Tooth movement to left with zones of compression along the advancing root surface and tension along the trailing root surface.

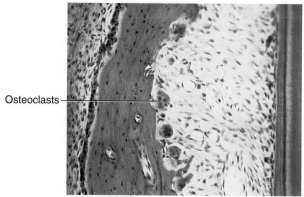

Fig. 12.16 Histology of compression zone of the periodontal ligament. Osteoclasts remove bone to relieve compression.

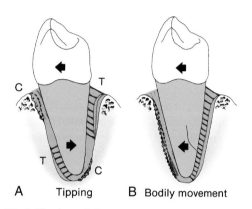

Fig. 12.15 A, Tipping of the tooth crown to the left causes the root to compress the ligament at the upper left and lower right. Tension then occurs at upper right and lower left *(T)*. **B,** Bodily movement of the crown and root to the left causes compression on the ligament *(C)*, bone resorption along the entire surface of the advancing root, and formation of a tension surface of bone and cement on the right.

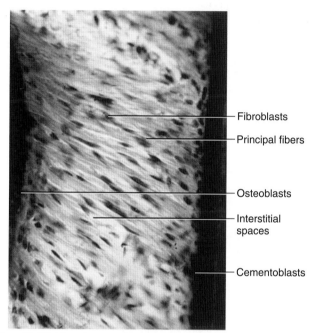

Fig. 12.17 Histology of tension zone of the periodontal ligament. Stretched fibers and a number of osteoblasts and cementoblasts are along the surface of hard tissue.

root and the bone. However, a tooth may need to be moved by **bodily movement**, in which case the root is moved in the same direction, affecting the entire surface of the socket. Compression changes occur in the ligament along the advancing root surface, and tension changes occur in the ligament fibers, bone, and cementum along the opposite surface (see Fig. 12.15B). The situation is the same whether a single-rooted tooth or a multiple-rooted tooth is involved. In the multiple-rooted tooth, movement is complicated by the bifurcation bone, which has the additional bony surface related to pressure and tension (see Fig. 12.4).

When compression is too great or too rapid, it causes **hyalinization** of the ligament. The vascularity is compromised, and the ligament appears colorless or "hyalinized." Tooth movement is limited by the rate of resorption, meaning that cells that respond to the needs of compression and tension must be mobilized. On the compression surface, bone removal is requisite, so the osteoclasts must become organized. These cells originate from monocytes in the bloodstream. The osteoclasts organize rapidly, appearing within a few hours after tooth movement begins (Fig. 12.16).

Bone loss may occur on the bony surface of the socket, the cementum of the root surface, or both. This action may be reversed by deposition of bone or cementum in the area of resorption. The process of deposition in a resorption zone is known as an **area of reversal**. The area where deposition begins, in this site, is termed a **reversal line**.

On the tension side of the root, collagen fibers appear stretched, and the cells become oriented in the direction of the tension (Fig. 12.17). As this occurs, the force of tension is transmitted into a biologic force characterized by the appearance of cells that are responsive to these needs. Fibroblasts, osteoclasts, and cementoblasts arise from the undifferentiated mesenchymal cells (stem cells) in this area and begin to function. Many fibroblasts are present that function in collagen renewal. Osteoblasts, in turn, synthesize bone proteins necessary for producing osteoid. These osteoblasts also mineralize the bone matrix and moderate the inflammatory response induced by the stretching or compression of the periodontal ligament fibers. As tension continues, bone develops along the alveolar bone and cemental surfaces around the stretched perforating fibers (Fig. 12.18).

Other types of tooth movement include **rotation** and a combination of tipping and rotation. In addition, **intrusion** or **extrusion** of a tooth may be necessary. Fig. 12.19 illustrates a case of tooth movement over the long term. Fingerlike projections of bone follow the path of tooth movement. This bone growth is a result of tension. The principles of compression and tension are similar in all cases. The plasticity of the alveolar process is remarkable.

CLINICAL COMMENTS

Patients may be concerned about tooth mobility, even when it is within normal limits. The mobility of individual teeth varies. Teeth are slightly more mobile in the morning than later in the day.

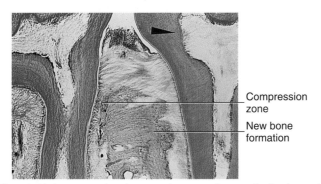

Compression zone

New bone formation

Fig. 12.18 Interproximal zone of two molar teeth. Both teeth moving to the right *(arrowhead)* cause compression of the ligament on the left and tension on the right. Bone formation appears along the alveolar bone on the right as a result.

AGING OF ALVEOLAR BONE AND CEMENTUM

A comparison of young and old alveolar bone reveals a shift with age from dense bone and smooth-walled sockets to osteoporotic bone and sockets with rough, jagged walls. Aging brings bone loss, with fewer fiber bundles inserted in the bone and cementum. Hard tissue then forms around the fibers in support of these bundles, thus creating a scalloped surface (Fig. 12.20). During aging, fewer viable cells are in the lacunae, and the marrow spaces become infiltrated with fat cells. Osteoporosis then becomes more apparent, and the support of the teeth is further diminished.

CLINICAL COMMENT

As in development, the interactions between the tooth and its supporting tissues are critical and ongoing throughout life. Loss of the teeth results in loss of the surrounding tissues, including the alveolar process.

EDENTULOUS JAWS

Several facts are known about the loss of teeth, although much remains to be learned about changes in the bony alveolar process after tooth loss. First, it is recognized that alveolar bone volume decreases. This is evident from the general loss of the alveolar process with tooth extraction. Next, some loss of the internal structure of the bone occurs, resulting in open spaces and fewer trabeculae in the cancellous supporting bone (Fig. 12.21). Osteoporosis may then become more evident. Little change occurs in the location of blood vessels, nerves, glands, and fatty zone in the aging edentulous jaws or in dense compact bone of the mandible beneath the alveolar bone (see Fig. 12.21).

Zones of tension and bone formation

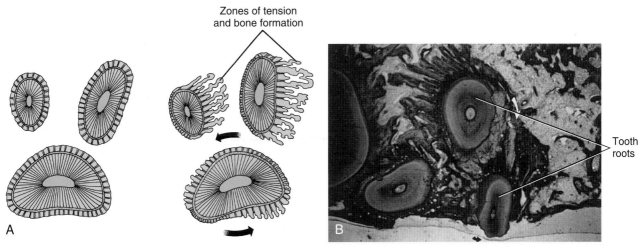

Tooth roots

Fig. 12.19 Rotation of a maxillary molar. A, The large lower root moves less than the two upper roots. Bone forms along trailing root surfaces, and resorption occurs on the advancing bony surface. **B,** Histology of rotation of a maxillary molar illustrating loss of bone along the advancing surfaces and bone formation along the tension (trailing) surfaces. In addition to rotation, the tooth is moving away from the zone of tension.

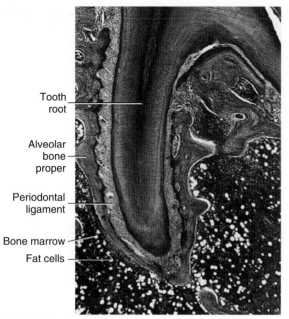

Tooth root

Alveolar bone proper

Periodontal ligament

Bone marrow

Fat cells

Fig. 12.20 Histology of aging alveolar bone, illustrating scalloping of alveolar bone proper and infiltration of fat cells in marrow spaces.

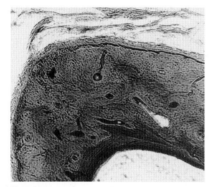

Fig. 12.21 Histology of an edentulous ridge after loss of tooth-bearing alveolar bone. The compact bone of the mandible is dense. This bone shows little evidence of osteoporosis.

CLINICAL COMMENT

Tooth movement can be monitored through radiographic examination, and changes in the interproximal bone density or dimension can also be evaluated. The orthodontist depends on this type of information to follow bone formation and resorption. Radiographs of the hard tissues are also useful in evaluating aging changes. Recognizing changes in the color of the gingival and alveolar mucosa is another valuable index of tissue health.

▌ SELF-EVALUATION QUESTIONS

1. The cortical plates are described as what type of bone?
2. What is the origin of osteoclasts and osteoblasts, and how rapidly can they be mobilized?
3. Define *mesial drift* and describe some consequences of its occurrence.
4. What is a reversal line and how is it evidenced?
5. Describe an aging periodontium and list the features seen.
6. Describe the difference in tipping and bodily movement.
7. Supporting bone comprises what parts of the mandible?
8. Describe the cells that function in compression and tension.
9. What is the life span of the alveolar bone?
10. In what manner do masticatory stress forces placed on bundle bone differ from those placed on Haversian bone?

CONSIDER THE PATIENT

Tooth movement, such as mesial drift or orthodontic treatment, could not occur. With tooth movement, cemental and root loss would occur.

QUANDARIES IN SCIENCE

The alveolar bone proper osteoblasts, periodontal fibroblasts, and cementoblasts are all derived from the dental follicle. Stem cells remain in the periodontium after maturation and functional occlusion. When needed, stem cells can be recruited to differentiate into the three cell types: osteoblasts, fibroblasts, and cementoblasts. Orthodontists can use differences in the remodeling of the periodontal structures to effectively move and align teeth for proper function. The periodontium remodels the quickest, followed by the alveolar bone proper, and finally the cementum. Because orthodontists understand the mechanics of bone remodeling and tooth movement, rarely are there problems. However, negative events can occur in the case of an undiagnosed disease such as diabetes or an unknown etiology that can result in tooth loss. When dental scientists can better understand how the alveolar bone proper, periodontium, and cementum interact, we will be able to maintain alveolar bone after tooth loss, thus allowing more clinical options for restorative treatments, including implant placement.

SUGGESTED READING

Bosshardt DD, Schroeder HE. Cementogenesis reviewed: a comparison between human premolars and rodent molars. *Anat Rec.* 1996;245(2):267–292.

Bosshardt DD, Schroeder HE. How repair cementum becomes attached to the resorbed roots of human permanent teeth. *Acta Anat (Basel).* 1994;150(4):253–266.

Grzesik WJ, Narayanan AS. Cementum and periodontal wound healing and regeneration. *Crit Rev Oral Biol Med.* 2002;13(6):474–484.

Indumathy P, Sai Prashanth P. Brief insight into the homeostasis of the periodontal ligament. *Indian J Dent Adv.* 2012;4(4):969–976.

Irie K, Ozawa H. Relationships between tooth eruption, occlusion and alveolar bone resorption: cytological and cytochemical studies of bone resorption on rat incisor alveolar bone facing the enamel. *Arch Histol Cytol.* 1990;53(5):497–509.

Pagni G, Pellegrini G, Giannobile WV, et al. Postextraction alveolar ridge preservation: biological basis and treatments. *Int J Dent.* 2012;2012:151030.

Rainsford KD. Fifty years since the discovery of ibuprofen. *Inflammopharmacol.* 2011;19:293–297. https://doi.org/10.1007/s10787-011-0103-7.

Ripamonti U, Heliotis M, Rueger DC, et al. Induction of cementogenesis by recombinant human osteogenic protein-1 (hop-1/bmp-7) in the baboon (Papio ursinus). *Arch Oral Biol.* 1996;41(1):121–126.

Roberts WE, Hartsfield Jr JK. Bone development and function: genetic and environmental mechanisms. *Semin Orthod.* 2004;10(2):100–122.

Schroeder HE. *Oral structure biology.* New York: Thieme Medical; 1991.

Seo BM, Miura M, Gronthos S, et al. Investigation of multipotent postnatal stem cells from human periodontal ligament. *Lancet.* 2004;364(9429):149–155.

Wikesjö UM, Lim WH, Thomson RC, et al. Periodontal repair in dogs: gingival tissue occlusion, a critical requirement for GTR? *J Clin Periodontol.* 2003;30(7):655–664.

Wikesjö UM, Sorensen RG, Kinoshita A, et al. Periodontal repair in dogs: effect of recombinant human bone morphogenic protein-12 (rhBMP-12) on regeneration of alveolar bone and periodontal attachment. *J Clin Periodontol.* 2004;31(8):662–670.

Temporomandibular Joint

OVERVIEW

This chapter discusses the articulation between the condyles of the mandible and temporomandibular fossa of the temporal bone. The temporomandibular joint (TMJ) allows the mandibular condyles to move in both gliding and hinge actions. Therefore instead of being a stationary hinge, the joint slides along the inclined plane while functioning also as a hinge joint. The complex motion of the joint can be observed during mastication. TMJ problems can be associated with pain in the related muscles of the jaws and neck.

The anatomy, histology, and function of the various structures related to jaw function are described in this chapter. The TMJ includes (1) the right and left condylar heads of the mandible, (2) the articulating surfaces of the mandibular condyles and the temporal fossae, (3) a disk that intervenes between the fossa and condyle, and (4) a capsule and supportive ligaments. The capsule enclosing this joint serves as a stabilizer, making complex function possible (Fig. 13.1).

The fibrous articular disk divides the joint in two. The upper half is involved in sliding action, and the lower functions as a hinge action. The joint is supported anteriorly by a tendinous attachment of the capsule and the lateral pterygoid muscle, laterally by the lateral or temporomandibular ligament, medially by the sphenomandibular ligament, and posteriorly by the stylomandibular ligament. The TMJ functions as a **ginglymoarthrodial** joint, indicating that it moves as a sliding and hinge joint.

Myofascial pain dysfunction (MPD) is a syndrome that has received recent attention. It has been defined as a complex problem relating to neuromuscular concepts, occlusal concepts, muscle balance, tooth morphology, and guidance and psychophysiologic factors. Much remains to be learned about the normal and abnormal stomatognathic system.

CLINICAL COMMENT

Because of the complexity of the TMJ, there are many ways to irritate it. Many different diseases can result in temporomandibular dysfunction (TMD), including bone and collagen disorders; neuromuscular diseases; and chronic inflammatory diseases such as fibromyalgia, lupus erythematosus, osteoarthritis, and rheumatoid arthritis.

STRUCTURE

Mandibular Condyle

The right and left heads of the mandibular condyles articulate in the temporomandibular or glenoid fossae. At birth, the heads of the condyles are round and covered with a thick layer of cartilage. The cartilage front is uneven, with spikes of cartilage projecting into the underlying marrow space. Bone forms around these spikes so the head of the condyle is porous (Fig. 13.2A). During development, the condyle grows in a lateral direction, changing into an ovoid shape by maturity, which is attained at age 25 years (see Fig. 13.2B). The oval condyle consists of a smooth, bony surface, which is covered with a layer of fibrous connective tissue in the adult. The cartilage serves as a growth site in the condyle.

New cartilage cells arise from the cellular layer of the perichondrium, which covers the condyle. The cartilage cells grow and divide, and the cells deeper in the cartilage die as the cartilage that surrounds these cells calcifies (Fig. 13.3A). The calcified cartilage is then replaced by bone from the underlying ramus (see Fig. 13.3B). This process continues during development with a gradual thinning of the cartilage layer, and, at maturity, the cartilage has been replaced by bone (see Fig. 13.3C).

The heads of the condyles and the heads of the long bones differ in that long bones form secondary ossification centers (Fig. 13.4). Secondary ossification centers produce cartilage–bone junctions termed *epiphyseal lines*, where the lengthening of long bone occurs. No epiphyseal line is formed in the condyles. The heads of the condyles, however, accomplish growth much like that of long bones. Differentiation of new cartilage cells appears first, then cartilage matrix around these cells develops, which is then replaced by bone. Another difference in long bones is that the cartilage cells are organized in long rows as they approach the bony junction, whereas in the condyles, the chondroblasts are scattered. The chondroblasts go through similar changes of cell enlargement, cartilage matrix calcification, and bony replacement (see Fig. 13.4). This ability to modify the shape of the condyles through cartilage–bone remodeling allows adaptation to functional stress.

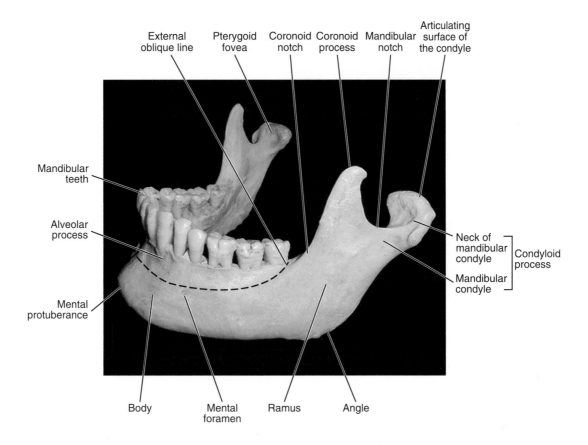

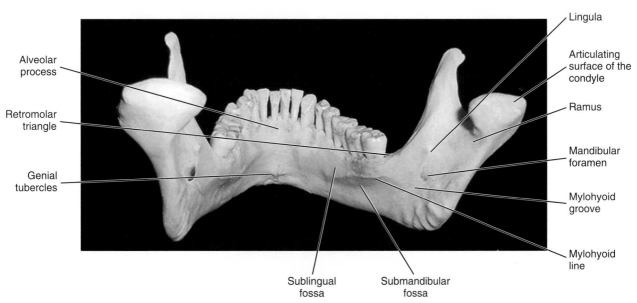

Fig. 13.1 Anatomic landmarks of the mandible. (Fehrenbach M, Popowics T. *Illustrated anatomy of the head and neck.* 4th ed. St. Louis: Saunders; 2016.)

Temporomandibular Fossa

The fossa is composed of an anterior part in the form of an eminence and a posterior part, a depression or cavity on the inferior part of the temporal bone. This fossa is located at the posterior medial aspect of the zygomatic arch (Fig. 13.5). The anterior wall of the fossa is smooth and forms a tubercle in which the condyles slide during articulation. On the posterior wall of the fossa is the petrotympanic fissure, which is the exit for the VII cranial nerve (facial).

The contents of the fissure include communications of cranial nerves VII and IX to the infratemporal fossa. A branch of cranial nerve VII, the chorda tympani, runs through the fissure to join with the lingual nerve providing special sensual (taste) innervation to the anterior two-thirds of the tongue. The tympanic nerve

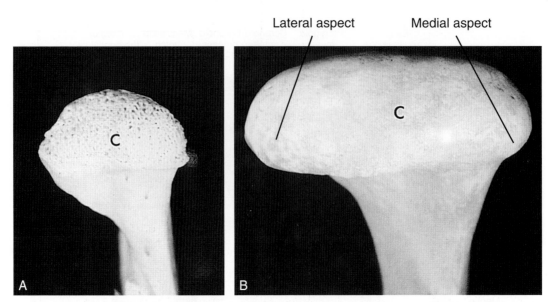

Fig. 13.2 A, Condyle *(C)* of a 6-year-old child. Perforations on surface are created by a cartilage cap, which is missing because of tissue preparation. **B**, In the adult, the smooth bony surface of condyle *(C)* illustrates lateral growth.

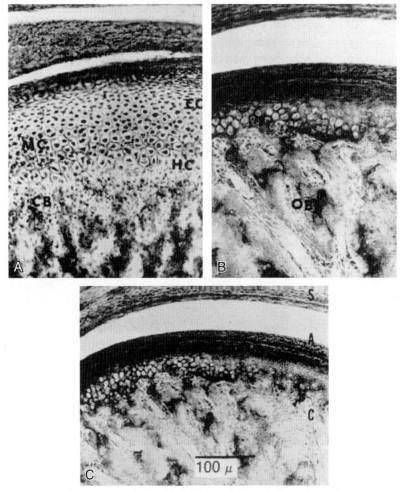

Fig. 13.3 Histology of condylar cartilage. A, The wide band of cartilage that appears during the postnatal period. *EC*, Reserve cartilage zone; *HC*, hypertrophy cartilage zone; *MC*, multiplication cartilage zone. **B**, Cartilage has thinned considerably. *OB*, Bone formation. **C**, Thin cartilage zone underlying the perichondrium in an 18-year-old patient. *S*, Synovial tissue; *A*, articular cartilage; *C*, cartilage.

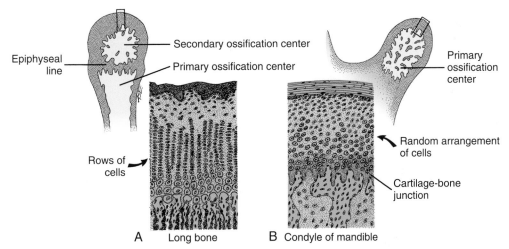

Fig. 13.4 Diagram comparing the head of a long bone and condyle. **A**, Cartilage of a long bone showing straight vertical rows of cartilage cells, young cells to maturing ones, top to bottom. Bone replaces cartilage at the junction of these two tissues. **B**, Random arrangement of cells in a condyle, which accomplishes same result as rows of cells. As in long bone, at the conclusion of this process in the condyle, bone replaces cartilage at the junction shown.

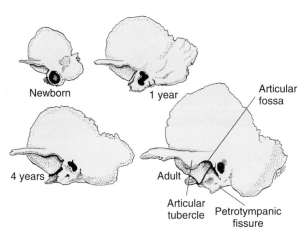

Fig. 13.5 Development of the glenoid (temporomandibular) fossa from birth to maturity. The articular fossa deepens during development to accommodate the growing condylar head as it enlarges laterally.

branches off of cranial nerve IX to pass through the fissure as the lesser petrosal nerve, which passes through the foramen ovale and joins V$_3$ of the trigeminal nerve, synapses in the otic ganglion, and provides parasympathetic innervation to the parotid gland.

This is the junction of the temporal and parietal bones. Some authors report that the origin of elastic fibers, which insert into the posterior part of the disk, is on the posterior wall of this fissure. These elastic fibers may function in retraction of the disk. The temporomandibular fossa is where the condyles are positioned at rest (see Fig. 13.5).

Upper and Lower Compartments

The TMJ cavity is divided into upper and lower compartments by the articular disk (Fig. 13.6). The upper compartment is bound by the articular fossa above and by the disk below. The lateral, medial, and posterior boundaries are enclosed by the capsule that outlines the TMJ. The lower compartment is bound superiorly by the disk and inferiorly by the head of the disk. The two compartments differ in action.

In the upper compartment is a gliding action between the condylar head and the articular eminence, and in the lower compartment is a hinge action between the undersurface of the disk and the rotating surface of the head of the condyle (see Fig. 13.6; Fig. 13.7).

Articular Disk

The articular disk is a dense, collagenous, fibrous pad between the condyle heads and the articular surfaces (see Figs. 13.6 and 13.7). The disk is composed primarily of fibrocartilage with abundant amounts of type I and III collagen. When the jaw opens, each condylar head moves from the articular fossa and slides along the articular plane to the articular eminence while resting on the intervening articular disk (Fig. 13.8A). The head of the condyle rotates during the sliding action (see Fig. 13.8B). This allows the two movements of the TMJ: a smooth, **gliding action** and a **hinge action**. The articular disk is a soft pad of fibrous tissue. It is thin and avascular in its center but thicker and vascular around the margin (Fig. 13.9). The articular disk attaches to the inner wall of the capsule anteriorly and posteriorly but not medially and laterally, which is where it attaches to the head of the condyle. This structural design requires the disk to be immobile when the head of the condyle moves.

The disk is covered with a thin layer of synovial fluid produced by synovial cells, which are positioned at the periphery of the disk and are not on the articulating surface. The structure that produces the synovial fluid is known as a **synovial membrane**. This membrane secretes a synovial fluid that moistens both the upper and lower surfaces of the articular pad and the lining of both compartments (Fig. 13.10). The synovial membrane lining is associated with numerous capillaries and lymphatics along

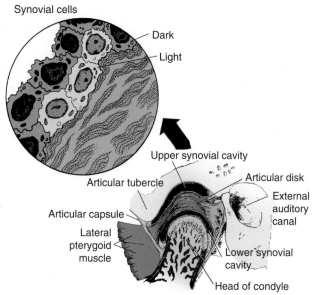

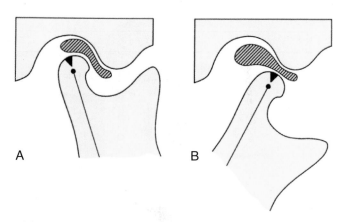

Fig. 13.8 The two actions of the temporomandibular joint. A, Pathway of movement of the condylar head along the slope of the articular eminence. **B,** Rotary movement of the condyle as the mouth is opened. Actions occur simultaneously.

Fig. 13.6 Temporomandibular joint with a thin anterior and thicker posterior articular disk. Observe the position of the capsule anteriorly and posteriorly and the upper and lower synovial compartments in relation to the lateral pterygoid muscle and external auditory canal. The upper and lower compartments that are not under shearing or compressive forces are lined with synovial cells. In the upper diagram are examples of light and dark synovial cells, which function to lubricate movements of condyles.

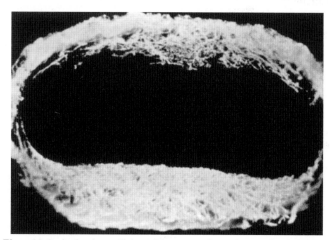

Fig. 13.9 Articular disk with vascular channels injected with latex and surrounding tissue removed. This preparation illustrates that the vascular network is only in the periphery of the disk and not to any extent in the center of the disk. (Avery JK. *Oral development and histology.* 3rd ed. Stuttgart: Thieme Medical; 2002.)

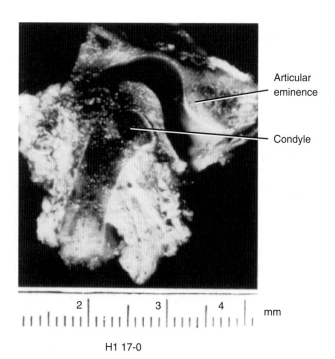

Fig. 13.7 Lateral view of the gross appearance of the temporomandibular joint at 17 years of age. This figure shows the size of the articular fossa and attachment of muscles to the condyle. (Avery JK. *Oral development and histology.* 3rd ed. Stuttgart: Thieme Medical; 2002.)

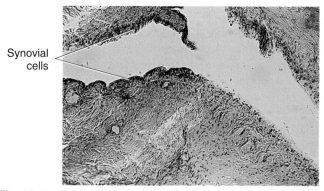

Fig. 13.10 Histology of lateral posterior aspects of the disk illustrating dark-stained synovial cells that line the joint cavity and disk.

the surface of the disk, especially in the periphery. Synovial fluid is a distillate of the blood, having a high viscosity that provides lubrication and allows freedom of condylar movement.

> ### CLINICAL COMMENT
>
> The TMJ is a complex and precisely integrated bilateral joint that functions in speech, mastication, and deglutition. You can perceive the downward and forward sliding action of the condylar heads by placing the fingers on them as you open the jaw. This sliding action can also be felt during symmetric protrusion and retrusion or asymmetric lateral shift.

Synovial tissue is sterile and composed of vascularized connective tissue that lacks a basement membrane. Two cell types (type A and type B) are present. Type A is derived from blood monocytes, and it removes the wear-and-tear debris from the synovial fluid. Type B produces synovial fluid. Synovial fluid is made of hyaluronic acid and lubricin, proteinases, and collagenases.

The disk can perforate in its center, or the center can contain a few cartilage cells and islands of cartilage, especially in older age.

Capsule and Ligaments

A fibrous capsule encloses the TMJ like a cuff. This capsule is composed of an inner lining, or synovial layer, and an outer loose ligamentous layer that is fibrous and tough and supports articulatory movements. The attachment superiorly is to the temporal bone around the limits of the articular eminence and the fossa, and the capsule attaches around the neck of the condyle (Fig. 13.11A). Fibers of the capsule fuse with the fibers of the lateral pterygoid muscle anteriorly; laterally, the capsule is strengthened by the **lateral ligament** or **temporomandibular ligament** (see Fig. 13.11B). Medially, the **sphenomandibular ligament** supports the joint (see Fig. 13.11C). This ligament arises superiorly from the spine of the sphenoid bone and extends downward on the medial side of the ramus to insert on the **lingula**, which is a spine of bone arising from the rim of the mandibular foramen (see Fig. 13.11C). Posteriorly, the **stylomandibular ligament** arises from the styloid process and inserts on the posterior border of the ramus (see Fig. 13.11B and C). The lateral ligament and the capsule work in concert to support the joint and limit excursions of the condyles to the normal range. The other two ligaments, the sphenomandibular and stylomandibular ligaments, also serve as support. Mandibular movements involve interplay of the morphology of the teeth and the action of muscles and ligaments surrounding the TMJ.

Vascular Supply

The blood supply to the TMJ is from four arteries: (1) branches of the **superficial temporal artery**, (2) the **deep auricular artery**, (3) the **anterior tympanic artery**, and (4) the **ascending pharyngeal artery** (Fig. 13.12). All these vessels converge on the joint, penetrate the capsule, and send branches into the network of vessels in the periphery of the disk and the posterior area of the joint. Fig. 13.8 shows that the disk is oval and has more blood vessels in the anterior and posterior areas than the lateral or medial surfaces. Interestingly, the blood vessels do not enter the fibrous covering of the head of the condyle (see Fig. 13.12) as do blood vessels in some other joints.

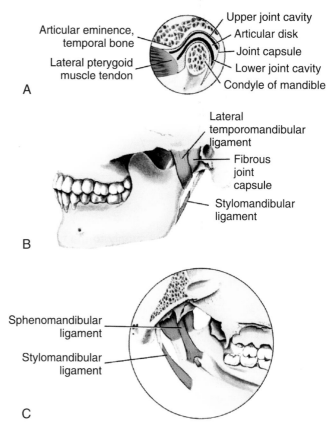

Fig. 13.11 Components of the temporomandibular joint (TMJ). **A,** Relationship of various TMJ compartments and the capsular ligament. **B,** Lateral view of the lateral fibrous joint capsule showing the relationship of the stylomandibular ligament to the mandible. **C,** Medial view illustrating the location and attachment of the sphenomandibular ligament of the TMJ.

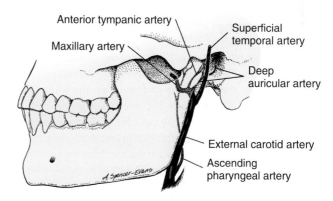

Fig. 13.12 Vascular supply of the temporomandibular joint (TMJ). The external carotid artery serves the TMJ through branches of the ascending pharyngeal and superficial temporal arteries. From the maxillary artery come the auricular and anterior tympanic arteries, which also supply the joint.

Innervation

The nerve supply to the TMJ arises from the branches of the mandibular division of the trigeminal nerve, specifically the **auriculotemporal, masseteric,** and **deep temporal** branches (Fig. 13.13). These are the same nerves supplying the muscles

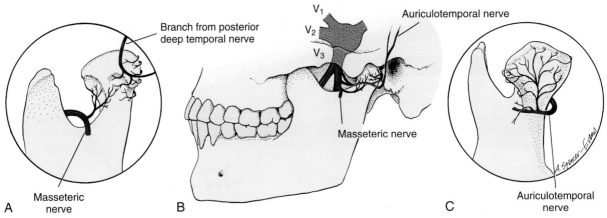

Fig. 13.13 Nerve supply to the temporomandibular joint (TMJ). Mandibular division of the fifth nerve supplies all surfaces of the TMJ through the auricular, temporal, masseteric, and deep temporal nerve branches. **A,** Anterolateral view. **B,** Lateral view. V_1, Ophthalmic branch; V_2, maxillary branch; V_3, mandibular branch. **C,** Posterior view.

of mastication that function with this joint movement, and they help to ensure coordination of function of the muscles and joint. Both large myelinated and smaller nonmyelinated nerves enter the capsule and disk, and they supply all surfaces of the condylar head, fossa, disk, and capsule (see Fig. 13.13). Pain, temperature, touch, deep pressure, and proprioceptive nerve terminals are found within the joint. Elaborate encapsulated terminals have been found in the connective tissue associated with the synovial folds and in the disk. Fig. 13.14 shows four types of nerve terminals located in the TMJ.

Muscles of Mastication

The eight powerful muscles of mastication include four on each side of the jaw. Each muscle has a different location, and therefore the direction of fiber contraction results in a different functional relationship. Three of the muscles on each side—the medial pterygoid, the masseter, and the temporalis—exert vertical forces in closing the jaw, whereas the lateral pterygoid muscles protract the mandible and stabilize the joint. These muscles do not function alone but work as a group with the suprahyoid muscles and tongue muscles. Free movements of the mandible relate to the interplay of masticatory muscles and the morphology of the teeth, whereas masticatory movement is the synergistic action of the three groups of muscles—the elevators, depressors, and protractors—that function together and at different times during mastication of food.

Following are more details about the muscles of mastication:

1. The **medial pterygoid** arises from the medial surface of the lateral pterygoid plate and inserts on the inferior surface of the ramus and on the angle of the mandible. The blood supply is from the maxillary artery, and the nerve supply is from the mandibular division of the trigeminal nerve. This muscle protracts and elevates the mandible (Figs. 13.15 and 13.16).

2. The **lateral pterygoid** has two heads, the upper arising from the greater wing of the sphenoid and the lower from the pterygoid plate. They insert into the front of the neck of the condyle and the capsule. The blood supply is from the maxillary

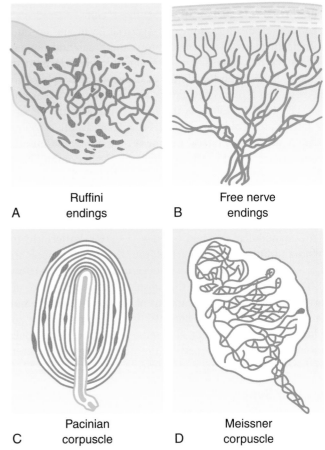

Fig. 13.14 Types of nerve endings in the temporomandibular joint. The four types are **(A)** Ruffini or temperature endings; **(B)** free nerve endings, which are pain endings; (C) the pacinian, which is a deep pressure receptor; and **(D)** Meissner corpuscles, which are touch receptors. These are representative of the variety of mechanoreceptors found in capsule, disk, and soft tissues of the joint that are also involved in proprioception. (Hall JE. *Guyton and Hall textbook of medical physiology.* 12th ed. St. Louis: Saunders; 2011.)

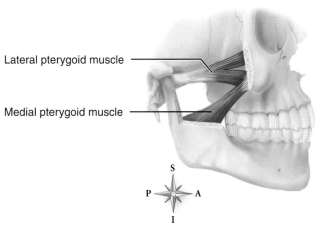

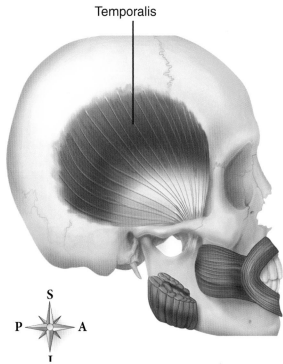

Temporalis

Fig. 13.17 Temporalis muscle of mastication. The temporalis muscle functions in elevation of the jaw, retraction of the mandible, clenching of the teeth, and side-to-side movements of the jaw. (Patton KT, Thibodeau GA. *Anatomy and physiology.* 9th ed. St. Louis: Mosby; 2016.)

Fig. 13.15 Lateral view of the medial pterygoid muscle of mastication. The medial pterygoid functions in elevation and protraction of the condyle. This muscle functions in concert with the masseteric muscle, forming a sling. (Patton KT, Thibodeau GA. *Anatomy and physiology.* 9th ed. St. Louis: Mosby; 2016.)

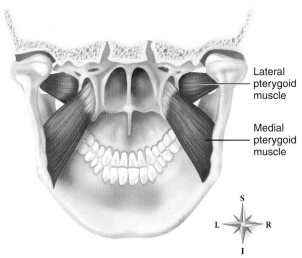

Lateral pterygoid muscle

Medial pterygoid muscle

Fig. 13.16 Inferior view of the medial and lateral pterygoids to illustrate attachments to the mandible and base of the skull. The medial pterygoid arises from the lateral pterygoid plate and inserts in the inferior angle of the mandible. The lateral pterygoid arises from the greater wing of the sphenoid and the lower head from the lateral pterygoid plate. These muscles insert in the neck of condyle and capsule. (Patton KT, Thibodeau GA. *Anatomy and physiology.* 9th ed. St. Louis: Mosby; 2016.)

artery, and the nerve supply is from the pterygoid branch of the mandibular nerve. Both heads of this muscle protrude the mandible and pull the articular disk forward (see Figs. 13.15 and 13.16). This muscle is sometimes referred to as the sphenomeniscus muscle because the superior head inserts into the articular disk.

3. The **temporalis** muscle fibers originate from the floor of the temporal fossa and temporal fascia. These muscle fibers insert on the anterior border of the coronoid process and anterior border of the ramus of the mandible (Fig. 13.17). The blood supply is from the superficial temporal and maxillary arteries,

and the nerve supply is from the deep temporal branches of the mandibular nerve. The temporalis muscle elevates and retracts the mandible and clenches the teeth.

4. The **masseter** muscle has a deep and superficial part. The superficial fibers originate from the anterior two-thirds of the lower border of the zygomatic arch, and the deep fibers originate from the medial surface of the same arch. The superficial fibers are at right angles to the occlusal plane of the posterior teeth, and the deep fibers are directed downward and slightly anteriorly. This muscle inserts into the lateral surface of the coronoid process of the mandible, the upper half of the ramus, and the angle of the mandible. The blood supply is from the superficial temporal and the maxillary arteries, and the nerve supply comes from the mandibular division of the trigeminal nerve. The masseter muscle elevates the jaw and clenches the teeth (Fig. 13.18).

CLINICAL COMMENT

A functional relationship of the occlusion of the teeth is expressed through the muscles of mastication. A detailed history and physical examination help the clinician provide an accurate diagnosis. Clinicians must rely on their own judgment in the treatment of patients with TMJ pain.

CONSIDER THE PATIENT

A patient is experiencing severe TMJ discomfort. What treatment is needed? What methods of pain alleviation could be employed during treatment?

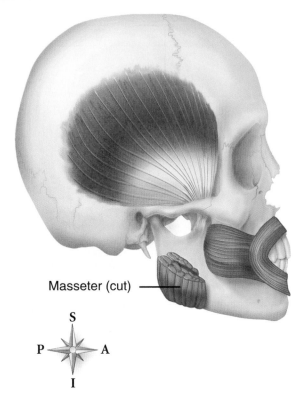

Masseter (cut)

S
P ⎯✦⎯ A
I

Fig. 13.18 Masseter muscle of mastication. The functions of the masseter muscle are to elevate the jaw, clench the teeth, and assist in side-to-side movement of the jaw. (Patton KT, Thibodeau GA. *Anatomy and physiology.* 9th ed. St. Louis: Mosby; 2016.)

REMODELING OF TEMPOROMANDIBULAR JOINT ARTICULATION

Articular remodeling is the morphologic adaptation of the joint in response to environmental stress. The articular surfaces of the TMJ have been shown to adapt to minimize the effects of stressful mandibular function. Presence of cartilage on the condyle and the fossa allows the TMJ to withstand stress better than other fibrous joints. Progressive remodeling occurs with proliferation of the articular cartilage and production of intercellular matrix, followed by its mineralization. The cartilage is then resorbed as it is replaced by bone (Fig. 13.19). This may happen in one or both of the condylar heads and articular eminences and may relate to any changes in structure of the articular surfaces. In some cases, remodeling may begin in the proliferative zone, causing an increase of cartilage on the surface, which may then become mineralized and be replaced by bone at the zone of resorption. Functional adaptation is the response of chondrogenesis and osteogenesis to withstand the effects of mastication resulting from compression. In aging, with decreased proliferation, these changes may be degenerative.

CLINICAL COMMENT

MPD continues to be an area of concern because of varying opinions about treatment. Because much remains to be learned about both the normal and abnormal functions of the TMJ, more progress in the treatment of MPD is expected.

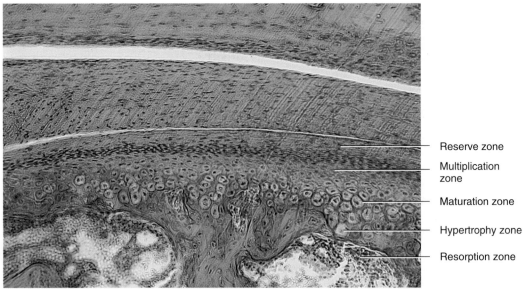

Reserve zone

Multiplication zone

Maturation zone

Hypertrophy zone

Resorption zone

Fig. 13.19 Histologic view of the head of the condyle and the overlying articular disk. The head of the condyle exhibits a perichondrium and zones of cartilage formation and resorption. The reserve cartilage cell zone overlies the multiplication zone, zone of cartilage cell hypertrophy, and zones of cartilage resorption and bone replacement. (Avery JK. *Oral development and histology.* 3rd ed. Stuttgart: Thieme Medical; 2002.)

CONSIDER THE PATIENT

Several approaches exist, but occlusal adjustment is usually the treatment of choice because of the prevalence of malocclusion. The administration of a mandibular anesthetic could help alleviate the pain. During this injection, the needle pathway is through the mucosa and the buccinator muscle and lateral to the medial pterygoid muscle, and the anesthetic is deposited near the mandibular foramen.

QUANDARIES IN SCIENCE

When functioning properly, the TMJ, the muscles of mastication, and the nerves innervating these structures are exquisitely sensitive; however, when changes occur in any one of these structures, TMD can occur. Patients with TMD are in chronic pain and have a poor quality of life. Because of the multifactorial nature of TMD and because there is usually more than one tissue or structure involved, diagnosis and treatment can be difficult. Often, there is a psychological component that further complicates the treatment and requires another team member. Treatment can be expensive, prolonged, and equivocal. There are, however, TMDs that have an organic component (e.g., osteoarthritis) and therefore have straightforward treatments.

SELF-EVALUATION QUESTIONS

1. Name the three supporting ligaments of the TMJ.
2. What is the role of the TMJ capsule?
3. Describe the two different functions of the upper and lower compartments of the TMJ.
4. How do the heads of the condyles change as a person grows and matures?
5. What are the functions of the two heads of the lateral pterygoid muscle?
6. What is the significance of the sling muscles? Is this a function of the muscles' location and innervation?
7. What are the location and function of the temporalis muscle?
8. What is the significance of the TMJ and the masticatory muscles having the same innervation?
9. What are the major blood vessels supplying the TMJ?
10. What is the function of the synovial cells?

CLINICAL CASE

A 20-year-old female student complains to the dentist that each morning after waking, she is experiencing pain in the muscles of mastication, and her TMJ is bilaterally painful. After a medical history and intra- and extraoral examination, the dentist suggests fabricating a bite splint because the stress the student is experiencing in her program of study is resulting in bruxism during her sleep and causing pain in her muscles, TMJ, and teeth. Some of the occlusal surfaces of her teeth are demonstrating wear facets, which are changing her functional occlusion and causing TMD.

The TMJ, periodontal ligament, and the muscles of mastication are exquisitely innervated by sensory and motor nerves and are under very fine neural control for proprioception, bite force, and muscular activity. Slight changes in occlusal forces or eccentric occlusion can cause asymmetric behavior in muscles and TMJ and lead to functional changes over time. Unilateral changes in occlusion can cause changes in contralateral occlusion, resulting in unusual wear and pain. Proper diagnosis from an experienced clinician knowledgeable in TMD can benefit the patient. Modern therapy often includes an interprofessional team including psychologists, neurologists, physicians, dentists, and others to treat this multifactorial disorder. In the case of this student, without any compounding factors, the bite splint and follow-up visits to her clinician should suffice and alleviate her pain.

SUGGESTED READING

Bravetti P, Membre H, El Haddioui A, et al. Histological study of the human temporomandibular joint and its surrounding muscles. *Surg Radiol Anat.* 2004;26(5):371–378.

Dimitroulis G. The role of surgery in the management of disorders of the temporomandibular joint: a critical review of the literature, part 2. *Int J Oral Maxillofac Surg.* 2005;34(3):231–237.

Hinton RJ, Jing J, Feng JQ. Genetic influences on temporomandibular joint development and growth. *Curr Top Dev Biol.* 2015;115:85–109. https://doi.org/10.1016/bs.ctdb.2015.07.008.

Honda K, Kawashima S, Kashima M, et al. Relationship between sex, age, and the minimum thickness of the roof of the glenoid fossa in normal temporomandibular joints. *Clin Anat.* 2005;18(1):23–26.

Kiga N. Histochemistry for studying structure and function of the articular disc of the human temporomandibular joint. *Eur J Histochem.* 2012;56(1):e11.

Kubein-Meesenburg D, Nägerl H, Schwestka-Polly R, et al. Functional conditions of the mandible: theory and physiology. *Ann Anat.* 1999;181(1):27–32.

La Touche R, Goddard G, De-la-Hoz JL, et al. Acupuncture in the treatment of pain in temporomandibular disorders: a systematic review and meta-analysis of randomized controlled trials. *Clin J Pain.* 2010;26(6):541–550.

Marbach JJ. Temporomandibular pain and dysfunction syndrome. History, physical examination, and treatment. *Rheum Dis Clin North Am.* 1996;22(3):477–498.

Mujakperuo HR, Watson M, Morrison R, et al. Pharmacological interventions for pain in patients with temporomandibular disorders. *Cochrane Database Syst Rev.* 2010;10:CD004715.

Nitzan DW, Kreiner B, Zeltser R. TMJ lubrication system: its effect on the joint function, dysfunction, and treatment approach. *Compend Contin Educ Dent.* 2004;25(6):437–471.

Nozawa-Inoue K, Amizuka N, Ikeda N, et al. Synovial membrane in the temporomandibular joint: its morphology, function, and development. *Arch Histol Cytol.* 2003;66(4):289–306.

Touré G, Duboucher C, Vacher C. Anatomical modifications of the temporomandibular joint during ageing. *Surg Radiol Anat.* 2005;27(1):51–55.

14

Oral Mucosa

LEARNING OBJECTIVES

- Describe the various types of oral mucosa, including lining, masticatory, and specialized.
- Describe the location and characteristics of each type of mucosa as well as the characteristics of nonkeratinocytes.
- Explain the various changes in oral mucosa that occur with aging.

OVERVIEW

The structure of stratified squamous epithelium of the oral mucosa includes both the nonkeratinized lining mucosa of the cheeks, lips, soft palate, and floor of the mouth, and the keratinized epithelium covering the palate and alveolar ridges. Masticatory mucosa consists of multiple layers of epithelial cells associated with the lamina propria, which contains blood vessels, nerve endings, and serous, mucous, or mixed glands. A third type of mucosa found on the surface of the tongue is specialized mucosa, consisting of four types of papillae, which are filiform, fungiform, foliate, and circumvallate.

Taste is associated with the latter three types of papillae, which are located on the tongue, soft palate, and pharynx. Traditionally, four types of taste are regionally associated with the tongue; however, a fifth taste modality, *umami*, is now accepted. Traditionally, sweet and salty tastes are perceived at the tip; sour taste is associated with the sides of the tongue; and bitter taste is at the back of the tongue. The tongue map is a traditional overview and is useful for determining broad regions of the tongue that are more sensitive to a specific taste modality. It is useful for a general understanding and not for specifics.

Masticatory mucosa includes the gingiva, which is composed of the tissue surrounding the cervicals (necks) of the teeth. The gingiva consists of three areas, which are free, attached, and interdental. The free gingiva is characterized by the gingival sulcus. The attached gingiva has junctional epithelium, which binds the gingiva to the cervicals of the teeth. The interdental area is the tissue between the teeth below their contact point. The hard palate is covered by masticatory mucosa, which is firmly attached to the underlying bone.

Cells of the oral mucosa, epithelial components, are termed *keratinocytes* and can be distinguished from the nonkeratinocytes, which are Langerhans cells, Merkel cells, and melanocytes. In case of inflammation, lymphocytes and leukocytes may appear in the mucosa. They are commonly found in gingival epithelium.

Four types of nerve receptors, heat, cold, pain, and touch, are located in the lips and oral cavity. They are most numerous in the lips and in the tip of the tongue. With age, the oral mucosa becomes thinner and may be lower on the cervicals of the teeth. Also, it can become less moist because of the decrease in activity of the salivary glands.

STRUCTURE OF ORAL MUCOSA

The oral cavity is lined with stratified squamous epithelium, which is divided into three types of tissue (Fig. 14.1). **Lining mucosa** covers the floor of the mouth and the cheeks, lips, and soft palate. It does not function in mastication and therefore has little attrition. **Masticatory mucosa** covers the hard palate and alveolar ridges and is so named because it comes in primary contact with food during mastication. **Specialized mucosa**, which covers the surface of the tongue, is quite different in structure and appearance from the two previous tissues.

Each type of tissue has structural differences. The lining mucosa is soft, pliable, and nonkeratinized. The masticatory mucosa is keratinized, indicative of the abrasion/attrition that takes place during mastication. Specialized mucosa on the tongue surface is composed largely of keratinized (cornified) epithelial papillae, which function in mastication. The mucosa of the oral cavity has several features common to epithelium elsewhere in the body. One of these features is the lamina propria, the connective tissue layer immediately below the epithelium. It is composed of the papillary layer and deeper reticular layer (Fig. 14.2). In the papillary layer, the connective tissue extends into pockets in the epithelium. This increases the surface of the epithelium for contact with vascular supply and nerves. The reticular layer contains the deeper plexus of vessels and nerves supported by the connective tissue. These two layers, papillary and reticular, contribute the lamina propria or dermis. Beneath this zone is the submucosa or subcutaneous tissue (Box 14.1).

Lining Mucosa

Lining mucosa is composed of a thin layer of epithelium and an underlying lamina propria. The epithelium is composed of a basal layer of cuboidal cells, termed the **stratum basale**. The next cell layer is called the **stratum intermedium** or **stratum spinosum**. The cells in this layer appear oval and somewhat flattened. The third or superficial layer is termed the **stratum superficiale**, and its cells are flattened, with many containing small oval nuclei (see Fig. 14.2). These three cell layers of the epidermis form the nonkeratinized epithelium of the oral mucosa and appear similar to the lining of the pharynx. Another component of the mucosa is the dermis or lamina propria, composed of the papillary and reticular connective tissue layers.

Lips

The inner oral surface of the lips is lined with moist surface, stratified squamous cells, and nonkeratinized epithelium and is associated with small, round seromucous glands of the lamina propria. These glands are part of the minor salivary glands found throughout the oral cavity. Beneath the lamina propria is the submucosa, in which fibers of the orbicularis oris muscle are located (Fig. 14.3). Nonkeratinized mucosa of the lips is distinguished by a red border known as the **vermilion border**. This area is at the junction between the oral mucosa and the skin of the lips, becoming modified into keratinized epithelium, which is different from skin or mucosa. There are three reasons the vermilion border is red: the epithelium is thin; this epithelium contains **eleidin**, which is transparent; and the blood vessels are near the surface of the papillary layer, revealing the red blood cells' color (Fig. 14.4). Also observable in the skin of the lips are hair follicles and their associated sebaceous glands, erector pili muscles, and sweat glands. **Ectopic** sebaceous glands can be seen at the angles of the mouth. They are not associated with hair follicles. These glands are known as **Fordyce spots** (Fig. 14.5).

Soft Palate

Lining mucosa of the highly vascularized soft palate is pinker than the mucosa of the keratinized epithelium of the hard palate

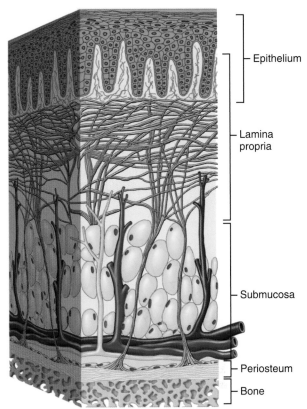

Fig. 14.2 Relationships among oral epidermis, dermis (lamina propria), and submucosal tissue. The names of layers of epidermis and dermis are noted on the right. (Nanci A. *Ten Cate's oral histology.* 9th ed. St. Louis: Saunders; 2018.)

Epithelium

Lamina propria

Submucosa

Periosteum

Bone

BOX 14.1   Some Selected Types of Collagen

Collagen occurs in many places throughout the body. More than 90% of the collagen in the body, however, is of type I.

So far, 28 types of collagen have been identified and described. The five most common types are:

- Collagen I: Skin, tendon, vascular ligature, organs, bone (main component of the organic part of bone)
- Collagen II: Cartilage (main component of cartilage)
- Collagen III: Reticulate (main component of reticular fibers), commonly found alongside type I
- Collagen IV: Forms bases of cell basement membrane
- Collagen V: Cell surfaces, hair, and placenta

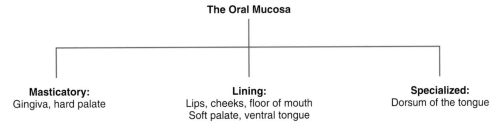

The Oral Mucosa

Masticatory:
Gingiva, hard palate

Lining:
Lips, cheeks, floor of mouth
Soft palate, ventral tongue

Specialized:
Dorsum of the tongue

Fig. 14.1 Structure of the oral mucosa.

(Fig. 14.6). This tissue is pink because the lamina propria contains many small blood vessels. Beneath the connective tissue of the lamina propria is the submucosa, which contains muscles of the soft palate and mucous glands.

Cheeks

The mucosa of the cheeks is like that of the lips or soft palate because each has stratified squamous epithelium that is non-keratinized, lamina propria, and underlying submucosa. In the cheeks, however, the submucosa contains fat cells and mixed glands (seromucous) located within and between the muscle fibers. The presence of these glands and fat cells is a unique feature of the cheeks (Fig. 14.7).

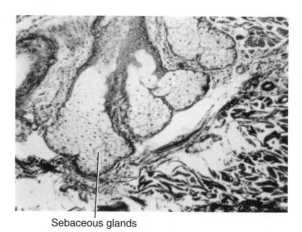

Sebaceous glands

Fig. 14.5 Fordyce spots, sebaceous glands not related to hair follicles, are found at the angles of the mouth.

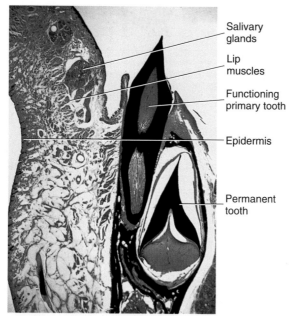

Salivary glands

Lip muscles

Functioning primary tooth

Epidermis

Permanent tooth

Fig. 14.3 Histology of the lip and alveolar bone, which contains functioning primary and developing permanent teeth.

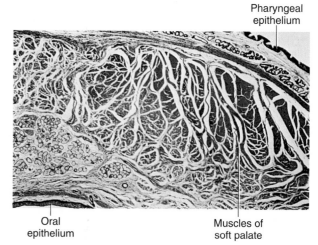

Pharyngeal epithelium

Oral epithelium

Muscles of soft palate

Fig. 14.6 Sagittal plane of the soft palate *(anterior on left)*. The nasal cavity is above, and respiratory epithelium covers the superior part of the soft palate. The oral cavity is below this tissue and is covered with stratified squamous epithelium. Observe the minor glands underlying the oral mucosa and muscle throughout the submucosa.

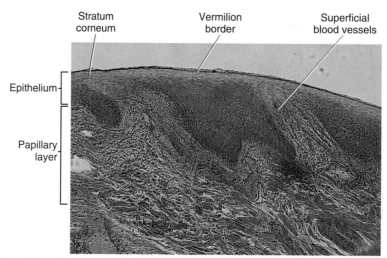

Stratum corneum

Vermilion border

Superficial blood vessels

Epithelium

Papillary layer

Fig. 14.4 Vermilion border of the lip illustrating the thin and lucent stratum corneum and the presence of capillaries in the papillary layer. Observe the close relationship of the blood supply to the surface of vermilion border epithelium.

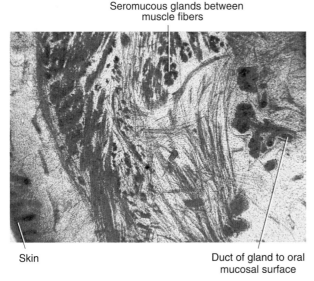

Seromucous glands between muscle fibers

Skin

Duct of gland to oral mucosal surface

Fig. 14.7 Histology of cheek tissues. Skin is on the far left, and oral mucosa on the far right. Observe the glands intermingling with muscle fibers in the subcutaneous zone of the cheek.

Ventral Surface of the Tongue

Lining mucosa also contains a lamina propria and submucosa. In the submucosa, muscle fibers are located under the surface of the tongue. The entire area exhibits dense, interlaced muscle and connective tissue fibers. Limits of the submucosa are not distinct because the submucosa continues with the deep muscles of the tongue along with connective tissue fibers (Fig. 14.8).

CLINICAL COMMENT

The ventral surface of the tongue is an area of well-vascularized lining mucosa of the oral cavity. This area is used for drug delivery in patients who suffer from cardiovascular disease and other systemic diseases.

Floor of the Mouth

Nonkeratinized mucous membrane covers the floor of the mouth and appears loosely attached to the lamina propria. In contrast, the adjacent undersurface of the tongue mucosa is firmly attached. In the floor of the mouth are minor salivary glands (Fig. 14.9) and the right and left major sublingual glands salivary glands, which produce a mostly mucous secretion.

Masticatory Mucosa

Masticatory mucosa is the epithelium covering the gingiva and hard palate. This mucosa is thicker than the nonkeratinized mucosa, with the addition of a keratinized surface of flat, keratinized cells offering resistance to attrition. The basal and intermediate stratum (stratum spinosum) layers are the same as those of nonkeratinized epithelium. The granular layer (**stratum granulosum**) and the surface layer (**stratum corneum**) are the two other layers (Fig. 14.10). The cells of the basal layer are cuboidal or columnar. Their nuclei are irregularly oval and exhibit numerous mitotic figures as they undergo constant cell division. These basal cells gradually migrate to the surface of the mucosa. Fig. 14.9 shows the differences in each cell layer. The second layer, stratum

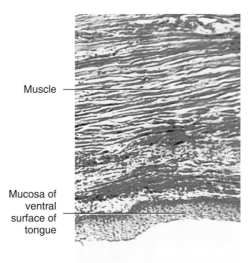

Muscle

Mucosa of ventral surface of tongue

Fig. 14.8 Histology of the ventral surface of the tongue showing the density of muscle fibers intermingling in the lamina propria.

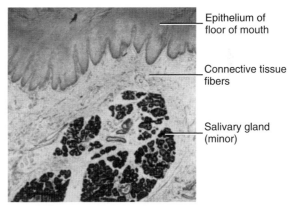

Epithelium of floor of mouth

Connective tissue fibers

Salivary gland (minor)

Fig. 14.9 Histology of mucosa lining the floor of the mouth. Observe the lack of muscle fibers and the delicate appearance of the connective tissue fibers. Scattered glands of minor serous and mucous salivary glands are near the tip of the tongue.

spinosum, is several cells thick. These cells are oval to polygonal, and mitotic figures can be seen in this layer. Occasionally, there will be mitotic figures in both the stratum basale and spinosum; combined, they are called stratum germinativum.

Basal cells interface with a membrane separating the epithelium and connective tissue. This membrane is called the **basal lamina**. The basal cells are attached to the basal lamina by minute disks termed **hemidesmosomes** (Fig. 14.11). These thickenings of the cell membrane are supported by filaments from within the cells, anchoring fibrils that attach the basal lamina and the epithelial cells to the collagen fibers of the lamina propria. Fig. 14.12 shows these structures.

The next layer of cells superficially is the stratum granulosum, so named because the cells contain many keratohyalin granules (Fig. 14.13). The surface layer of cells, the stratum corneum, is characterized by thin, flattened, nonnucleated cells. These cells are filled with a soft keratin that replaces the cell cytoplasm. This soft keratin may be compared with hard keratin of the nails and hair. Keratin is tough, nonliving material that is resistant to friction and impervious to bacterial invasion.

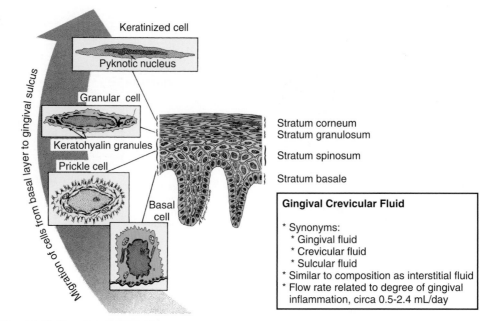

Fig. 14.10 **Keratinized stratified squamous epithelium of the oral cavity.** Observe the characteristics of four cell types of this epithelium from basal to surface layers. In the box on the right, gingival crevicular fluid helps maintain the health of the gingival by washing food debris, desquamated cells, and bacteria out of the sulcus, thereby preventing the initial inflammation that can lead to pocket formation and eventually periodontal disease.

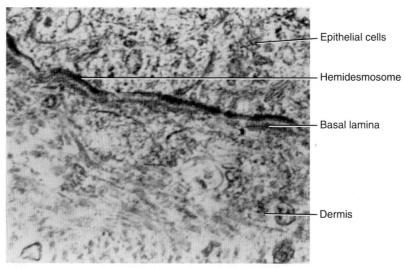

Fig. 14.11 **Ultrastructure of the junction of epithelium and lamina propria, as seen in an electron micrograph.** Extending across the field from left to right is basal lamina, to which epithelial cells are attached by hemidesmosomes.

To permit cell movement and loss of individual cells along the surface, the superficial layers have surface interdigitations rather than desmosomes. These cells are continually being lost and replaced by cells of the underlying layers.

As each cell moves to the surface of the epithelium, it does so by means of cell attachments to neighboring cells that hold until the cell has reached a specific stage of development. When that stage occurs, the cell attachment releases, allowing that cell to move to a higher level, where it reattaches. All epithelial cells function with **desmosomes**. In the oral mucosa, desmosomes are discoid and are called **macula adherens** (Fig. 14.14). The junctions are composed of thin protein adhesion disks located between the cells. These disks are anchored by means of intracellular filaments, termed **tonofibrils**, which arise in the cell and project to the surface, where they attach to the cell junction.

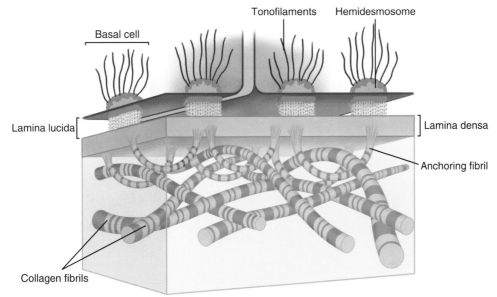

Fig. 14.12 Diagram of hemidesmosomes of oral mucosa showing how hemidesmosomes of epithelial cells attach to the basal lamina membrane. Anchoring collagen fibers of connective tissue attach to the basal lamina and fibers of the hemidesmosome. (Nanci A. *Ten Cate's oral histology.* 8th ed. St. Louis: Saunders; 2013.)

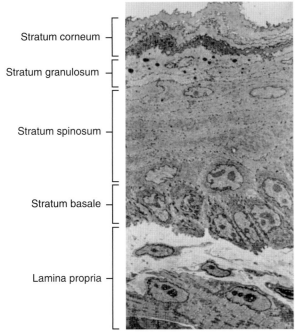

Fig. 14.13 An electron micrograph of oral epithelium. This is a view of keratinized oral epithelium that shows the relative thickness of each cell layer from stratum basale to stratum corneum and lamina propria beneath the epithelium.

The disks temporarily hold the cells in contact but later release them, allowing the cells to move superficially and reattach to a cell in another location (see Figs. 14.13 and 14.14).

Gingiva and Epithelial Attachment

In the oral mucosa, the gingiva surrounds the cervicals of the teeth and extends apically to the mucogingival junction (Fig. 14.15). The gingiva develops as a coalescence of the oral and reduced enamel organ epithelium when the tooth first emerges into the oral cavity (Fig. 14.16A–C). The reduced-enamel organ epithelium makes contact with the undersurface of the oral epithelium, and the two fuse. Then the tooth penetrates this combined layer to enter the mouth and produces the gingiva as the epithelium continues to separate from the enamel surface (see Fig. 14.16C) until occlusion of the teeth is reached (see Fig. 14.16D). At this point, the gingiva covers only the cervical area of the enamel where it is attached (see Fig. 14.16D).

The gingiva is divided into three zones: (1) the **free** or **marginal zone**, which encloses the tooth and defines the gingival sulcus; (2) the **attached gingiva**, that portion of the epithelium attached to the neck of the tooth by means of junctional epithelium; and (3) the **interdental zone** (groove), the area between two adjacent teeth beneath their contact point (see Fig. 14.15). The free and attached gingivae have an indistinct groove on the surface of the epithelium separating them. This groove is termed the **free gingival groove** (see Fig. 14.15; Fig. 14.17).

Free and Attached Gingiva

The free or marginal gingiva is bound on its inner margin by the gingival sulcus, which separates it from the tooth; on its outer margin by the oral cavity; and apically at its free surface by the free gingival groove (Fig. 14.18). This groove separates the free and attached gingivae. Therefore the attached gingiva lies adjacent to the free gingiva and is separated from the alveolar mucosa by the **mucogingival junction** (see Fig. 14.18). The free and attached gingivae are keratinized, but the alveolar mucosa is not. The attached gingiva is stippled due to attachment sites to the underlying alveolar bone, but the free gingiva has a smooth surface (Fig. 14.19). In some instances, the free gingiva may be covered with parakeratinized mucosa, which contains

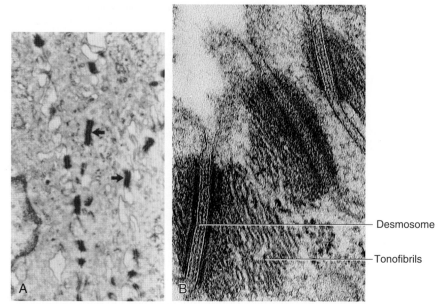

Fig. 14.14 Electron micrographs of cell junctions of oral epithelial cells; these are termed desmosomes or macula adherens. **A**, At low magnification, *arrows* indicate attachments between each cell. **B**, At higher magnification, multilayer arrangement of desmosomes can be seen. Tonofibrils from individual cells attach to these platelike junctions.

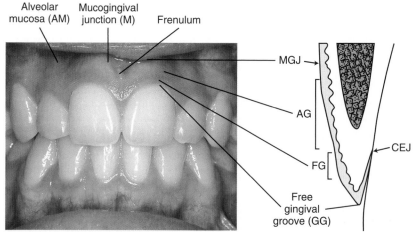

Fig. 14.15 Diagram of gingiva showing both facial and lateral views. Shown are free gingiva *(FG)* along the crest of gingiva; free gingival groove *(GG)* at junction between free and attached gingiva; stippled attached gingiva *(AG)*; mucogingival junction *(M)*, which separates gingiva from alveolar mucosa; and alveolar mucosa *(AM)* above attached gingiva. The frenulum and interdental zones *(grooves)* are also shown. *MGJ*, 5 mucogingival junction; *CEJ*, 5 cementoenamel junction; *FG*, 5 free gingiva. (Graber LW, Vanarsdall RL, Vig KWL, et al. *Orthodontics: current principles and techniques.* 6th ed. St. Louis: Elsevier; 2017.)

keratinized cells modified by the presence of nuclei in the cells of the surface layer. The unique feature of attached gingiva is the junctional epithelium.

Junctional Epithelium

Junctional epithelium provides attachment for the gingiva to the tooth in the cervical area and forms the epithelium-lined floor of the gingival sulcus (Fig. 14.20). Cells of the attached epithelium are cytologically different from other cells of the gingival epithelium. They have fewer desmosomes (cell attachment buttons). This indicates a higher rate of turnover than occurs in the other gingival epithelial cells (see Fig. 14.20). These cells have been reported to turn over in approximately 6 days (from the time of their appearance in the stratum basale to the time when they are sloughed in the free surface). The cells have many organelles, such as rough-surface endoplasmic reticulum, Golgi apparatus, and mitochondria, indicating high metabolic activity.

Stratum basale cells also contain hemidesmosomes, the mechanism for the attachment of cells to the salivary protein layer, which covers the cervical area of the enamel (Fig. 14.21).

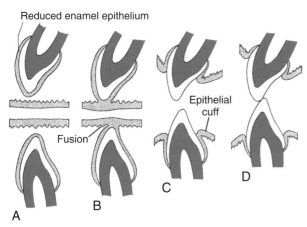

Fig. 14.16 Diagram of gingiva developing from reduced enamel epithelium (including the developmental cuticle) of the tooth combined with oral epithelium. The two meet, fuse, and rupture to allow the tooth to erupt.

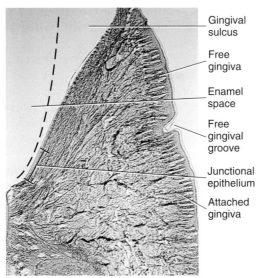

Fig. 14.17 Histology of gingiva illustrating the gingival sulcus, junctional epithelium, and free gingiva. Enamel space is created by loss (decalcification) of enamel.

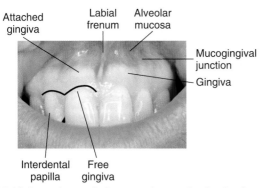

Fig. 14.18 Location of free and attached gingivae and location of the mucogingival junction. This junction separates keratinized gingiva from nonkeratinized alveolar mucosa. (Berkovitz BKB, Holland GR, Moxham BJ. *Oral anatomy, histology, and embryology.* 4th ed. St. Louis: Mosby; 2009.)

The half of a desmosome in these junctional epithelial cells is like the hemidesmosome of the basal cells of the squamous epithelium, which attaches to the basal lamina and lamina propria of the gingiva (see Fig. 14.13). Disturbance of this attachment to the tooth by infection, food impaction, calculus, or other irritants results in a deepening of the gingival sulcus that results from loss of epithelial attachment to the tooth surface (initially enamel but as the defect becomes deeper, the cementum of the root surface) and then reattachment at a more apical location.

CLINICAL COMMENT

In examining the gingiva, keep in mind its normal appearance. From this viewpoint, conditions other than normal ones can be more easily recognized.

Interdental Papilla and Col

Gingiva located between the teeth and extending high on the interproximal area of the crowns on the labial and lingual surfaces is known as the **interdental papilla** (see Fig. 14.19). This tissue fills the space created by the constricted cervical areas of the adjacent crowns. In the interproximal area between the lingual and vestibular papilla is a concave zone of the gingiva that follows the contour of each crown (Fig. 14.22). The junctional epithelium of this zone is known as the **col**, characterized as a thin, nonkeratinized epithelium. These basal epithelial cells invade the connective tissue where inflammatory cells of the lamina propria may appear (Figs. 14.23 and 14.24). The col is more inclined in a sharp peak between anterior teeth and more flattened or concave between posterior teeth. When the interproximal gingiva becomes inflamed or hyperemic, the col is exaggerated and is positioned higher on the neck of the tooth (see Fig. 14.23). Because of the location of the col below the contact points, it is a difficult area to keep free of debris and therefore exhibits signs of inflammation unless the individual takes meticulous care in keeping the area as clean as possible.

Hard Palate

The roof of the mouth, or hard palate, is covered with keratinized stratified squamous epithelium. This epithelium is similar to that of the gingiva in the midline, where there is no submucosa. The midline is known as the **median raphe**, which may only be barely discernible, except anteriorly, where an incisive papilla can be seen. On each side of the median raphe are ridges of tissue called **rugae** (Fig. 14.25). These folds of epithelium are supported by dense lamina propria (Fig. 14.26). In the anterior lateral palate, a zone of fatty tissue is located in the submucosa. However, in the posterior lateral hard palate is mucous glandular tissue (see Fig. 14.25). Both the hard and soft palates have mucous glands. **Traction bands** (Fig. 14.27) exist in the lamina propria of the rugae. These bands also exist between the lobules of fatty tissue and glands of the anterior and posterior hard palate. Traction bands are bundles of collagen fibers that insert into the papillary fibers of the lamina propria and extend into the bony palate. These collagen fibers anchor the palatal mucosa to the underlying bone, and the hard palate assists in mastication.

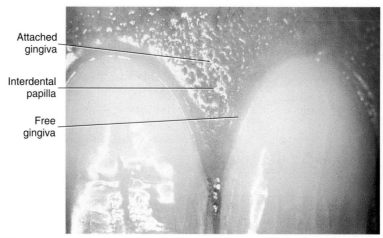

Fig. 14.19 View of normal gingiva, illustrating free and attached (stippled) gingivae.

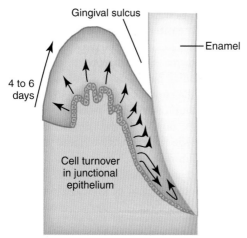

Fig. 14.20 Epithelial cell turnover in gingiva. Note the direction of epithelial cell maturation from basal cell to surface in attachment zone and in the margin of gingiva.

Specialized Mucosa

Types of Papillae

The dorsum or superior surface of the tongue (anterior two-thirds) is covered with a specialized mucosa. This mucosa consists of four types of epithelial structures called **papillae** (Fig. 14.28). Most of these papillae are **filiform papillae**, which are slender, threadlike keratinized extensions of the surface epithelial cells. The entire roughened surface of the tongue is covered with these papillae (Figs. 14.29 and 14.30), which project about 2 to 3 mm high from the surface of the tongue. These papillae facilitate mastication and movement of the food on the surface of the tongue.

Interspersed between the filiform papillae are the **fungiform papillae**, which are few in number but more numerous near the tip of the tongue. The fungiform papillae are mushroom shaped, with the cap usually larger than the stalk (Fig. 14.31). The covering epithelium of the fungiform papillae is thin and nonkeratinized, so the papillae appear pink or reddish because blood vessels are near the surface. Taste buds are found on the superior surface of the fungiform papillae (see Fig. 14.31; Fig. 14.32B). A third type of papilla is the **circumvallate papilla**.

Only 10 to 14 in number, the circumvallate papillae are located along the V-shaped sulcus between the body and base of the tongue (see Fig. 14.32). These papillae are level with the surface of the tongue, and each has a surrounding groove or sulcus. They are large—3 mm in diameter.

Ducts of the underlying serous glands (von Ebner glands) are seen opening into the grooves surrounding these papillae. Taste buds line the walls of the papillae (see Fig. 14.32B). The serous or watery secretion of these glands washes out substances so that new tastes can be recognized. On the lateral posterior sides of the tongue are 4 to 11 vertical grooves or furrows containing taste buds (see Fig. 14.32A). Within these furrows are **foliate papillae**. Like circumvallate papillae, they contain serous glands underlying the taste buds, which cleanse the trenches surrounding the foliate papillae.

Taste Buds

Taste buds are microscopically visible, barrel-shaped bodies found in the oral epithelium. These discrete sense organs contain the chemical sense of taste. They are generally associated with the papillae of the tongue—the circumvallate, foliate, and fungi formal—though some are distributed in the soft palate, epiglottis, larynx, and pharynx (Figs. 14.33–14.35; Box 14.2).

Taste buds are easily recognized under the microscope as barrel-shaped structures; their epithelial cells appear ovoid (see Fig. 14.33). Although they have been referred to as neuroepithelial structures, they are more correctly referred to as epithelial cells closely associated with club-shaped sensory nerve endings. These nerves arise from branches of cranial nerves VII, IX, and X, and come to lie among the taste cells.

CLINICAL COMMENT

The distribution of nerve endings in the oral cavity is greatest in the lips and anterior oral mucosa and least in the more posterior regions of the oral cavity. Therefore the mouth tastes food and beverages before they are taken farther into the alimentary canal. The one exception to this anterior sensitivity is that of cold and pain nerve endings, which are numerous in the posterior palate.

Several types of taste cells are found among the 10 to 14 cells in a taste bud. Each taste bud contains a few **supporting**

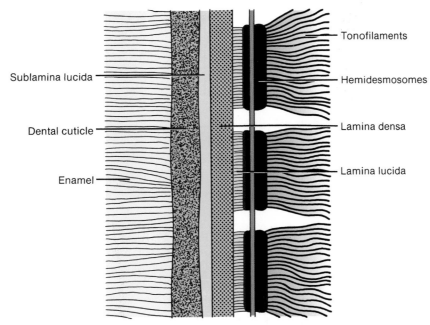

Fig. 14.21 The means of gingival attachment with tooth's surface. Diagram of a hemidesmosome, which is a specialized attachment plaque that attaches a cell to the protein of cuticle or pellicle on a tooth's surface. Protein of enamel surface is composed of dense and lucent layers. If the hemidesmosome is disturbed, reattachment can occur.

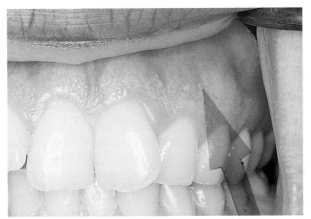

Fig. 14.22 Clinical view of gingiva showing free and attached gingiva and the interdental groove *(arrow)*. The col is found in the interdental area.

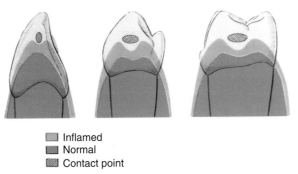

Inflamed
Normal
Contact point

Fig. 14.23 Positional relationship of the col in health and disease. The col is accentuated in inflammation and swelling of gingiva. The col is pointed in anterior teeth and flat or concave posteriorly. The contact point on each crown is represented by an oval above the col.

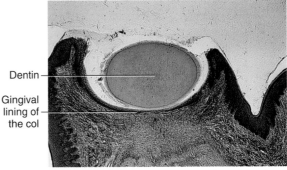

Fig. 14.24 Histology of a col, a concave, nonkeratinized epithelial lining of gingiva between teeth.

or **sustentacular cells** (several types) that lie in the periphery of the taste bud. Most **taste cells** bear either elongated microvilli that project into the taste pore or ones with shortened villi that open into the base of the pore. Each cell is associated with nerves that penetrate the taste bud. Another type of cell found in the taste bud is the **basal cell**. These basal cells are in close contact with the basal lamina (see Fig. 14.35). There is a rapid turnover of these cells approximately every 10 days. They are believed to arise from the surrounding epithelial cells.

Five types of taste sensation can be detected, and evidence of regional sensitivity for these tastes is on the tongue and palate. The five taste sensations are **sweet, salty, sour, bitter**, and **umami**. Sensations of sweet and salty are perceived at the tongue's tip, sour on the sides, and bitter in the region of the circumvallate papillae (Fig. 14.36). Umami is recognized by taste buds throughout the oral cavity and is activated by glutamate (glutamic acid, an amino acid). These areas overlap, and evidence indicates that all papillae respond to all four types of taste

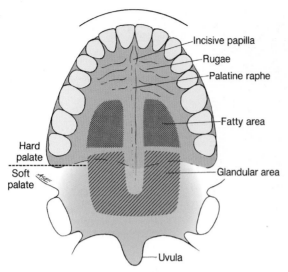

Fig. 14.25 Diagram of the palate indicating location of the fatty zone anteriorly and the glandular zone posteriorly. These tissues are found in subcutaneous tissue underlying the lamina propria. In the midline of the palate, there is no subcutaneous zone; only lamina propria exists, as in the gingiva of the lateral palate.

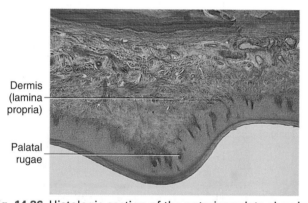

Fig. 14.26 Histologic section of the anterior palate showing rugae. Rugae are epithelium-covered ridges in the lamina propria of the anterior palate.

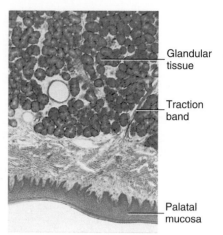

Fig. 14.27 Histologic section of the palate in the glandular zone. Traction bands of collagen fibers bind palatal epithelium to the underlying bone.

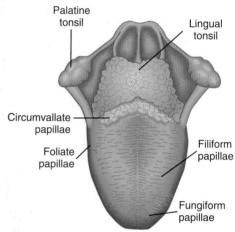

Fig. 14.28 Diagram of the dorsal surface of tongue showing papillae. Filiform papillae are scattered over the surface of the tongue body. Fungiform papillae are few in number, round, and pink but larger than filiform papillae. Foliate papillae are 4 to 11 in number along the posterior sides of the tongue. Circumvallate papillae are 8 to 10 in number along the junction of the body and base of the tonsillar area of the tongue.

sensations. However, the levels of sensitivity differ. For example, with higher concentrations of a bitter taste, the sensation is perceived most notably on the posterior segment of the tongue. This indicates a regional selectivity of taste in the mouth, which may be caused in part by the origin of the nerve supply or evolutionary considerations.

Nerves for taste buds of the anterior two-thirds of the tongue pass to the chorda tympani branch of the facial nerve (VII), those of the posterior one-third pass to specific branches of the glossopharyngeal nerve (IX), and those from the epiglottis and larynx pass to branches of the vagus nerve (X).

Mixing the five basic modalities of taste cannot explain all the flavors that humans are capable of experiencing. Factors such as odors and temperature also contribute to flavors. In addition, taste buds can discriminate between subtleties in flavor, such as the difference between citric or acetic acid. This enables taste buds to identify specific substances even when they are mixed.

Umami Taste Modality

Early in the 20th century, a new taste modality called *umami* was suggested. This distinctive taste was associated with the amino acid glutamate (glutamic acid). Glutamate is an amino acid and a building block of protein. This molecule commonly is combined with sodium to make monosodium glutamate (MSG) and is used to flavor foods in many restaurants and kitchens. However, some people can develop severe allergies to MSG and at least in the United States, many restaurants have discontinued its use.

NERVES AND BLOOD VESSELS

The nerves and blood vessels appear in the lamina propria. Terminal endings of nerves and loops of blood vessels appear in the dermal papillae. There, blood vessels consist of a deep

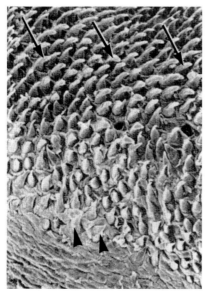

Fig. 14.29 A scanning electron micrograph of the tongue's surface showing filiform papillae *(arrows)*. These pointed papillae *(arrowheads)* are directed toward the throat and assist in moving food in that direction as the tongue moves.

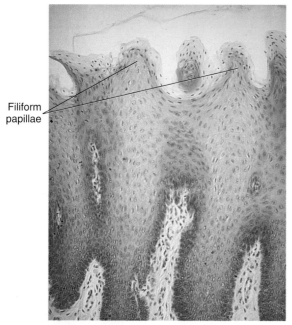

Fig. 14.30 Histologic picture of the filiform papillae of the tongue's dorsal surface. Pointed keratinized projections are shown.

Filiform papillae

plexus of larger vessels in the submucosa underlying the lamina propria, and capillary loops extend into a secondary plexus in the dermal papillae. The overlying epithelium is avascular, and its metabolic needs come from the vessels of the lamina propria. Nutrition passes from these vessels through the connective tissue and basal lamina and then enters the epithelium. Throughout the gingiva, nerves and nerve endings are prevalent. The encapsulated touch and temperature endings are located in the papillary tissue of the lamina propria and axons associated with Merkel cells (Fig. 14.37). Free endings associated with pain can be seen entering the epithelium between the cells. Table 14.1 shows the areas and levels of sensitivity.

EPITHELIAL NONKERATINOCYTES

In contrast to the epithelial cells or keratinocytes, the nonkeratinocytes (or dendritic cells) constitute about 10% of the mucosal cell population. These cells have a clear halo around their nuclei and have been called *clear cells*. All three types of nonkeratinocytes also have long dendritic processes and are sometimes referred to as *dendritic cells*. The three types of these cells are **Langerhans cells, Merkel cells**, and **melanocytes**. Two other nonkeratinocytes—lymphocytes and polymorphonuclear leukocytes—appear in the epithelium in cases of inflammation.

Langerhans Cells

Langerhans cells are a type II antigen-processing cell found in the stratum spinosum that functions in the processing of antigenic material. They are, therefore, in an ideal location to make contact with invading bacteria and establish response mechanisms to protect the body. The cells have processes but do not have desmosomes or tonofilaments. This type of cell has unique, racket-shaped organelles (Fig. 14.38). Langerhans cells are migratory and can move in and out of the epithelium in response to an antigenic challenge.

Merkel Cells

Merkel cells are located in the basal layer of the gingival epithelium. Unlike keratinocytes, these cells are associated with the terminal axon. However, they may contain round, electron-dense granules in their cytoplasms adjacent to their axons. These cells and their axons function as touch and pressure receptors and are slowly adaptive (Fig. 14.39).

Melanocytes

Melanocytes are melanin-producing cells in the basal layer of the gingival epithelium. Melanocytes lack desmosomes and tonofilaments and are dendritic. A characteristic feature of the melanocyte is the melanin granules (melanosomes) in the cytoplasm. Such cells may inject melanosomes into nearby keratinocytes (Fig. 14.40). Melanocytes are derived from neural crest cells that migrated to the epithelium during development.

Lymphocytes and Leukocytes

Lymphocytes, leukocytes, and mast cells, which are associated with gingival inflammation, may be found in the gingival epithelium and connective tissue. They may be located anywhere in the gingiva but most often underlie the junctional epithelium. Their appearance is different from keratinocytes because they have no desmosomes, tonofilaments, or organelles. These lymphocytes appear typical, with a large oval nucleus occupying most of the cytoplasmic space (Fig. 14.41). Granule-bearing mast cells may also be seen in the gingival mucosa during inflammation.

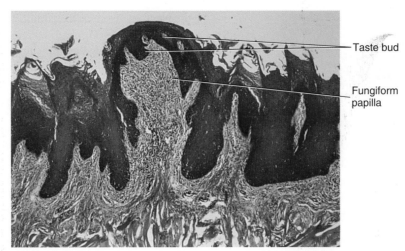

Fig. 14.31 Histologic section of the fungiform papilla, with a connective tissue core and epithelial covering. Two taste buds are located on the superior surface of the papilla.

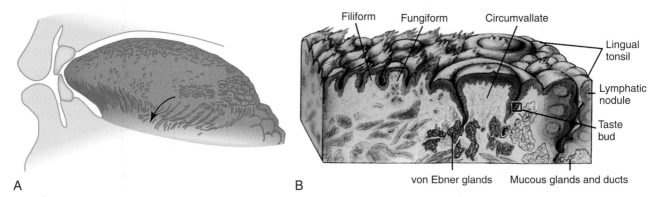

Fig. 14.32 Circumvallate papillae. **A**, Note the large (2-mm) papillae, with a trench around each and underlying serous (von Ebner) glands, which wash out tasteable substances from the area of the taste buds. **B**, Rectangle in **A** enlarged. Dorsal appearance of the tongue, with filiform, fungiform, and circumvallate papillae. A taste bud is shown within the *small square*.

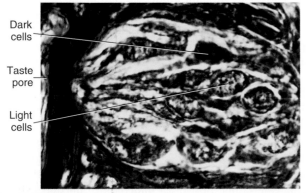

Fig. 14.33 Light microscope picture of a taste bud, with its dark and light cells. The taste pore on the left opens into the wall of a trench, as seen in Fig. 14.34.

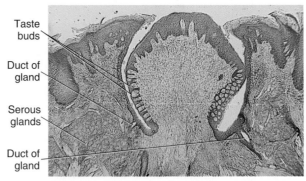

Fig. 14.34 Histology of the circumvallate papilla, with taste buds located in its walls in a trench. von Ebner gland (pure serous secretion) and its ducts are emptying into a trench located in the lower left and right.

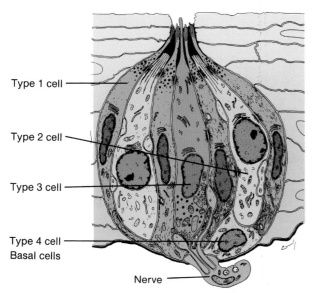

Fig. 14.35 Diagram of typical taste bud, with four types of cells. Type 1, dark cells, represents 60% of the cells; type 2, light cells, represents 30%; type 3 represents 7%; and type 4, basal cells, represents 3%.

BOX 14.2 Number of Taste Buds in the Human Adult

Tongue: 10,000
Soft palate: 2500
Epiglottis: 900
Larynx and pharynx: 600
Oropharynx: 250

CLINICAL COMMENT

Halitosis can be caused by multiple factors. If the ingestion of certain foods (e.g., garlic) is ruled out as a cause, possible food impaction, plaque, or the need for oral prophylaxis should be considered. Disease of tooth origin or the periodontium is another factor. Diseased tonsils or sinuses and systemic factors, such as lung problems, are also possible causes.

CHANGES WITH AGING

Recognition of changes in the oral mucosa associated with aging is important. With age, the oral epithelium becomes thinner and more fragile. A flattening of the surface ridges and surface cells causes the oral mucosa to appear smoother. Because of gradual atrophy of the minor salivary glands and less activity of the major glands, the oral mucosa appears less moist. In aging, cellular activity decreases and fibrosis increases. Also, calcifications appear in the lamina propria of the gingiva and the periodontal ligament. The ability to repair is reduced, and the length of healing time is increased. Apical migration of the gingiva usually is associated with periodontal disease but appears routinely in the aging oral mucosa. Some patients may be taking blood thinners or other medications that affect gingival bleeding. Compare Figs. 14.42 and 14.43.

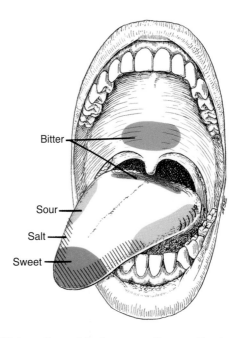

Fig. 14.36 Location of taste perception on the tongue and soft palate. The tip of the tongue has sweet receptors, along the front sides are salty receptors, on the posterior sides are sour receptors, and on the posterior center of the tongue and soft palate are bitter receptors. (Courtesy Dr. R. Murray, University of Indiana School of Medicine.)

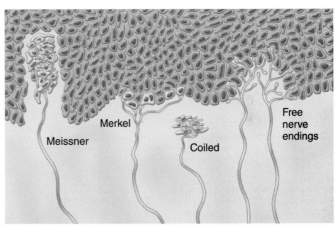

Fig. 14.37 Nerve endings in oral mucosa showing the location of various types in epithelium or lamina propria.

TABLE 14.1 Levels of Sensitivity of the Oral Region

Sensation	Greatest Sensitivity	Moderate Sensitivity
Pain	Lips, pharynx, base of tongue	Anterior tongue
Heat	Lips	Tip of tongue
Cold	Lips, posterior palate	Base of tongue, ventral tongue
Touch	Lips, tip of tongue	Gingiva

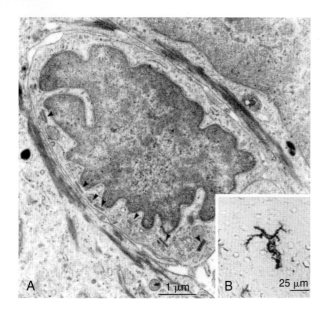

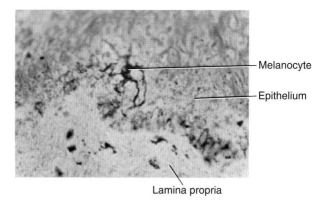

Fig. 14.40 Histology of another type of nonkeratinocyte. A dendritic melanocyte is in the stratum basale of the oral epithelium.

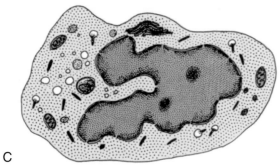

Fig. 14.38 Three histologic views of a nonkeratinocyte. **A**, In an electron micrograph of Langerhans cell, the rodlike granules are indicated by *arrows*. **B**, Appearance of cell under light microscopy. **C**, Diagram of Langerhans cell.

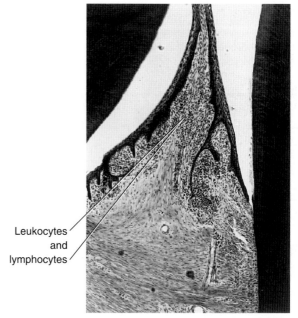

Fig. 14.41 Inflamed gingiva with many leukocytes and lymphocytes in the connective tissue of the gingiva.

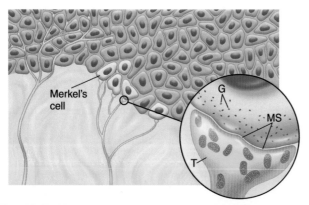

Fig. 14.39 Merkel cells that are located in basal cell layer and are associated with a nerve ending **(MS)**. They function as touch receptors. The inset shows nerve terminals *(T)* and secretory granules in Merkel cell *(G)*.

CONSIDER THE PATIENT

The floor of the mouth is an appropriate area for absorption of some medications, such as for the relief of angina, because it is a rapid route. The epithelium is thin and nonkeratinized, with capillaries present in the dermis, which is near the surface of the mucosa.

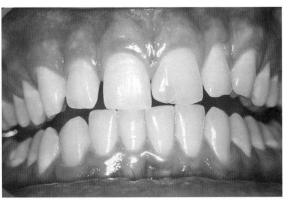

Fig. 14.42 Healthy gingiva in young adult showing normal color, form, and density. (Newman MG, Takei H, Klokkevold P, et al. Carranza's clinical periodontology. 12th ed. St. Louis: Saunders; 2015.)

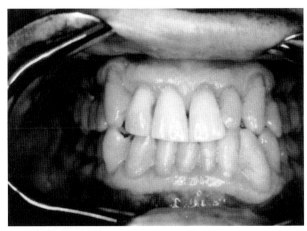

Fig. 14.43 Healthy gingiva of an 80-year-old person differs from that of the young adult shown in Fig. 14.42. Normal form and contours are altered in older persons.

SELF-EVALUATION QUESTIONS

1. Describe the three areas of the gingiva and the characteristics of each.
2. Name the areas covered with lining mucosa and masticatory mucosa.
3. Where are taste buds most numerous in the oral cavity and in what other areas are they located?
4. What are the locations and functions of traction bands?
5. Describe junctional epithelium and state its turnover time.
6. What are the location and function of Langerhans cells?
7. Name four types of nerve sensation found in the oral cavity and their location.
8. What taste sensations are located on the tip, anterior sides, posterior sides, and posterior center of the tongue?
9. What is the name and type of gland found at the corners of the mouth?
10. Describe the structure and function of a hemidesmosome.

QUANDARIES IN SCIENCE

The oral mucosa is a complex tissue, with a multitude of functions. One of its major functions is protective because it prevents foreign materials from entering the body. When foreign materials do penetrate the tightly adherent mucosa, there are a series of mechanisms in place that quickly scavenge the antigens and mount the appropriate response. Langerhans cells, dendritic type II antigen-processing cells, have the ability to migrate through the connective tissue and the epithelium, uptake and process antigens, and present them to T lymphocytes. An emerging field of medicine called personalized medicine has introduced a procedure that uses a person's own Langerhans cells that have been removed, exposed to the person's own tumor cells in a culture dish, and replaced to fight cancer. This work by Bruce A. Beutler, Jules A. Hoffmann, and Ralph M. Steinman won the Nobel Prize in Physiology or Medicine in 2011. The oral mucosa presents many mysteries that will someday be better understood to improve a person's overall quality of life. What other aspects of the biology of the oral mucosa can be used to benefit people?

CLINICAL CASE

A 20-year-old college student presents at the dentist's office with painful, open vesicular sores on his lower lip. The patient tells the dentist that there was redness and itching before the lesions formed, and that he experienced a sore throat and inflamed lymph nodes associated with lymphatic drainage of the lower lip. After a complete medical and dental history, an extra- and intraoral exam is performed. Submental and submandibular lymph nodes draining the lower lip were enlarged and tender. Open vesicular lesions were located at the midline of the lower lip extending toward the right side. A clear exudate could be seen emanating from the lesions that tested positive for herpes simplex virus (HSV) type I. The patient was given a prescription for acyclovir and left the office. He was instructed to call the dentist if the lesions did not heal within 7 to 10 days.

HSV type I is a virus that resides in neuronal ganglia and will travel via anterograde axoplasmic transport to a nerve terminal where the virus replicates and infects surrounding epithelial cells. Herpes is transmitted via direct contact with an infected person, or can be transferred via utensils such as a spoon or fork and toothbrushes.

Once infected, a person will have the virus for life, and it can exist in the body in an active or latent form. Activation of the virus can be caused by stressful situations, including going to the dentist's office. Modern treatments include a variety of antiviral drugs, which can shorten the healing time.

SUGGESTED READING

Bhaskar SN, ed. *Orban's oral histology and embryology*. 11th ed. St. Louis: Mosby; 1991.

Borgnakke WS. Does treatment of periodontal disease influence systemic disease? *Dent Clin North Am*. 2015;59:885–917.

Fischer A, Gilad Y, Man O, et al. Evolution of bitter taste receptors in humans and apes. *Mol Biol Evol*. 2005;22:432–436.

Hajishengallis G. Periodontitis: from microbial immune subversion to systemic inflammation. *Nat Rev Immunol*. 2015;15:30–44.

Kessler HR. Herpes virus infections: a review for the dental practitioner. *Tex Dent J*. 2005;122(2):150–165.

Kvidera A, Mackenzie IC. Rates of clearance of the epithelial surfaces of mouse oral mucosa and skin. *Epithelial Cell Biol*. 1994;3(4):175–180.

Nakamura E. One hundred years since the discovery of the umami taste from seaweed broth by Kikunae Ikeda, who transcended his time. *Chem Asian J*. 2011;6(7):1659–1663.

Nunzi MG, Pisarek A, Mugnaini E. Merkel cells, corpuscular nerve endings, and free nerve endings in the mouse palatine mucosa express three subtypes of vesicular glutamate transporters. *J Neurocytol.* 2004;33(3):359–376.

Risso D, Tofanelli S, Morini G, et al. Genetic variation in taste receptor pseudogenes provides evidence for a dynamic role in human evolution. *BMC Evol Biol.* 2014;14:198.

Roper SD. Signal transduction and information processing in mammalian taste buds. *Pflugers Arch.* 2007;454(5):759–776.

Spruance SL, Stewart JC, Rowe NH, et al. Treatment of recurrent herpes simplex labialis with oral acyclovir. *J Infect Dis.* 1990;161(2):185–190.

Wheller L, Carman N, Butler G. Unilesional self-limited Langerhans cell histiocytosis: a case report and review of the literature. *J Cutan Pathol.* 2013;40:595–599. https://doi.org/10.1111/cup.12121.

Zhang Y, Venkitasamy C, Pan Z, et al. Novel umami ingredients: umami peptides and their taste. *J Food Sci.* 2017;82(1):16–23.

15

Salivary Glands and Tonsils

LEARNING OBJECTIVES

- Discuss the classification of the major and minor salivary glands.
- Explain the composition and function of saliva.
- Describe the location and purpose of salivary gland duct systems.
- Discuss the classification of tonsillar tissue.
- Explain the function of the tonsils.

OVERVIEW

This chapter discusses the structure and function of the salivary glands, saliva, and tonsils. Despite different structures and functions, these soft tissues all contribute significantly to oral health. Saliva is a balanced secretion resulting from both the composition of the secretion and the location of the salivary gland secretions into the oral cavity. The two cell types are serous, which is high protein and low carbohydrate, and mucous, which is low protein and high carbohydrate. Glands of the lips, cheeks, and anterior floor of the mouth produce a watery mixture of a serous and mucous secretion, whereas other glands of the posterior palate, pharynx, and tongue contribute a viscous mucous solution that protects the membranes in those regions. The major salivary glands contribute 85% to 90% of the saliva into the more anterior area of the mouth. In addition to protein and carbohydrate, the parotid gland, which is the largest gland, secretes the enzyme amylase, which aids in digestion of carbohydrates. Therefore the buffering ability of saliva results from ionic secretions by the salivary glands. These secretions are collected and modified through an elaborate secretory duct system.

Tonsils, like the salivary glands, have locations that maximally affect and protect the oral environment. These lymph node–like organs are positioned in the oropharynx at the entrance to the alimentary canal. They produce lymphocytes and, with the assistance of macrophages, protect against microbes, foreign cells, and cancer cells. Lymphocytes can recognize foreign cells and respond to them either by becoming T cells, which destroy the foreign cells directly, or by forming B cells, which transform into plasma cells that secrete antibodies to eliminate the foreign cells.

CLASSIFICATION OF SALIVARY GLANDS

Salivary glands are classified as either major or minor, depending on their size and the amount of their secretion. The **major glands** carry their secretions some distance to the oral cavity by means of a main duct. The smaller **minor glands** empty their products directly into the mouth by means of short ducts. Both are composed, however, of the same type of cells, either **serous** or **mucous cells** or a combination of the two called **serous demilunes** (Fig. 15.1).

The functional unit of the salivary gland is the **alveolus** or **acinus**. An acinus is a cluster of pyramidal cells, either mucous or serous or a combination of the two, that secretes into a terminal collecting duct (see Fig. 15.1). The collecting duct is termed the **secretory end piece** or **intercalated duct**. Both the large and small glands are composed of many acini, although the larger glands contain more acini or units arranged in lobules and lobes (Fig. 15.2). Each cell type provides a different type of secretion. Serous cells secrete mostly proteins and small amounts of carbohydrates. Their secretion also contains **zymogen granules**, precursors of the enzyme **amylase**, which functions in the breakdown of carbohydrates. Serous cell secretion has a watery consistency. Mucous cells are high in carbohydrates and low in proteins and discharge a viscous product called **mucin** (Fig. 15.3). When mucin mixes with watery oral fluids, it becomes mucous, causing the saliva to be thick and viscous.

CLINICAL COMMENT

The salivary glands are also important for the production of growth factors, including nerve growth factor and epidermal growth factor, which belongs to a family of growth factors that stimulate cell growth, proliferation, and differentiation.

Both types of acinar cells are pyramidal. The nucleus of the serous cell is oval to round, and that of the mucous cell is oval to spindleshaped (see Fig. 15.1). In each of these cell types, the nuclei appear in the basal part of the cell. The cytoplasm of the serous cell stains deeply because it is filled with albumin, whereas the mucous cell appears light and foamy because of the presence of carbohydrates in mucin (see Fig. 15.3; Fig. 15.4).

Ultrastructurally, the serous cell is filled with secretory granules in the apical region, rough-surface endoplasmic reticulum, a Golgi apparatus, mitochondria, and an oval nucleus (Fig. 15.5). The mucous cells contain larger droplets of mucin apically

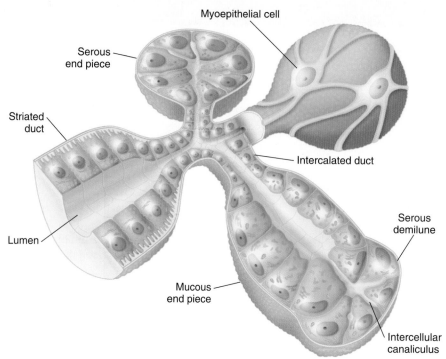

Fig. 15.1 Salivary acinar cells. The serous, mixed, and mucous alveoli are displayed. Observe cell size, shape, and position relative to collecting tubules and intercalated duct.

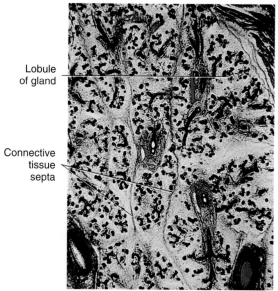

Fig. 15.2 Histology of the developing salivary gland at a stage in which lobules can be seen outlined by connective tissue fibers (septa).

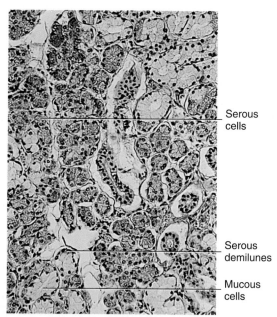

Fig. 15.3 Histologic features of the submandibular gland. Serous cells are at the upper left and mucous cells are at the lower left. A few mucous cells are capped with serous cells (serous demilunes).

and a prominent Golgi apparatus and rough endoplasmic reticulum around the flattened nucleus (Fig. 15.6). A third cell type arrangement is a terminal alveolus of mucous cells with a cap of serous cells (see Fig. 15.4). This configuration is termed a *serous demilune*, with the secretion of the serous cells passing down a duct between the terminal mucous cells to the lumen of the alveolus (see Fig. 15.1).

Salivary glands are termed **merocrine glands** because the basic mode of product excretion is through membrane vesicles passing to the cell's apex. These vesicles fuse with the cell plasma membrane, and their contents are released by **exocytosis**, the process by which a cell can release substances to the extracellular milieu (see Fig. 15.6).

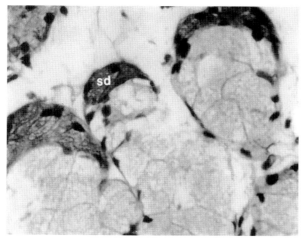

Fig. 15.4 Histology of a serous demilune *(sd)* cap on mucous cells in mixed acinus of the submandibular gland.

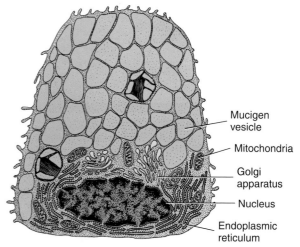

Fig. 15.6 Ultrastructural design of a mucous cell. Compare the shape of this cell and its nucleus with those of the serous cell. Shown are the Golgi apparatus, rough-surface endoplasmic reticulum, and mucous accumulation (mucigen vesicles) in the cell.

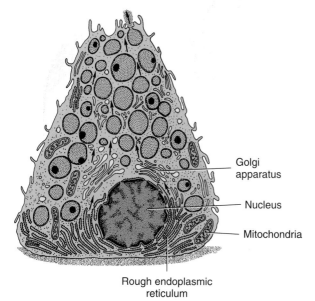

Fig. 15.5 Ultrastructure of a serous cell with vesicles developing and migrating to the cell apex above. Note the round nucleus, Golgi apparatus, and rough endoplasmic reticulum that are characteristic of a protein-secreting cell. *Arrows* point to vesicles arising from the Golgi zone and migrating to the cell surface.

CLINICAL COMMENT

The serous and mucous cells of the major glands secrete 85% to 90% of saliva. Their combined secretions produce the viscosity and the important buffering actions of saliva. These properties result from the actions of protein, carbohydrate, carbonate, and phosphate that are contributed by the secretory ducts of the glands.

MAJOR SALIVARY GLANDS

The major salivary glands are present as three bilateral pairs. The **parotid glands** are located on the sides of the face in front of the ears; the second pair, the **submandibular glands**, are inside the angle of the mandible; and the third pair, the **sublingual glands**,

are on either side of the midline beneath the mucosa of the anterior floor of the mouth (Fig. 15.7; Table 15.1).

Each major gland secretes a different product. The parotid glands produce a nearly pure serous secretion, the submandibular gland produces a mixed serous and mucous secretion, and the sublingual gland's secretion is nearly pure mucous.

The parotids are the largest glands, although they contribute only 25% of the total saliva. The submandibular glands are intermediate in size, but they produce 60% of the saliva. The sublingual glands are the smallest, contributing 10% to the total salivary flow. The minor salivary glands located throughout the oral cavity contribute about the same amount as the sublingual glands.

These salivary glands are organized like grapes on a vine. The acini are the grapes, and they are arranged in groups or **lobules** invested in connective tissue. These groups of lobules form larger **lobes**. In turn, the lobes are surrounded by connective tissue containing the ducts that drain the glands and the blood vessels and nerves that supply the glands (Fig. 15.8).

The parotid ducts extend anteriorly across the masseter muscles and then bend toward the mouth, opening adjacent to the crowns of the second maxillary molar teeth (see Fig. 15.7). The ducts of the submandibular and sublingual glands have a common opening in the anterior floor of the mouth, located at the sublingual papillae on either side of the frenulum and at the tongue's tip (see Fig. 15.7).

MINOR SALIVARY GLANDS

The minor salivary glands are classified as serous, mucous, and mixed types, the same as the major glands (Table 15.2). These glands are located throughout the oral cavity and are named for their location. The glands of the cheeks and lips are termed the **buccal** and **labial glands**. They contain a combination of serous and mucous secretions and are thus known as **mixed glands**.

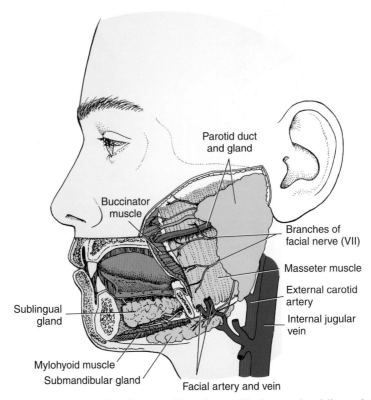

Fig. 15.7 Location of major glands: parotid, submandibular, and sublingual. The diagram demonstrates the relationship of facial nerves and blood vessels to oral structures.

TABLE 15.1	**Major Salivary Glands and Contribution to Saliva**				
Gland	**Size**	**Location**	**Type Cells**	**Amount Secretion (%)**	**Duct Type: Striated/ Intercalated**
Parotid	Largest	Anterior ear	Serous	25	Long/long
Submandibular	Intermediate	Angle of mandible	Mixed serous demilune	60	Long/short
Sublingual	Smallest	Anterior floor of mouth	Mucous	5	Short/none

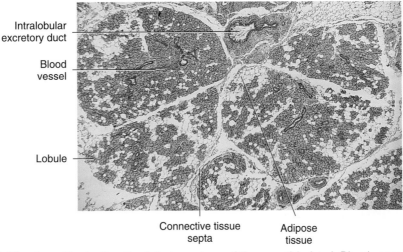

Fig. 15.8 Histology illustrating the lobular nature of the parotid gland. Blood vessels can be seen within the lobule. Light lines that surround each lobule are connective tissue fibers that support lobules. The parotid gland contains many adipose cells (light-stained cells).

TABLE 15.2 Minor Salivary Glands and Contribution to Saliva

Name	Location	Type Secretion
Labial	Lips	Mixed
Buccal	Cheeks	Mixed
Palatine	Hard and soft	Pure mucous
Lingual	Anterior	Mixed
	Middle	Serous
	Posterior	Pure mucous

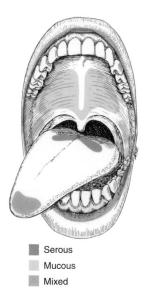

■ Serous
■ Mucous
■ Mixed

Fig. 15.9 Location of the minor salivary glands in the oral cavity. Serous glands are located in the mid-tongue, mucous glands in the palate, and mixed glands in the lips, cheeks, and tongue tip.

The glands of both the posterior hard palate and soft palate are called **palatine glands**, and those of the tonsillar folds are the **glossopalatine glands**. These glands are referred to as **pure mucous glands**. The tongue contains **lingual glands**, which are mixed glands at the tongue's tip. **Serous glands** of von Ebner are located at the junction of the tongue's body and base, where the watery secretion washes off the taste buds of the circumvallate papillae. The tongue also has mucous glands in the posterior region under the lingual tonsillar tissue. Fig. 15.9 shows all these minor glands. Each minor gland is small, consisting of a cluster of acini, and each is drained by a short duct.

SALIVA

Composition

All of the major and minor salivary glands contribute to the composition of saliva (Fig. 15.10). This composition varies according to the rate of secretion, which is low during sleep and high (±1 mL per minute) during stimulation. Secretion is controlled by the salivary center in the brain, and flow is generated by taste (gustatory). Masticatory function is controlled through receptors in the periodontium and muscles of mastication. Oral and pharyngeal pain and irritation can also induce secretion.

Saliva has fewer proteins and ions than blood. Saliva contains potassium, sodium chloride, calcium, magnesium, phosphorus, carbonate, urea, and traces of ammonia, uric acid, glucose, and lipids. The major salivary protein is amylase, which is present in the parotid gland and to a lesser extent (20%) in the submandibular gland. The sublingual or minor glands do not have any amylase. Saliva also contains the proteins lysozyme and albumin. The viscous nature of saliva results from the presence of salivary mucin, which is a mixture of glycoproteins. Saliva contains epithelial cells shed by the oral epithelium as well as leukocytes from the gingival crevices and lymphocytes from the tonsils. The latter two are known as **salivary corpuscles** (Box 15.1).

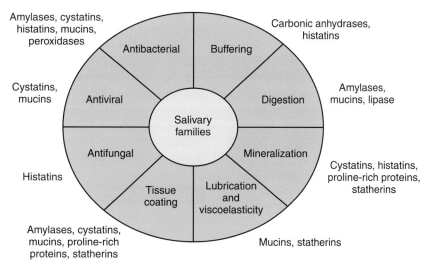

Fig. 15.10 Components of saliva.

BOX 15.1 Composition of Saliva

Cells
- Desquamated epithelial cells
- Neutrophils
- Small amount of lymphocytes and monocytes
- Bacteria

Inorganic Ions
- Similar to plasma
- Potassium 2× higher than in plasma (cell breakup)
- Calcium higher than in oral fluid

Organic Components
- Similar to plasma: serum albumin, globulins, complement, protease inhibitors
- Small organic molecules: lactate, urea, hydroxyproline
- Enzymes

CLINICAL COMMENT

The locations of various minor glands in the oral cavity are important to oral functions. In the palate, where keratinized epithelium is present, mucous glands provide adequate lubrication to the epithelium. The lips and cheeks have similar mixed glands that assist in mastication, swallowing, and speech. These minor glands assist in swallowing and speech. Contributions of the three bilateral major glands provide the other 90% of oral fluids.

Functions

The 1.4 L (3 pints) of saliva secreted each day serve several important functions, some of which are the following:

1. Washing the surfaces of the teeth and reducing the possibility of acid etching the enamel surface and leading to dental caries
2. Keeping the oral tissues moist and protecting against irritants and desiccation
3. Aiding in mastication and swallowing of food
4. Providing antibacterial action
5. Assisting in the formation of the pellicle, which is a protective membrane on the tooth's surface
6. Providing protection in acid-neutralizing and acid-buffering actions, which prevent dissolution of enamel

The presence of calcium and phosphate ions in saliva increases the enamel surface hardness of newly erupted teeth and assists in enamel remineralization. Through the action of amylase, starches are broken down to more easily digestible carbohydrates. Saliva is necessary for taste by breaking down food molecules into a solution that is then brought into contact with the taste buds.

CLINICAL COMMENT

Saliva is important in mastication, swallowing, and speech. In addition, saliva contains amylase, an important enzyme that functions in the breakdown of carbohydrates and initiates digestive action in the oral cavity. Saliva also contains secretory immunoglobulin A, which is an immunoglobulin important during the immune response.

Saliva has numerous proteins—such as lysozymes, lactoperoxidase, and lactoferrin—that have antimicrobial properties.

Additionally, saliva has antibodies or immunoglobulin, such as immunoglobulin A (IgA). Saliva also contains epidermal growth factor (EGF) and nerve growth factor (NGF), which may assist in the healing of injured oral mucosa.

During most of the day and night, salivary flow is minimal. Secretion depends on gustatory and masticatory stimulation. Both taste and smell perform a major role in determining salivary flow, as do the nerve endings in the periodontal ligament and the muscles of mastication.

Duct Systems

Ducts of the smallest diameter are in direct contact with salivary acini. They become much larger as other acini empty into a collecting duct, which continues increasing in size until it enters the oral cavity. The ducts of the major glands are long, and various types of ducts are found within the glands. Many of these ducts are so small that it is difficult to visualize them microscopically.

The duct system consists of a **secretory portion**, which lies among the acinar cells, and an **excretory portion**, which lies in the connective tissue septa between the lobules and lobes of the glands. These ducts continue beyond the glands, emptying into the oral cavity (Fig. 15.11). The difference between the secretory and excretory ducts is that substances enter and leave the cells of the secretory duct by ion exchange with the adjacent blood vessels, whereas the excretory duct is simply a saliva-collecting tube. Acinar cells drain directly into **intercalated ducts**, which are low cuboidal cells (see Fig. 15.10). These secretory cells have metabolic function and contain mitochondria, rough endoplasmic reticulum, and secretory granules. Intercalated ducts also produce two growth factors, including EGF and NGF.

The intercalated duct opens directly into a larger duct called the **striated duct**. The cells of the striated duct are slightly taller and more columnar than those of the intercalated duct (see Fig. 15.11). These cells have striations caused by enfolding of the basal membrane, which increases the surface area of the cell and allows increased absorption of fluids and exchange of ions with the nearby blood vessels (Fig. 15.12). Sodium resorption and potassium secretion occur in these cells, causing changes in the saliva composition.

Both intercalated and striated ducts are part of the **intralobular duct system** located inside the lobules. In contrast, the remaining **interlobular excretory ducts** are located in the connective tissue septa between the lobules and lobes of the gland (see Fig. 15.11). As the ducts enlarge, their walls contain larger and more numerous cells, such as stratified columnar cells. Near its orifice, the duct becomes lined with stratified squamous epithelium, which is continuous with the oral epithelium. The **Stensen duct** drains the parotid gland, and the **Wharton duct** drains the submandibular gland.

CLINICAL COMMENT

The action of saliva provides an important protective function on the tooth's surface and the oral epithelium, where acids contribute to changing conditions. Saliva also contains calcium and phosphate, which aid in the remineralization of the enamel surface and reverse the action of dental caries.

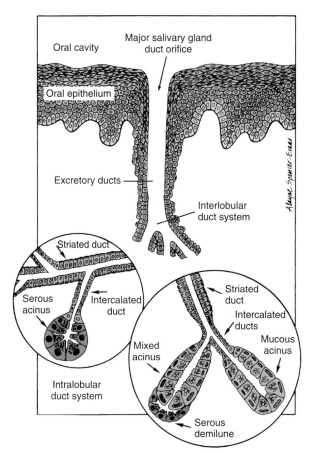

Fig. 15.11 Duct system of the salivary glands. Circles show the duct system of intralobular ducts, that is, intercalated and striated secretory ducts located within the lobule. Above are interlobular and multicelled excretory ducts located outside the lobules and lobes.

CONSIDER THE PATIENT

A patient complains of pain and tenderness on the right side of the floor of the mouth. What is the best approach in determining the cause?

Innervation of the Salivary Glands

Salivary gland secretion is regulated mostly by the postganglionic sympathetic and parasympathetic autonomic nervous system, with cell bodies located within specific ganglia of the head and neck. Histologically, stimulation of the salivary glands by sympathetic nerves results in an organic secretion (protein rich), and stimulation by the parasympathetic nerves results in a watery secretion (Fig. 15.13).

MYOEPITHELIAL CELLS

Myoepithelial cells originate from the oral epithelium at the time that the oral epithelial cells of the salivary gland grow into the mesenchyme. The cells remain on the outside of the secretory end pieces and function as muscle cells to contract and squeeze the acinus, facilitating secretion. The term *myoepithelial cells* is

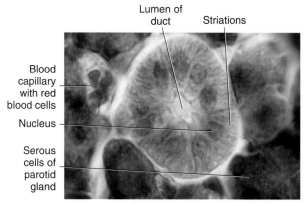

Fig. 15.12 Histology of a striated duct in center of field surrounded by parotid acinar cells. In the duct cell is the centrally located nucleus with basal striations on the periphery of each cell. These striations result from enfolding of the outer cell membrane, which provides a larger area for exchange of nutrients with adjacent vascular supply. A blood capillary can be seen on the left.

used because these cells have an epithelial origin and a muscle function. These cells have long processes that wrap around the acinar and intercalated duct cells (Figs. 15.14 and 15.15). Their large nuclei and abundant cytoplasm, containing α-smooth muscle actin, enable them to act as muscle cells. Myoepithelial cells can respond to both neurotransmitters such as acetylcholine and to hormones such as oxytocin.

CLINICAL COMMENT

Because the salivary glands can secrete proteins directly into the bloodstream and/or, using the ducts, into the mouth or gut, they provide an ideal model for showing how the insertion of a gene (e.g., that turns on a hormone) into the glandular tissue will allow the cells to synthesize a protein that the glands do not normally secrete.

CLINICAL COMMENT

Drugs such as tranquilizers, barbiturates, and antihistamines, as well as chemotherapeutic drugs and radiation therapy, decrease salivary flow. In some older patients who may already have deficient salivary flow, this could be a cause of dry mouth (xerostomia).

CLASSIFICATION OF TONSILLAR TISSUE

Tonsillar tissue surrounds the oropharynx in a ring called the **Waldeyer ring**. In the oropharyngeal midline is the single **pharyngeal tonsil** or **adenoid**, adjacent to the posterior molars are the bilateral **palatine tonsils**, and in the floor of the mouth are the bilateral **lingual tonsils** (Fig. 15.16). Tonsils are part of the lymphatic system, which also includes lymph nodes, thymus, spleen, and diffuse lymphatic tissue. Each tonsil is composed of lymphatic tissue or nodules. The lymphatic nodules, in turn, may have **germinal centers**, which are active sites of lymphocyte formation. These centers are common in the lingual and palatine tonsils. The tonsils are covered with epithelium. In the

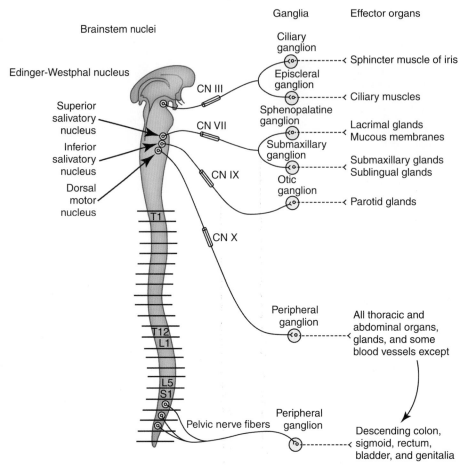

Fig. 15.13 Preganglionic and postganglionic parasympathetic innervation of various structures of the body and their target organs.

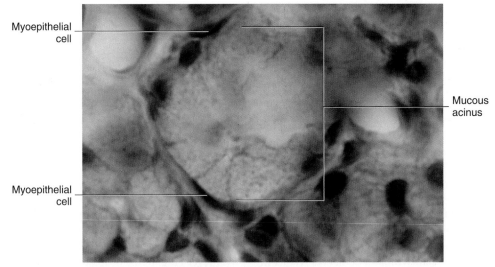

Fig. 15.14 Histology of a light-stained mucous acinus that contains mucous cells. The mucous acinus is surrounded by a myoepithelial cell.

pharyngeal tonsil, the epithelium is respiratory because the tonsil is in the nasopharynx. In the orally located palatine and lingual tonsils, it is stratified squamous epithelium. This epithelial covering lines the grooves or clefts of each gland. Unlike lymph nodes, tonsils have no afferent lymphatic vessels that lead to them. However, both tonsils and lymph nodes do have efferent

lymphatic vessels draining them. Each tonsil is supported by connective tissue and has associated glands underlying it.

Palatine Tonsils

The palatine tonsils are large in children, and these structures are best recognized when they become infected and bulge into

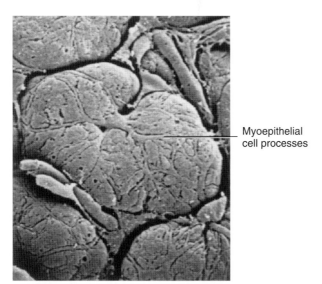

Fig. 15.15 Scanning electron micrograph of a myoepithelial cell and its cytoplasmic processes wrapping around the acinus of the submandibular gland.

Myoepithelial cell processes

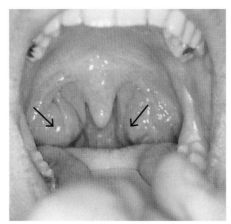

Fig. 15.17 Oral view of palatine tonsils *(arrows)*. These inflamed, swollen tonsils project into the oropharyngeal cavity.

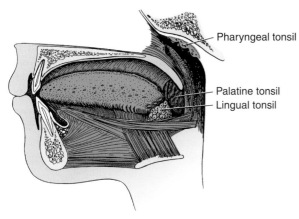

Pharyngeal tonsil

Palatine tonsil
Lingual tonsil

Fig. 15.16 Location of three tonsillar groups. The palatine tonsil is in the lateral wall of the oropharynx, the lingual tonsil is in the posterior of the tongue, and the pharyngeal tonsil is in the midline of the posterior pharyngeal wall.

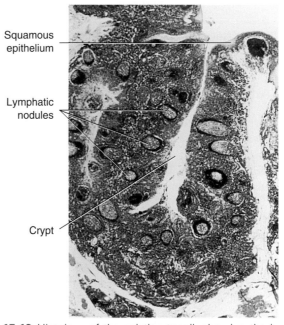

Squamous epithelium

Lymphatic nodules

Crypt

Fig. 15.18 Histology of the palatine tonsil, showing the investing squamous epithelium, deep branching crypts, and organized lymphatic nodules.

the throat, causing difficulty in swallowing. When the tonsils are infected and swollen, they appear red, with streaks of white, purulent material on their surfaces (Fig. 15.17). They become infected largely as a result of their structure. Because palatine tonsils have deep, branching crypts in which oral bacteria may become lodged, these crypts may become plugged with lymphocyte discharge and desquamated epithelial cells. Beneath the palatine tonsils are seromucous glands, which assist in flushing out these crypts. Their ducts, however, do not open into the tonsillar crypts but onto the surface of the glands. This lack of flushing action in the crypts may account for the accumulation of foreign debris and bacteria that causes tissue inflammation. Structurally, these are the largest tonsils of the three types and are divided into lobules by the crypts. Each lobule contains numerous lymphatic nodules, which contain germinal centers

(Fig. 15.18). Septa of connective tissue support the nodules of lymphatic tissue and invest the gland in a capsule.

Lingual Tonsils

Lingual tonsils are located on the surface of the posterior third of the tongue (see Fig. 15.14). The tonsillar mass is bilateral because it is divided in the midline, reflecting the bilateral origin of the tongue. The lingual tonsils are composed of wide-mouthed crypts and are nonbranching. They form rows of lymphatic nodules supported by connective tissue septa that are present in each lobule of the gland (Fig. 15.19). These tonsils also have a connective tissue capsule investing them. The capsule is covered with nonkeratinized stratified squamous epithelium. Underlying these tonsils, between the mucous glands, are skeletal muscles and adipose tissue of the tongue. These mucous

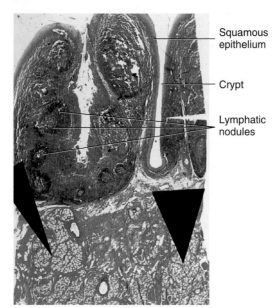

Fig. 15.19 Histology of the lingual tonsil on the posterior tongue. Observe the investing squamous epithelium, short crypts, and lymphatic nodules. *Arrows* denote underlying mucous glands.

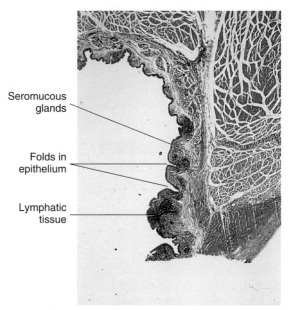

Fig. 15.20 Histologic appearance of the pharyngeal tonsil. Observe the folds in the epithelium rather than crypts in tissue, diffuse lymphatic tissue rather than nodules, and seromucous glands underlying the tonsillar tissue.

glands, with their ducts opening into the crypt, function in a cleansing action. Also, because these tonsils are located in the posterior floor of the mouth, the washing action of saliva provides effective cleansing. Therefore this tonsillar mass is rarely inflamed.

Pharyngeal Tonsil

The pharyngeal tonsil, or **adenoid**, is located in the posterior wall of the superior portion of the nasopharynx. It is subject to infection in childhood. The pharyngeal tonsil may grow laterally from the midline location to surround the opening of the eustachian tubes. Tonsillar tissue at this location is called the *tubal tonsil* and can be the source of infection to the eustachian tubes. The pharyngeal tonsil is unlike the other tonsils in that it is an aggregation of lymphocytes that does not have crypts but has occasional folds that appear as clefts in the mucosa (Fig. 15.20). This tonsil is variable in structure because only occasionally are there lymphoid nodules, which are usually only on a surface accumulation of diffuse lymphoid tissue. The covering epithelium is transformed either into respiratory or stratified squamous epithelium. Underlying the tonsil are mixed glands that drain the surface of the epithelium overlying the gland tissue. This tonsil overlies the muscles of the pharynx.

FUNCTION OF TONSILS

The most notable function of tonsils is the production of lymphocytes that protect the body from foreign microorganisms inhaled or swallowed. Allergens may be sensed by these cells, which start the complex process of coding for antibody production. Because of their ability to retain this information, the lymphocytes have been called **memory cells**. Some lymphocytes transform into **T cells** and engulf bacteria or discharge

substances to destroy them. Other lymphocytes become **B cells**, which differentiate into plasma cells. Plasma cells secrete antibodies that destroy antigens. Plasma cells and lymphocytes are found in chronic infections, such as periodontal disease. Plasma cells found in the area of the salivary glands produce IgA, which joins in the end piece of the intercellular area to form secretory IgA. Some foreign substances are absorbed from the crypts of the glands into the gland proper and are then destroyed.

SELF-EVALUATION QUESTIONS

1. Discuss the location and function of the myoepithelial cells.
2. Describe the types of secretory duct cells and their functions.
3. What are the contributions of the major and minor salivary glands to the total volume of saliva?
4. Compare the appearance and function of serous and mucous cells.
5. Where are most serous demilune cells found?
6. What is the origin of secretory IgA?
7. Name and describe the various types of minor salivary glands.
8. Describe the gland type underlying each tonsil.
9. How does gland structure relate to the causes of tonsillitis?
10. What is the function of B and T cells in the tonsils?

CLINICAL COMMENT

Tonsils are ideally positioned around the entrance to the alimentary canal to aid in protecting the body from invasion of microorganisms. They are important in the antibacterial action of the B and T lymphocytes and in the action of the plasma cells in the formation of secretory IgA, which neutralizes viruses and can be an antibody to food antigens.

CONSIDER THE PATIENT

The dentist must examine the mouth carefully, and radiographs should be taken. Radiographs may reveal a stone in the submandibular duct, which is the most common site for a stone. Such a stone will interfere with salivary gland function and should be removed. Palpation by the dentist could assist the stone in passing through the duct.

QUANDARIES IN SCIENCE

In addition to saliva, salivary glands are important for providing many other substances that help maintain and protect the various structures in the oral cavity. Growth factors synthesized and secreted by the submandibular gland—EGF, fibroblast growth factor, and NGF—have a multitude of functions at the local level and at distant sites. In addition to growth factors, salivary glands, in combination with the tonsils, play a major role in mounting an effective immunologic response to the invasion of foreign substances. During radiation treatment for cancer in the orofacial region, salivary function is often reduced, and the patient experiences many negative sequelae. With proper diagnosis and treatment, many of the concerns (e.g., reduced saliva production and increased caries) can be alleviated. However, the immunologic and growth factor functions are usually not restored. Whether the introduction of bioengineered organs will be able to restore function and therefore provide a higher quality of life is a question that only the future can answer.

CLINICAL CASE

A 35-year-old man presents at the dentist's office with swelling in the region of the submandibular gland that he first noticed 2 weeks earlier. The swelling was initially asymptomatic but became increasingly tender with time and prompted the appointment. The extraoral exam confirms swelling and tenderness over the submandibular gland upon palpation. An obvious redness at the external orifice of the submandibular gland and an apparent reduced amount of salivary secretion were demonstrated on completion of the intraoral exam. Radiographs showed a radiodense structure within the submandibular duct. When palpated, a hard, slightly movable lump was found, suggestive of a sialolith (salivary stone) lodged in the submandibular duct. The patient was told to remain hydrated and return if the pain increased.

The patient presented again with increased swelling and pain. The patient was referred to an oral surgeon, who cannulated the duct and was able to extract the stone without further complications. When the patient returned to the oral surgeon in a week, the swelling and inflammation had subsided, as had the pain, and the patient was discharged.

Salivary stones are more prevalent in males than females in patients between the ages of 30 and 60. The exact etiology of sialoliths is unknown, but some predisposing factors include diet, Sjögren syndrome, and dehydration concomitant to the use of particular pharmaceuticals. Complications can include bacterial infection due to stasis of the salivary secretion contaminated with pathogenic bacteria from the oral cavity. The submandibular gland is the most susceptible to sialoliths, followed by the parotid and sublingual salivary glands. Treatment can vary from increased water intake to surgical extraction and/or lithotripsy (breakup of the salivary stones by focused external ultrasonic therapy). Recurrence of salivary stones is unusual except in cases of underlying systemic diseases associated with mineral, especially calcium and phosphate, metabolism.

SUGGESTED READING

Arens R, Marcus CL. Pathophysiology of upper airway obstruction: a developmental perspective. *Sleep.* 2004;27(5):997–1019.

Arvidsson A, Löfgren CD, Christersson CE, et al. Characterisation of structures in salivary secretion film formation. An experimental study with atomic force microscopy. . *Biofouling.* 2004;20(3):181–188.

Bradley RM. Salivary secretion. In: Getchell TV, et al., ed. *Smell and taste in health and disease.* New York: Raven Press; 1991.

Castle D. Cell biology of salivary protein. In: Dobrosielski-Vergona K, ed. *Biology of the salivary glands.* Boca Raton, FL: CRC Press; 1993.

Drummond JR, Chrisholm DM. A qualitative and quantitative study of the ageing human labial salivary glands. *Arch Oral Biol.* 1984;29:151–155.

Ekström J. Autonomic control of salivary secretion. *Proc Finn Dent Soc.* 1989;85(4-5):323–331. [discussion: 361–363].

Emmelin N, Gjörstrup P. On the function of myoepithelial cells in salivary glands. *J Physiol.* 1973;230(1):185–198.

Field A, Scot J. Changes in the structure of salivary glands with age. In: Dobrosielski-Vergona K, ed. *Biology of the salivary glands.* Boca Raton, FL: CRC Press; 1993.

Fukami H, Bradley RM. Biophysical and morphological properties of parasympathetic neurons controlling the parotid and von Ebner salivary glands in rats. *J Neurophysiol.* 2005;93(2):678–686.

Gershan LA, Durham PL, Skidmore J, et al. The role of salivary neuropeptides in pediatrics: potential biomarkers for integrated therapies. *Eur J Integr Med.* 2015;7(4):372–377.

Haberman AS, Isaac DD, Andrew DJ. Specification of cell fates within the salivary gland primordium. *Dev Biol.* 2003;258(2):443–453.

Jaskoll T, Zhou YM, Chai Y, et al. Embryonic submandibular gland morphogenesis: stage-specific protein localization of FGFs, BMPs, Pax6 and Pax9 in normal mice and abnormal SMG phenotypes in FgfR2-IIIc(+/Delta), BMP7 (–/–) and Pax6(–/–) mice. *Cells Tissues Organs.* 2002;170(2-3):83–98.

Joraku A, Sullivan CA, Yoo JJ, et al. Tissue engineering of functional salivary gland tissue. *Laryngoscope.* 2005;115(2):244–248.

Kagami H, Hiramatsu Y, Hishida S, et al. Salivary growth factors in health and disease. *Adv Dent Res.* 2000;14:99–102.

Kim M, Chiego Jr DJ, Bradley RM. Ionotropic glutamate receptor expression in preganglionic neurons of the rat inferior salivatory nucleus. *Auton Neurosci.* 2008;138(1-2):83–90.

Kim M, Chiego Jr DJ, Bradley RM. Morphology of parasympathetic neurons innervating the lingual salivary glands. *Auton Neurosci.* 2004;111:27–36.

Ozbilgin MK, Polat S, Mete UO, et al. Antigen-presenting cells in the hypertrophic pharyngeal tonsils: a histochemical, immunohistochemical and ultrastructural study. *J Investig Allergol Clin Immunol.* 2004;14(4):320–328.

Passàli D, Damiani V, Passàli GC, et al. Structural and immunological characteristics of chronically inflamed adenotonsillar tissue in childhood. *Clin Diagn Lab Immunol.* 2004;11(6):1154–1157.

Quissell DO. Stimulus exocytosis coupling mechanism in salivary gland cells. In: Dobrosielski-Vergona K, ed. *Biology of the salivary glands.* Boca Raton, FL: CRC Press; 1993.

Rice DH, Becker TS. *The salivary glands.* New York: Thieme Medical; 1994.

Richards AT, Digges N, Norton NS, et al. Surgical anatomy of the parotid duct with emphasis on the major tributaries forming the duct and the relationship of the facial nerve to the duct. *Clin Anat.* 2004;17(6):463–467.

Riva A, Puxeddu R, Loy F, et al. Serous and mucous cells of human submandibular salivary gland stimulated in vitro by isoproterenol, carbachol, and clozapine: an LM, TEM, and HRSEM study. *Eur J Morphol*. 2003;41(2):83–87.

Shear M. The structure and function of myoepithelial cells in salivary glands. *Arch Oral Biol*. 1966;11(8):769–778.

Ship JA, Hu K. Radiotherapy-induced salivary dysfunction. *Semin Oncol*. 2004;31(6 suppl 18):29–36.

Skinner LJ, Winter DC, Curran AJ, et al. Helicobacter pylori and tonsillectomy. *Clin Otolaryngol Allied Sci*. 2001;26(6):505–509.

Turner RJ. Mechanisms of fluid secretion by salivary glands. *Ann N Y Acad Sci*. 1993;694:24–35.

Webb CJ, Osman E, Ghosh SK, et al. Tonsillar size is an important indicator of recurrent acute tonsillitis. *Clin Otolaryngol Allied Sci*. 2004;29(4):369–371.

Zhang PC, Pang YT, Loh KS, et al. Comparison of histology between recurrent tonsillitis and tonsillar hypertrophy. *Clin Otolaryngol Allied Sci*. 2003;28(3):235–239.

16

Biofilms

LEARNING OBJECTIVES

- Define the origin and components of cuticle.
- Discuss the composition of acquired pellicle and plaque.
- Describe the location and composition of calculus.
- Explain why saliva is important in determining oral health.

OVERVIEW

This chapter describes substances that form on the surface of the teeth and explains how they develop. Microbial biofilms are a major concern today because they are also associated with implantable medical devices. The dental plaque is composed of a biofilm. It is important that this biofilm is characterized because it exists on the surface of the body and is capable of being analyzed, characterized, and treated with known agents. The primary cuticle is of cellular origin and is formed before tooth eruption. All other products originate from saliva. The primary cuticle forms the zone of junctional epithelium; the remaining epithelium is lost soon after the teeth erupt into incisal or occlusal contact. Saliva contains salivary proteins and glycoproteins that attach to enamel or exposed cementum or dentin. Saliva then deposits a thin protein coat or membrane, called a *pellicle*, on the surface of the tooth. The pellicle, although protective to the tooth, allows plaque to form on the surface of the tooth. This plaque is composed of bacteria and salivary proteins that will become a dense layer that gradually accumulates on the tooth's surface if not removed. The bacteria in plaque may produce acid that can cause etching and disintegration of the tooth's surface. This leads to the initiation of dental caries. Dental caries therefore develops in areas where brushing or washing of the tooth's surface does not occur. In other instances, plaque may not produce acid but may become mineralized into calculus. Calculus forms by mineralization of the remaining plaque bacteria into a hydroxyapatite deposit on the enamel and exposed cementum surfaces. Continuous acquisition of calculus forms a thick deposit that should be removed because the potential for inflammation or infection of gingival tissue could lead to destructive periodontal disease.

ORAL BIOFILMS

Biofilms are highly complex and heterogeneous communities of microbial organisms that colonize living and nonliving surfaces in specific and predictable ways. These communities develop and change in character, and microbial inhabitants dependent on time, nutrient availability, waste exchange, pH, temperature, oxygen availability, type of substrate, and other factors. Biofilms are significant in dentistry, medicine, the food industry, and aquaculture.

In the oral cavity, biofilms, or dental plaque, form on hard and soft tissues such as the teeth and oral mucosal surfaces. However, they also form on dental restorative materials such as composite resin, gold alloys, glass ionomer, porcelain, and amalgam alloys. Oral biofilms are multispecies aggregates of microorganisms embedded in an extracellular polymeric substance, or exopolysaccharide (EPS), layered onto a surface. The EPS is a matrix of biopolymers consisting of polysaccharides, proteins, glycolipids, glycoproteins, and, in some cases, extracellular DNA. The EPS influences the immediate surroundings of the biofilm residents by modifying the porosity, density, stability, water content, and other properties of the matrix. In contrast, the sum total of microorganisms in the oral cavity is referred to as the oral microbiome or as "all microorganisms that are found on or in the human oral cavity and its contiguous extensions" (Dewhirst 2010).

Generally, oral biofilms are beneficial to oral health. Oral biofilms maintain the balance of healthy oral flora, limit the growth of pathogenic flora, aid in the host immune recognition of foreign substances, and provide a potential reservoir for fluoride. However, oral biofilms can also pose challenges for the host, such as increased antimicrobial resistance.

Microbial organisms are dependent on the salivary pellicle to begin the process of biofilm formation. The salivary pellicle is formed by the adsorption of salivary constituents such as proteins, lipids, and carbohydrates to teeth, mucosa, and dental restorative materials. The salivary pellicle mediates biofilm initiation by attachment of microbial components to the pellicle constituents. Early microbial adhesion is reversible and not very specific, but later microbial adhesion is irreversible due to specific mechanisms, such as those involving adhesin binding.

There are four main criteria used to describe a biofilm: constituents, quantity, structure, and function. These four criteria can be used to characterize a biofilm and predict its behavior in response to changes in the environment or the host (Lin 2004).

Constituent microorganisms include archaea, viruses, bacteria, and fungi, delicately balanced with environmental and host conditions to maintain health. However, if the balance is disrupted, one constituent can increase in number, change its genetic expression, or alter its metabolic activity to modify pathogenicity and facilitate disease. Indeed, the biofilm is the source of organisms implicated in the two most common infectious diseases in dentistry: dental caries and periodontal disease. Identifying the constituents of human oral biofilms is complex; some common methods used include culture-based and biochemical methods. The challenge remains to identify those organisms that are viable but not culturable (VBNC), or persister cells, particularly those persister cells that may be involved in local or distant pathology.

Quantity can refer to an absolute count or relative amount, and it can be measured directly or indirectly. An *absolute count* of cells in the biofilm can be extrapolated from a count of cells in a given, known area. An *indirect count* refers to an extrapolation from a count of a specific cellular component in aggregate. There is also a *differential count*, both absolute and relative, typically used when comparing constituent populations of cells within a biofilm, particularly in response to an environmental or host change. *Viable cell count* is also used but may exclude cells such as persister cells, depending on the detection method utilized. Overall measurement of the oral biofilm (biomass) is typically the easiest because it does not discriminate for the more challenging organisms, such as VBNC cells. Biomass measurements are used when investigating methods of biofilm elimination or dispersal.

The structure of the biofilm reflects the constituent microorganisms and characteristics, such as cell-to-cell proximity, thereby influencing interactions such as gene transfer, quorum sensing, and resource allocation and competition. Oxygen tension, substrate type, time, and nutrient availability are some conditions that affect the population and therefore the structure of the biofilm. In fact, oral biofilm constituents are characterized into early and late colonizers as components of a multispecies architecture that matures over time. The structure also influences the ability of antimicrobials to penetrate the structure to successfully target the intended organisms.

Functions of the oral biofilm include viability, metabolic activity, chemical signaling, gene expression, and acid production, among others. Many of these functions are affected by nutrient availability, waste elimination, oxygen tension, temperature, and pH. In oral biofilms, acid production has been highly studied in caries susceptibility and formation in tooth enamel.

CUTICLE

The **primary** or **developmental cuticle** is deposited on the enamel's surface by the ameloblasts as their last function shortly before the tooth crown erupts into the oral cavity. At this time, the formed enamel has reached a thickness of 2 to 2.5 mm over the cusps and is fully mineralized. In their final action, the ameloblasts secrete a thin, structureless protein membrane on the tooth's surface. On the outer surface of this cuticle is the remainder of the enamel organ cells, termed the **reduced enamel epithelium**. This cellular membrane on the tooth's surface includes the ameloblasts and other remnants of the enamel organ. Ameloblasts form the primary cuticle.

The reduced enamel epithelium is lost during eruption of the teeth in the oral cavity (Fig. 16.1). Only the developmental cuticle remains on the surface of the tooth as it erupts into occlusal function. However, this cuticle is not present long on the enamel, because abrasion from contact of the opposing teeth causes it to wear away. Only the part covering the enamel in the gingival crevice remains (Fig. 16.2). This membrane serves as an attachment of the gingival junctional epithelial cells to the tooth. The sulcular epithelium is continually forming protein, which renews the gingival attachment throughout its life. **Cuticular protein**, which initiates attachment of the junctional epithelium to enamel, is the most important function of the primary cuticle.

ACQUIRED PELLICLE

When the tooth's surface is cleansed, salivary proteins and glycoproteins are quickly deposited with their strong attraction for the enamel surface. The resulting layer forms a thin, structureless membrane about 0.5 to 1.0 mm thick, which is in contrast to the previously formed cuticular layer. This membrane is termed the **pellicle** or **acquired pellicle** (Fig. 16.3). Although the pellicle is bacteria-free when formed, bacteria rapidly attach to its surface. The pellicle covers the entire free surface of the enamel and may penetrate any convenient defect in the tooth's surface, such as a crack, a pit, or an overhanging restoration (Fig. 16.4). Normally, surface layers of enamel rods are straight and at right angles to the tooth surface. The zone is about 30 mm thick, with the long axis of the apatite crystals oriented nearly perpendicular to the enamel surface. This area is termed the **prismless zone**

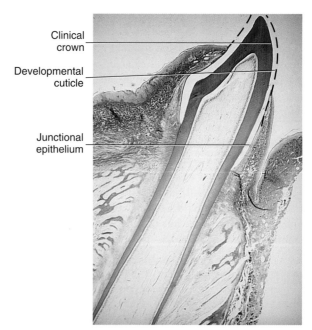

Fig. 16.1 Histology of an erupting crown. Enamel is covered with a developmental cuticle at that time.

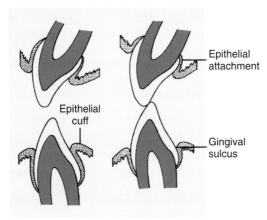

Fig. 16.2 Diagram of an erupting tooth showing the position of the gingiva and epithelial attachment on the cervical enamel.

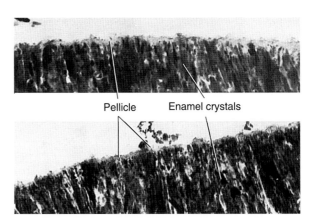

Fig. 16.4 Electron micrograph showing two areas of newly formed bacteria-free acquired pellicle on the enamel's surface (prismless zone of enamel).

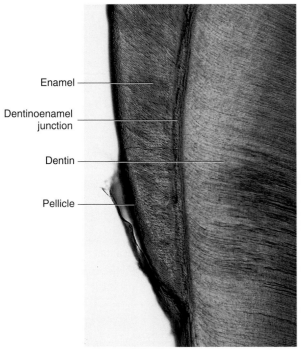

Fig. 16.3 Histology of an enamel surface and structureless organic pellicle, which covers enamel rods, in this case, at the cervical area.

of enamel. The acquired pellicle overlying this zone has a fine, granular appearance and is approximately 500 Å thick when viewed in ultrastructure (see Fig. 16.4). If the pellicle is lost as a result of an oral prophylaxis, it forms again in a few minutes. Although the acquired pellicle is considered protective to the enamel surface, it does provide an attachment site for bacteria, which form plaque.

> **CLINICAL COMMENT**
>
> The acquired pellicle provides an ideal location for attachment of bacteria. During early adherence, the bacteria are mostly aerobic cocci, but over time, the ecology changes to rods and filamentous forms.

> **CLINICAL COMMENT**
>
> The bathing of the tooth's surface with saliva causes formation of a thin organic membrane, the pellicle, which in part protects the tooth's surface from the action of oral bacteria. Oral bacteria lodge anywhere there is a crevice or other defect and can attach and penetrate the pellicle, causing enamel dissolution by acid production.

PLAQUE

The central fissure of a molar, premolar, or cervical margin of any tooth is the site for accumulation and colonization of oral organisms (Fig. 16.5). In addition to bacteria that attach to the pellicle, lymphocytes, leukocytes, desquamated epithelial cells, and clumps of mucin may lodge in any of these sites (Figs. 16.6 and 16.7). Organisms attach to the pellicle and utilize the presence of debris in acid formation.

In gingival or tonsillar inflammation, the number of lymphocytes and leukocytes increases (Fig. 16.8). If microscopic analysis of a saliva sample reveals many lymphocytes, tonsillitis is present. However, an increase in leukocytes in saliva is indicative of gingival inflammation. These cells are called **salivary corpuscles** (Fig. 16.9). At first, only a few bacteria are on the pellicle, but they rapidly grow into a thick **plaque** that contains a variety of microorganisms. The initial plaque quickly changes in composition to include rods and filamentous organisms. These appear after a few days, as shown in Fig. 16.10.

The composition of plaque depends also on the extent of gingival disease and whether the location of the plaque is supragingival or subgingival. The initial carious lesions affect the prismless zone of enamel because plaque bacteria cause dissolution of these surface crystals. A breakdown of enamel crystals is seen clinically as a brown spot on the tooth's surface. Fig. 16.11 shows a microscopic view of the loss of enamel rod structure. The enamel pellicle may overlie the area of an early lesion on the tooth's surface and may be covered by plaque bacteria. Such a lesion may become filled with organic debris and bacteria (Fig. 16.12). Crystals appear to dissolve in one area and be intact in an adjacent area of enamel. Plaque can best be seen when a **disclosing solution** (0.2% basic fuchsin or erythrosine red No. 3 dye) is used to determine whether all the plaque has been removed. The advantage of using No. 3 dye is that it does not permanently discolor composite restorations or clothing. The stain left after a quick rinsing reveals any remaining plaque deposits, as observed in Fig. 16.13. These visible deposits can be removed by further polishing.

CALCULUS

Calculus is a stonelike concretion that forms on teeth or dental prostheses. It is primarily composed of calcium phosphate in the form of **hydroxyapatite**, which develops on the organic cell walls of bacterial plaque. Calculus formation is the reverse of enamel surface demineralization.

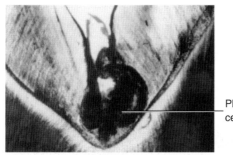

Plaque in central fissure

Fig. 16.5 Incipient carious lesion in a central fissure of enamel in a human molar. Plaque has accumulated in this area.

CLINICAL COMMENT

Deposition of calculus can occur when the bacteria become calcified, forming a stonelike deposit. A disclosing agent can expose plaque bacteria to facilitate their removal, but plaque will reappear unless appropriate preventive oral hygiene is practiced. The removal of plaque is therefore important in the prevention of gingival and periodontal disease.

Calculus appears on the teeth most often near the opening of the parotid excretory duct on the buccal surfaces of maxillary molars and on the lingual surfaces of the lingual incisors near the openings of the submandibular and lingual ducts. After plaque accumulates, mineralization begins in the inner layer of the pellicle and then spreads into the overlying plaque. Plaque

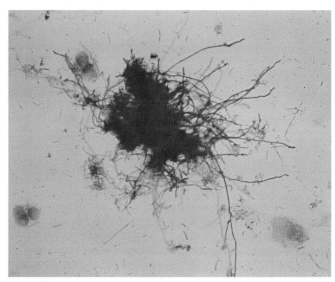

Fig. 16.7 Clumps of mucin from saliva that may adhere to crevices or imperfections in enamel's surface.

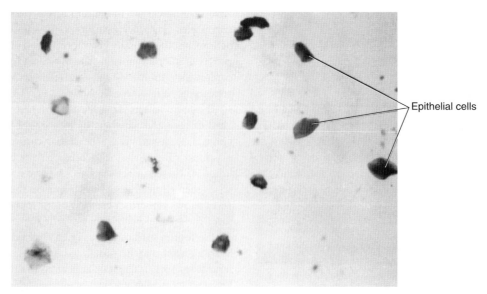

Epithelial cells

Fig. 16.6 A salivary smear viewed microscopically showing the presence of desquamated epithelial cells.

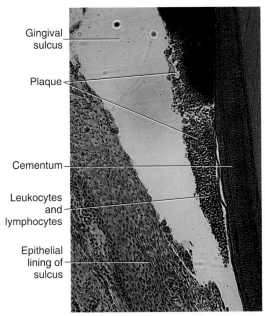

Fig. 16.8 The gingival sulcus viewed microscopically. Leukocytes and lymphocytes appear along the surface of the sulcus and tooth.

Gingival sulcus

Plaque

Cementum

Leukocytes and lymphocytes

Epithelial lining of sulcus

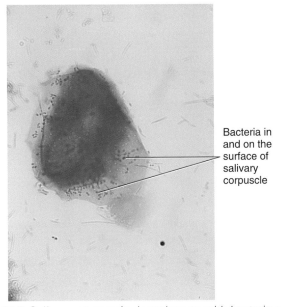

Bacteria in and on the surface of salivary corpuscle

Fig. 16.9 Salivary corpuscle. Lymphocyte with bacteria on its surface as present in saliva.

continues to thicken, with further deposition of plaque protein. The calcified bacteria appear as circular profiles (Fig. 16.14) and are known as bacterial ghosts.

CLINICAL COMMENT

Salivary calculus is damaging to the gingival tissues and should be removed by scaling. This scaling is frequently accompanied by bleeding of the gingival tissues. The gingiva heals rapidly, however, and the bleeding soon abates.

Calculus deposition follows any surface irregularity of the tooth, such as enamel or cementum (Fig. 16.15). Therefore

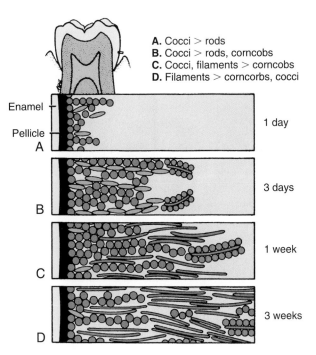

A. Cocci > rods
B. Cocci > rods, corncobs
C. Cocci, filaments > corncobs
D. Filaments > corncorbs, cocci

Enamel

Pellicle

A — 1 day

B — 3 days

C — 1 week

D — 3 weeks

Fig. 16.10 Changes in plaque composition over a 3-week period. A, At 1 day. **B,** At 3 days, the cocci and a few filaments characterize the plaque. **C,** After 1 week, the filamentous organisms increase in number. **D,** By 3 weeks, the filamentous organisms predominate in the plaque. (Avery JK. *Oral development and histology.* 3rd ed. Stuttgart: Thieme Medical; 2002, with modification.)

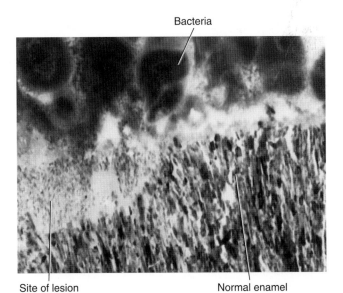

Bacteria

Site of lesion   Normal enamel

Fig. 16.11 Electron micrograph of bacterial effects on the enamel surface. An initial lesion is shown in the enamel surface *(at left)*. Notice the loss of enamel crystals. (Avery JK. *Oral development and histology.* 3rd ed. Stuttgart: Thieme Medical; 2002.)

calculus forms in a calcospherite manner as the calcium salts derived from saliva organize in the organic skeletons of plaque bacteria. As the plaque calcifies, it loses its ability to produce an acid environment.

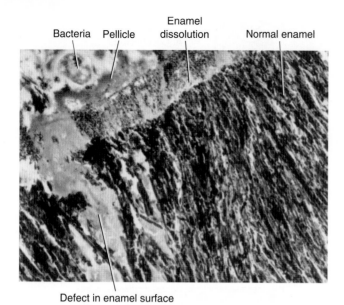

Fig. 16.12 Electron micrograph of a penetrating carious lesion appearing in the enamel *(left)*. Initial enamel dissolution and normal enamel under the pellicle and plaque are shown *(upper right)*. (Avery JK. *Oral development and histology*. 3rd ed. Stuttgart: Thieme Medical; 2002.)

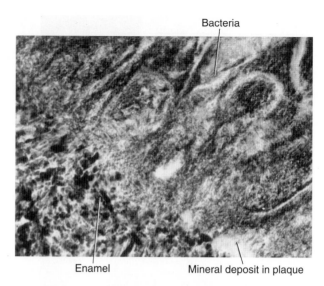

Fig. 16.14 Calculus formation viewed by electron microscopy. Minute mineral crystals fill circular bacterial ghosts on enamel surface. (Avery JK. *Oral development and histology*. 3rd ed. Stuttgart: Thieme Medical; 2002.)

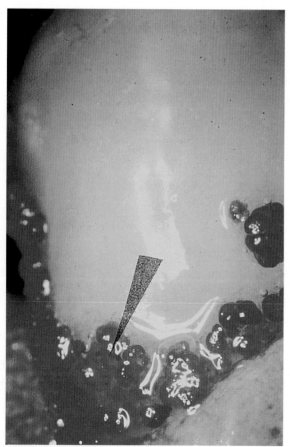

Fig. 16.13 View of gingival crevice area and tooth surface after use of disclosing solution, with areas of stained plaque indicated by the *arrowhead*.

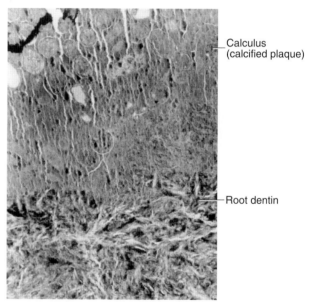

Fig. 16.15 Calculus on an irregular surface of dentin. Minute mineral crystals are in calculus *(above)*, with larger crystals in dentin *(below)*. (Avery JK. *Oral development and histology*. 3rd ed. Stuttgart: Thieme Medical; 2002.)

Calculus varies in both composition and hardness. Harder calculus contains more mineral matter. Calculus may develop above the gingival margin or within the gingival crevice. Subgingival calculus is much harder and forms more slowly than supragingival calculus. Subgingival calculus is referred to as **serumal calculus** and is usually darker because it contains serum and blood pigments.

Typical bacteria and calculus appear in the gingival crevice (Fig. 16.16). Gram-positive organisms appear in the supragingival area, and gram-negative organisms are in the subgingival area (Fig. 16.17). This is because gram-positive organisms are aerobic, or live in air, whereas gram-negative organisms are anaerobic, or function best without air. Bacterial action and the deposits result in gingival inflammation, affecting the location of the gingival attachment to the cementum rather than the cervical enamel.

A List (some but not all) of Viral Infections Affecting the Oral Facial Region and is based after Thakkar P, Banks J, Rahat R, et al. Viruses of the oral cavity: prevalence, pathobiology and association with oral diseases. *Rev Med Virol.* 2022;32(4):e2311. https://doi.org/10.1002/rmv.2311

HERPES SIMPLEX VIRUS

Herpes simplex virus (HSV) is one of the most prevalent and common viral infections of the orofacial region. The infection can be induced by many different factors, including stress, fever, cold, and systemic disease. HSV resides predominantly in the trigeminal ganglion and can travel down the axon to affect the mucosa by causing ulcerations, which can be severe. Most cases are resolved in 5 to 7 days, but recurrent infections are common and usually manifest at the vermilion border of the lips.

HUMAN CYTOMEGALOVIRUS

Human cytomegalovirus (HCMV) can be found residing in the cells of the salivary glands and endothelium when in an inactive form. When active, the infection is often asymptomatic, but it can induce fever and joint and muscle pain, among other symptoms. HCMV is commonly associated with patients with acquired immunodeficiency syndrome (AIDS) and/or patients

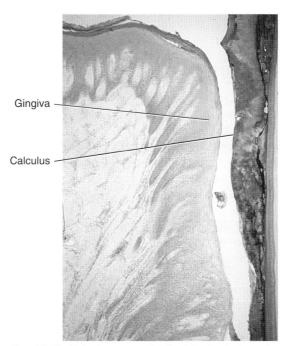

Gingiva

Calculus

Fig. 16.16 Calculus appearing in this gingival crevice will relate to pocket formation.

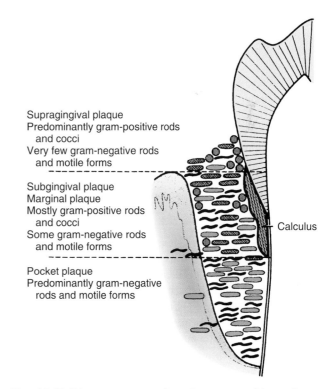

Supragingival plaque
Predominantly gram-positive rods and cocci
Very few gram-negative rods and motile forms

Subgingival plaque
Marginal plaque
Mostly gram-positive rods and cocci
Some gram-negative rods and motile forms

Pocket plaque
Predominantly gram-negative rods and motile forms

Calculus

Fig. 16.17 Diagram comparing the composition of supragingival plaque organisms with subgingival organisms. Deep in the pocket are gram-negative rods and motile spirochetes. Gram-positive rods are in the area of the supragingival and gingival margin. (Avery JK. *Oral development and histology.* 3rd ed. Stuttgart: Thieme Medical; 2002, with modification.)

who are immunocompromised. Oral lesions are prevalent in the above patients.

PAPILLOMAVIRUSES 16 AND 18

Papillomaviruses have been shown to induce cervical carcinoma, anal carcinoma, oropharyngeal carcinoma, and penile carcinoma. Human papillomavirus (HPV) is the most common often sexually transmitted virus in the world. Due to the development of a vaccine against HPV, which prevents approximately 80% of the cases, there has been a significant decline in diseases caused by HPV.

SEVERE ACUTE RESPIRATORY SYNDROME CORONAVIRUS 2

SARS-CoV-2 is a virus that causes COVID-19. SARS-CoV-2 is one of the members of the *Coronaviridae* family. This virus can spread rapidly and can invade many different species besides humans. SARS-CoV-2 is very contagious and can rapidly spread from an infected to uninfected person. SARS-CoV-2 is responsible for the latest pandemic, which as of 2023 is ongoing but diminishing.

The viral genome is large and contains genetic information used for synthesizing viral structural proteins and viral replication. The viral genome encodes for proteins, including the spike and membrane glycoproteins and envelope and nucleocapsid proteins. The S protein of the virus allows interactions with target host cells through a transmembrane, cellular receptor, and regulator protein called angiotensin-converting enzyme 2 (ACE2). Some of the most innovative vaccines have targeted the spike protein and ACE2.

Children under the age of 12 can be asymptomatic, although some display mild, flulike symptoms. Some symptoms of SARS-CoV-2 include fever, headache, cough, difficulty breathing, sore throat, loss of taste or smell, diarrhea, and confusion. Individuals with preexisting medical conditions are at greater risk for experiencing more severe symptoms. Some patients exhibit more severe symptoms and require hospital intensive care.

HIV

Human immunodeficiency virus (HIV) is divided into types 1 and 2 (HIV-1 and HIV-2). The genome contains twin single-stranded RNA molecules. The surface molecule on the mature HIV particle binds to the CD4 receptor on the host cell, which can include T helper cells, macrophages, dendritic cells, and astrocytes. HIV enters the human body through intact mucous membranes, injured skin, or mucosa, or by injection. Symptoms after 3 to 6 weeks include fever, lymph node enlargement, fatigue, malaise, rash with small slightly raised lesions, and gastrointestinal issues. These symptoms usually last around 2 to 6 weeks. After initial symptoms, the second phase is largely asymptomatic and can last for several years.

People with HIV are susceptible to chronic dry mouth, gingivitis, periodontitis, canker sores, oral warts, oral candidiasis, dental caries, herpetic ulcers, HPV lesions, and diseases of the salivary glands. Chronic dry mouth is common and can lead to increased caries and tooth decay. Aphthous ulcers can be found on the tongue, cheeks, and lips. Oral warts can also be found on the inside of the lips and the oral cavity.

ENTEROVIRUS

Human enteroviruses (EV) induce ulcers and blisters on the soft palate, tonsils, and posterior pharynx within the oral cavity. Current research on EV has not shown any positive correlations between EV and specific oral disease.

COXSACKIEVIRUS

Coxsackieviruses consist of single-stranded positive-sense RNA viruses. Coxsackievirus infections are common during early childhood and can range from being asymptomatic and mild to life-threatening. Symptoms include aseptic meningitis, febrile rash, respiratory tract disease, epidemic myalgia, acute hemorrhagic conjunctivitis, and severe sepsis illness in newborns.

Regarding the oral cavity specifically, coxsackievirus is the most common cause of hand, foot, and mouth disease (HFMD), specifically coxsackievirus A16 and enterovirus A71.

ECHOVIRUS

Echoviruses are single-stranded RNA viruses that belong to the *Picornaviridae* family, of which echoviruses make up the largest subgroup. Echoviruses cause many common human illnesses, such as meningitis, encephalitis, and rashes. Despite being widespread and having clinical importance, little is known about their pathobiology. HFMD is a common illness, with symptoms like fever, oral sores, and rashes with blisters, often seen in children under the age of 10.

ENTEROVIRUS

EVs are the most common human viruses. EVs are known to be transmitted through the fecal–oral route. These viruses are also responsible for several diseases in humans, including the common cold, HFMD, myocarditis, acute hemorrhagic conjunctivitis, encephalitis, and poliomyelitis. HFMD is most commonly caused by an enteroviral infection and can be characterized by stomatitis with ulcers on the tongue, gums, and inside buccal mucosa.

SUMMARY

The presence of viruses and their persistence in oral tissues suggest that viruses have a predilection for oral cells. Our understanding is limited regarding cells that are critical to viral tenacity in oral diseases like periodontitis, periapical periodontitis, pulpitis, and periimplantitis, which have multimicrobial etiology.

Despite the prevalence and number of viral infections and oral diseases worldwide, we still are not fully cognizant of how viruses affect oral diseases. Many virus families have not been studied in depth in the context of oral diseases. Though we still lack knowledge surrounding viral activity and mechanisms of action, we must not underestimate the role that viruses play in perturbing oral tissue structure. To gain a better understanding of how viruses in the oral cavity behave, we will need to have a stronger commitment to basic and translational research efforts to develop new drugs and therapeutic methods.

SELF-EVALUATION QUESTIONS

1. Describe the changes that occur in plaque from 1 day to 3 weeks.
2. Define salivary corpuscles.
3. On what matrix does calculus form?
4. Name and characterize the outermost layer of enamel.
5. What types of bacteria are seen supragingivally and subgingivally?
6. Where does plaque usually form?
7. What are the components of a pellicle?
8. How long does it take an acquired pellicle to form?
9. What is one way to determine if all plaque has been removed from the teeth?
10. What is the difference between serumal and salivary calculus?

CLINICAL CASE

A 56-year-old man presents with acute, sharp pain in the upper right quadrant of the maxilla. After appropriate diagnostic procedures and a thorough health history, the dentist determines that the second maxillary molar could have pulpal involvement. The patient also demonstrates poor dental hygiene and has significant accumulations of plaque and calculus on the lingual and palatal surfaces of his maxillary and mandibular arches. Radiographs demonstrate a large periapical radiolucency surrounding the root apices of the second maxillary molar. The patient also has periodontal pocket formation, inflammation, and edema of his periodontium. Significant bleeding was demonstrated upon probing. A thorough cleaning and scaling of the teeth was accomplished, followed by an endodontic procedure on the second maxillary molar. The patient was also prescribed an antibiotic regimen to prevent any systemic sequelae due to aspiration or blood septicemia. He was sent home and scheduled for quarterly appointments to ensure the hygienic phase is adhered to.

Biofilms (e.g., plaque and calculus) on teeth frequently have been reported to be associated with systemic disease, including cardiovascular disease, diabetes, and pregnancy complications. Also, periodontal disease has been linked to other diseases, including respiratory disease, chronic kidney disease, rheumatoid arthritis, metabolic syndrome, erectile dysfunction, and cancer. It is important that the dental practitioner be cognizant of the current literature on the treatment of periodontal disease and the adverse consequences that can develop if left untreated and prescribe the appropriate antibiotic regimen if necessary, especially if the patient has any predisposing health issues.

ACKNOWLEDGMENT

The author wishes to thank Dr. Dominica Sweier for her contributions to the fifth edition of this book.

SUGGESTED READING

Chetruș V, Ion IR. Dental plaque: classification, formation, and identification. *Int J Med Dentistry*. 2013;3:139–143.

Dewhirst FE, Chen T, Izard J, et al. The human oral microbiome. *J Bacteriol*. 2010;192(19):5002–5017.

Dietrich T, Jimenez M, Krall Kaye EA, et al. Age-dependent associations between chronic periodontitis and edentulism and risk of coronary heart disease. *Circulation*. 2008;117:1668–1674.

Flemming HC, Neu TR, Wozniak DJ. The EPS matrix: the "house of biofilm cells. *J Bacteriol*. 2007;189(22):7945–7947.

Fowler EB, Breault LG, Cuenin MF. Periodontal disease and its association with systemic disease. *Mil Med*. 2001;166:85–89.

García-Godoy F, Hicks MJ. Maintaining the integrity of the enamel surface: the role of dental biofilm, saliva, and preventive agents in the enamel demineralization and remineralization. *J Am Dent Assoc*. 2008;139:25S–34S.

Kolenbrander PE. Oral microbial communities: biofilms, interactions, and genetic systems. *Annu Rev Microbiol*. 2000;54(1):413–437.

Li J, Helmerhorst EJ, Leone CW, et al. Identification of early microbial colonizers in human dental biofilm. *J Appl Microbiol*. 2004;97(6):1311–1318.

Lin NJ. Biofilm over teeth and restorations: What do we need to know? *Dent Mater*. 2017;33(6):667–680.

Marsh PD, Devine DA. How is the development of dental biofilms influenced by the host? *J Clin Periodontol*. 2011;38(suppl 11):28–35.

Moutsopoulos NM, Madianos PN. Low-grade inflammation in chronic infectious diseases: Paradigm of periodontal infections. *Ann N Y Acad Sci*. 2006;1088:251–264.

Paquette DW. The periodontal infection-systemic disease link: A review of the truth or myth. *J Int Acad Periodontol*. 2002;4:101–109.

Rudney JD. Saliva and dental plaque. *Adv Dent Res*. 2000;14:29–39.

Rudney JD, Pan Y, Chen R. Streptococcal diversity in oral biofilms with respect to salivary function. *Arch Oral Biol*. 2003;48(7):475–493.

Takeuchi Y, Baehni PC. Anti-plaque agents in the prevention of biofilm–associated oral diseases. *Oral Dis*. 2003;9(suppl 1):23–29.

Thakkar P, Banks J, Rahat R, et al. Viruses of the oral cavity: prevalence, pathobiology and association with oral diseases. *Rev Med Virol*. 2022;32(4):e2311. https://doi.org/10.1002/rmv.2311

Vats N, Lee SF. Active detachment of Streptococcus mutans cells adhered to epon-hydroxylapatite surfaces coated with salivary proteins in vitro. *Arch Oral Biol*. 2000;45(4):305–314.

Willershausen B, Kasaj A, Willershausen I, et al. Association between chronic dental infection and acute myocardial infarction. *J Endod*. 2009;35:626–630.

Zaura E, Ten Cate JM. Dental plaque as a biofilm: a pilot study of the effects of nutrients on plaque pH and dentin demineralization. *Caries Res*. 2004;38(suppl 1):9–15.

GLOSSARY

Absorption   The passage of substances across and into tissues; a vital process carried out by cells in the body.

Accessory root canal   Secondary canal extending from the pulp to the surface of the root, usually found near apices of the root.

Acellular cementum   That part of the cementum covering one-third to one-half of the root of a tooth adjacent to the cementoenamel junction. It consists of collagenous fibers and ground substance.

Aciniform   Fine pain receptors in the periodontal ligament.

Acinus (alveolus)   A small, terminal, saclike dilation particular to glands such as the salivary glands.

Acquired pellicle   An acellular, organic, thin skin or film deposited on the surface of teeth from salivary proteins (saliva) that bathe the surface of the teeth after eruption.

Actin   Protein of the myofibril, localized in the I band; acting along with myosin particles, it is responsible for the relaxation and contraction of muscle.

Adsorption   The adhesion of a substance to a surface or substrate.

Adventitia   Outer layer of vessels within the pulp organ.

Afferent (sensory) system   Nerve processes that carry information and convey it from the peripheral nervous system in muscles and glands to the central nervous system.

Agranulocyte   A nongranular leukocyte.

Alveolar bone   Ridge of bone; refers to tooth-bearing part of the mandible and maxilla because it contains the tooth sockets.

Alveolar bone proper   A thin lamina of bone that lines the tooth sockets, supports the roots of the teeth, and gives attachment to principal fibers of the periodontal ligament.

Alveolar crest fibers   Principal fibers of the periodontal ligament extending between the crest of the alveolar bone and the neck of the tooth.

Alveoli   *See* dental alveoli.

Ameloblast   One of the differentiated cells of the inner layer of the enamel organ; from these cells comes the enamel of the teeth.

Ameloblastin   A protein found in tooth enamel.

Amelogenesis   The process of production and development of enamel.

Amelogenin   Protein found in newly deposited enamel matrix. Amelogenins are lost during maturation of enamel.

Amylase   Enzyme that catalyzes the hydrolysis of starch into smaller water-soluble carbohydrates.

Anaphase   That stage in mitosis and meiosis following the metaphase in which the centromeres divide and the chromatids lined up on the spindle begin to move apart toward the poles.

Anatomic crown   That portion of the tooth covered by enamel.

Angioblast   The mesenchymal cells of an embryo that form blood cells and vessels.

Angiogenic clusters   Origin of angioblasts located in the visceral mesoderm during the third week of prenatal life.

Angstrom   Unit of wavelength equivalent to 0.1 millimicron (1027 mm). Abbreviated Å.

Ankylosis   A fusion of two mineralized tissues without an intervening periodontal ligament, usually due to trauma.

Anlage   The initial condensation of embryonic cells from which an organ or body part develops.

Anterior tympanic artery   One of the main vessels supplying blood to the temporomandibular joint.

Antibody   A protein that is produced in the body in response to invasion by a foreign agent or antigen and that has a specific reaction.

Aortic arches   A series of arterial channels encircling the embryonic pharynx within the mesenchyme of the branchial arches.

Aortic arch vessel   Vessel contained in each of the five pharyngeal arches that leads from the heart through the arches to the face, brain, and posterior regions of the body.

Apical fiber group   Part of the dentoalveolar fiber group that extends perpendicular from the surface of the root apices to the adjacent fundic alveolar bone.

Apical foramen   Opening at the apex of the tooth's root giving passage to the nerves and blood vessels.

Appositional growth (exogenous)   Deposition of successive cell products laid down upon those already present.

Area of reversal   The process of deposition in a resorption zone.

Articular disk (of the temporomandibular joint)   The fibrous disk that separates the upper and lower joint cavities.

Ascending pharyngeal artery   One of the main vessels supplying blood to the temporomandibular joint.

Assimilation   The transformation of food into living tissue.

Astral rays/asters   Those fibers that form around the centrioles during the prophase step of mitosis.

Attached gingiva   The part of the oral mucosa that is firmly bound at the neck of the tooth and the alveolar process.

Attached pulpal stones or denticles   Mineralized tissues that are partly fused with the dentin of the coronal pulp or root canal.

Auditory capsule   The cartilage of the embryo that develops into the bony labyrinth of the inner ear.

Auditory tube   The ear canal.

Auricular hillocks   Six small hillocks of tissue grouped around the external ear canal during development.

Auriculotemporal artery   Branch of the trigeminal nerve supplying the temporomandibular joint.

Autonomic nervous system   That part of the efferent system that produces responses involuntarily and is divided into sympathetic and parasympathetic divisions.

Axon   That process of a neuron by which impulses travel away from the body of the neuron.

Axon terminals   Synaptic end bulbs at the branch ends of axons.

Axoplasmic transport   The continuous pulsing, undulating movement of the cytoplasm between the cell body of a neuron, where protein synthesis occurs, and the axon fiber to supply it with the substances vital for the maintenance of activity and for repair.

B cells   Lymphocytes that have differentiated into plasma cells. Plasma cells secrete antibodies that destroy antigens.

Basal cell   Type of cell found in the taste bud, in close contact with the basal lamina, that has a turnover rate of approximately 10 days. They are believed to arise from the surrounding epithelial cells.

Basioccipital cartilages   One of the earliest formed skeletal elements in the craniofacial area, located behind the sphenoid cartilage.

Basion   A craniometric landmark located at the midpoint of the anterior border of the foramen magnum in the midsagittal plane.

Basophilic   Related to structures that stain with a basic dye including the nucleus and ribosomes, of which the most common dye is hematoxylin.

Basophils   Granulocytic white blood cells found in pulp blood vessels.

Basal lamina   Membrane separating the epidermis and dermis that is a product of both.

Bell stage   Developmental stage of the tooth characterized by the differentiation of inner enamel epithelial cells into ameloblasts and the differentiation of neural crest cells to odontoblasts and includes the formation of the outline of the future crown by these cells.

Blastocyst   The postmorula stage of development; a blastula with a fluid-filled cavity.

Bone   Mineralized animal tissue consisting of an organic matrix, cells, and fibers of collagen impregnated with mineral matter, chiefly calcium phosphate and calcium carbonate. *See also* **bundle bone, cancellous bone, compact bone,** and **haversian bone.**

Branchial arch (pharyngeal arch)   One of a series of mesodermal bars located between the branchial clefts. During embryonic stages, the arches contribute to the formation of the face, jaws, and neck. They appear in higher forms only vestigially.

Branchial arch cartilages   The cartilages found in the branchial arches of the embryo.

Branchial barlike   Resembling the gills of a fish.

Buccal and labial glands   The minor salivary glands of the cheeks and lips.

Bud stage   Initial stage of tooth development; the enamel organ develops from this structure.

The dental papilla lies adjacent to the epithelial bud, and the dental sac encloses both.

Bundle bone Specialized bone lining the tooth socket into which the fibers of the periodontal ligament penetrate. The radiographic term *lamina dura* is synonymous with bundle bone.

C

Calcification See diffuse calcification.

Calcospherite One of the small globular bodies formed during the process of calcification by chemical union between the calcium particles and the albuminous organic matter of the intercellular substance.

Calculus An abnormal concretion within the body, usually formed of mineral salts and often deposited around a minute fragment of inorganic material, the nucleus. See also **dental calculus, serumal calculus.**

Canals See haversian canals.

Cancellous bone Spongy or latticelike structure composed mainly of bone tissue.

Capillaries Endothelium-lined tubes that form a network among the odontoblasts.

Cap stage Part of tooth development; an early stage in enamel organ formation following the bud stage.

Cardiac muscle Involuntary muscle of the heart that pumps blood through some 50,000 miles of blood vessels.

Cartilage Fibrous connective tissue characterized by nonvascularity and a firm consistency. Forms most of the temporary skeleton of the embryo. See also **hyaline cartilage.**

Cell Smallest unit of living structure capable of independent existence.

Cell body Part of the neuron that contains the nucleus and the cytoplasm.

Cell cycle A series of discrete steps by which the cell divides.

Cell-free zone Relatively cell-free layer of the dental pulp adjacent to odontoblasts and overlying the cell-rich zone. Composed of delicate fibrils in ground substance.

Cell-rich zone Layer of the dental pulp situated between the pulp core and the cell-free zone that is richly supplied with cellular elements, blood vessels, and nerves.

Cell signaling A system of effectors, modulators, and receptors through which cells interact.

Cellular cementum That part of the cementum covering the apical one-half to two-thirds of the root of a tooth. This cementum is most abundant on the root tip.

Cementicles Calcified spherical bodies composed of cementum lying free within the periodontal ligament, attached to the cementum, or embedded within it.

Cementoblast A large cuboidal cell lying on the surface of the bone that is active in cementum formation.

Cementocyte A cell found in the lacuna of cellular cementum. Numerous cytoplasmic processes extend from its free surface.

Cementoid layer See intermediate cementum.

Cementum Bonelike connective tissue that covers the tooth from the cementoenamel junction to and surrounding the apical foramen. Cementum does not contain blood vessels (avascular) and does not have a nerve supply (aneural). See also **acellular cementum, cellular cementum.**

Central nervous system (CNS) Composed of the brain and spinal cord.

Centriole Either of two short cylinders appearing near the nucleus that migrate to opposite poles of the cell during cell division.

Centromere The constricted portion of the chromosome where the chromatids are found.

Cerebellum The part of the brain located behind the brainstem, responsible primarily for coordinating voluntary muscular activity.

Cerebral hemispheres The two halves of the cerebrum.

Cervical loop Growing free border of the enamel organ. Here, the outer and inner enamel epithelial cell layers are continuous with each other.

Chondroblasts Cells that arise from the mesenchyme and form the cartilage.

Chromatids The paired chromosome strands, joined at the centromere, that make up a metaphase chromosome.

Chromosomes In animal cells, a rodlike structure in the nucleus containing a linear thread of DNA that transmits genetic information.

Circular or circumferential fibers Type of fiber within the gingival fiber group that is continuous around the neck of the tooth and resists gingival displacement.

Circumpulpal dentin Inner portion of the dentin located near the pulp organ of the tooth.

Circumvallate papilla 10 to 14 large, 3-mm diameter papillae located along the V-shaped sulcus between the body and base of the tongue.

Cleft lip The most common facial malformation, affecting one or both sides of the lip.

Clinical crown That portion of the crown exposed and visible in the oral cavity.

CNS See central nervous system (CNS).

Col Valleylike depression in the facial lingual plane of the interdental gingiva. It conforms to the shape of the interproximal contact area.

Collagen White fibers of the corium of the skin, tendon, and other connective tissue. The fiber is composed of fibrils bound with interfibrillar cement.

Collagen fiber High-molecular-weight protein composed of several structural types that vary in diameter and usually are arranged in bundles.

Common carotid arteries Third aortic arch vessels that later supply the neck, face, and brain with blood.

Compact bone Dense bone more highly calcified than cancellous (spongy) bone.

Conductivity The ability of an electric or other system to transmit sound, heat, light, or electromagnetic energy; a vital process carried out by cells in the body.

Condyle See mandibular condyle.

Connective tissue proper Tissues composed of cells, fibers, and intercellular material that function in tissue support and protection of the body parts, in areas of fluid exchange, and in storage of adipose (fat) tissue.

Coronal pulp Pulp present in the crown of a tooth.

Coronoid process Unit of the mandible that responds to the temporalis muscle development and attachment.

Cranial Pertaining to the cranium, specifically those bones covering the brain.

Cranial base Lower portion of the skull constituting the floor of the cranial cavity.

Cranial base cartilages Cartilages that arise to support the brain, from which come the auditory and olfactory sense capsules.

Crypts Pitlike depressions or tubular recesses on a free surface.

Cuticle See primary cuticle.

Cuticular protein The most important function of the primary cuticle, which initiates attachment of the junctional epithelium to enamel.

Cytoplasm Protoplasm of a cell located in the area surrounding the nucleus.

Cytosol Semifluid part of cytoplasm in which organelles are suspended and solutes dissolved.

D

Dead tracts Empty dentinal tubules resulting from the death of the odontoblasts and loss of the odontoblastic processes.

Deciduous dentition Primary teeth (20) that function during the first 8 years of life and then exfoliate, providing space for the permanent teeth.

Deep auricular artery One of the main vessels supplying blood to the temporomandibular joint.

Deep temporal artery One of the branches of the maxillary artery on each side of the head.

Deep temporal nerve Branch of the trigeminal nerve supplying the temporomandibular joint.

Dehiscence Alveolar bone loss in the coronal root.

Demilune A crescent-shaped structure or cell. See also **serous demilune.**

Dendrite Component of the neuron that receives impulses and conducts them to the cell body.

Dental alveoli The alveoli or sockets in which the roots of teeth are embedded.

Dental calculus Stonelike concretion formed on the teeth, on a prosthesis, or in salivary ducts. It varies in color from creamy yellow to black and is composed mostly of calcium phosphate.

Dental lamina Horseshoe-shaped epithelial bands that traverse the upper and lower jaws and give rise to the ectodermal portions of the teeth.

Dental papilla Part of the formative organ of the teeth that forms the dentin and the pulp.

Dental plaque Organic deposit on the surface of teeth. Site of bacterial growth and formation of dental calculus.

Dental pulp The soft tissue contained within the pulp chamber. Consists of connective tissue, blood vessels, nerves, and lymphatics.

Dental sac (follicle) Area of mesenchymal cells and fibers that surround the dental papilla and the enamel organ of the developing teeth. It produces the periodontal ligament, alveolar bone, and cementum.

Denticles   Pulp stones.

Dentin   Yellowish body of the tooth. It surrounds the pulp and underlies the enamel on the crown and the cementum on the roots of the teeth. Composed of 20% organic matrix, which is mostly collagen, and 10% water. The inorganic fraction (70%) is hydroxyapatite, with some carbonate, magnesium, and fluoride. *See also* **intratubular** or **peritubular dentin** and **mantle dentin**.

Dentinoenamel junction   Interface of the enamel and dentin of the crown of a tooth.

Dentinogenesis   The process of dentin formation in the development of teeth.

Dentoalveolar group   Principal fiber group that surrounds the roots of the teeth.

Deoxyribonucleic acid (DNA)   The nucleic acid constituting the primary genetic material of all cellular organisms.

Dermatomes   Dorsal lateral portion of the somite of the embryo. These cells form the dermis, subcutaneous tissue, and supporting tissue of the gastrointestinal tract.

Dermis   Arises from the mesoderm underlying the epidermis. The dermis and the epidermis together form the skin.

Desmosome   Cell junction. It consists of a dense plate near the cell surface that relates to a similar structure on an adjacent cell, between which are thin layers of extracellular material.

Developmental cuticle   *See* primary cuticle.

Diaphysis   The shaft of the long bone.

Differentiation   Process by which cells acquire individual cellular characteristics from an undifferentiated state, that is, specialization.

Diffuse calcification   Irregular calcified deposits along collagen fiber bundles or blood vessels in the pulp or elsewhere. It is considered a pathologic condition.

Diphyodont   Species that develops two separate dentitions during a lifetime.

Direct innervation   Theory based on the belief that nerves may extend to the dentinoenamel junction from the pulp.

Disclosing solution   Formula of 0.2% basic fuchsin or erythrosin red #3 dye used to determine if all plaque has been removed from teeth.

Drift   Movement of a tooth to a position of greater stability.

Duct   Tube with well-defined walls for passage of excretions or secretions.

Dystrophy   A disorder arising from defective or faulty nutrition.

E

Ear   Organ composed of three parts: the external ear receives sound waves, the middle ear translates these waves into mechanical vibrations, and the internal ear receives the vibrations and changes them into specific impulses that are transmitted by the acoustic nerve to the brain.

Ectodermal cells   Cells that will form the outer body covering (epithelium) of the embryo.

Ectomesenchyme (neural crest cells), mesoderm   Forms spinal ganglia and many other structures in the body.

Edentulous jaw   Alveolar bone without teeth.

Efferent (motor) system   Nerve process consisting of neurons that convey responses from the central nervous system to muscles and glands.

Elastic or fibrous cartilage   Cartilage containing elastic fibers.

Eleidin   A protein allied to keratin and protoplasm but more transparent than protein keratin.

Embryonic disk   A small disk, to become the embryo, formed after implantation when two small cavities develop on either side of the inner cell mass and meet in the center.

Embryonic period   The second to eighth weeks of prenatal life.

Enamel   *See* gnarled enamel.

Enamel crystals   Hydroxyapatite crystals found in enamel rods. They are formed during tooth mineralization.

Enamel lamellae   Thin, leaflike spaces that extend from the enamel surface toward the dentinoenamel junction. They represent defects or organically filled spaces in the enamel.

Enamel organ   Originates from the dental lamina and consists of four distinct layers.

Enamel pearls   Enameloma, a developmental anomaly in which a small nodule of enamel is formed near the cementoenamel junction, usually at the bifurcation zone of molar teeth.

Enamel rod   One of the structural units of enamel, extending from the dentinoenamel junction to the surface of the tooth and normally having a translucent crystalline appearance.

Enamel spindles   Dentinal tubules in enamel extending from the dentin crossing the dentinoenamel junction and terminating in the enamel caused by disoriented odontoblasts during induction.

Enamel tuft   Narrow, ribbonlike structures whose constricted inner end arises at or near right angles to the dentinoenamel junction and extends a third of the way into the thickness of the enamel. Tufts consist of hypocalcified spaces that may be filled with organic substance.

Enamelin   One of the organic protein components of enamel.

Enameloid   A thin, structureless layer of substance that may be a form of enamel that is deposited by the root sheath.

Endochondral   Relating to the type of bone formation that occurs within cartilage and replaces it.

Endocrine   Refers to glands of internal secretion that release their secretory product(s), hormones, directly into the bloodstream rather than through a duct system.

Endoderm (entoderm)   The innermost of the three primary germ layers of the embryo.

Endometrium   The mucous membrane lining the uterus.

Endomysium   Individual muscle fiber covering.

Endoplasmic reticulum (ER)   An ultrastructural organelle consisting of membrane-bound cavities in the cytoplasm of the cell.

Eosinophils   Granulocytic bilobed leukocytes, somewhat larger than a neutrophil, that constitute 1% to 3% of the body's white blood cells.

Epidermal growth factor (EGF)   Element in saliva that may assist in the healing of injured oral mucosa.

Epidermis   The surface nonvascular cell layer of the skin that develops from the surface ectodermal cells. It consists of five layers; they are, from the inner to the outer layer, (1) basal, (2) spinous, (3) granular, (4) clear (lucidum), and (5) horny (corneum).

Epimysium   Muscle fascicle (a group of muscle fibers) covering.

Epiphysis   The extremity of a long bone as opposed to the shaft (diaphysis).

Epithelial attachment (junctional epithelium)   Attachment of the gingival epithelium to the tooth's surface at the dentogingival junction.

Epithelial cell rests   Origin from the epithelial root sheath that covers the roots during root development. As the sheath develops further, it breaks up into epithelial cell rests, which migrate into the periodontal ligament. Occasionally, they may develop into dental cysts. The cell groups are of these types: (1) resting, (2) proliferating, and (3) degenerating.

Epithelial diaphragm   Inward-turning portion of the root sheath at the beginning of root development, important during root formation. It narrows the width of the cervical opening of the root.

Epithelial pearls   Discrete, rounded or ovoid groups of epithelial cells, frequently keratinized, found in the lamina propria.

Epithelial root sheath   A double layer of cells (inner root sheath cells and outer root sheath cells) formed from the fusion of the outer and inner enamel epithelium that function in root formation and induction of cells of the dental follicle to form periodontal structures.

Epithelium   Cellular avascular layer covering all the free surfaces of the body, internal and external, and the lining of vessels. Consists of cells and small amounts of intercellular substance. *See also* **inner enamel epithelium**.

Equatorial plate   The central area of the cell.

Equilibrium   Sense of balance controlled by the vestibular organs, which are located in the internal ear.

ER   *See* endoplasmic reticulum.

Eruption pathway   The altered tissue area of decreased blood vessels and degenerated nerve fibers overlying the teeth, visible as an inverted triangular area formed by tissue lysis and bone resorption.

Erythrocytes   The red blood cells.

Ethmoid   Cartilaginous nasal capsule.

Ethmosphenoid and sphenoccipital articulations   Interposing bands of cartilage that exist between the ethmoid and sphenoid and the occipital bones in the midline during the period of craniofacial growth.

Etiology   To study the origin or cause of a disease.

Eustachian tube   Part of the ear that develops from the corresponding first pharyngeal pouch.

Excretion   The process of eliminating, shedding, or getting rid of substances by the cells of the body.

Exfoliate To shed or eliminate something from the surface of the body, as in the loss of teeth from the jaws.

Exocrine Denotes glands that release their secretory product(s) into a duct system.

Exocytosis Discharge of secretory product(s) from the cell, preserving the cell membrane through fusion of the secretory vesicles with the cell membrane.

External auditory canal The canal leading to the middle ear, developed from the deepening of the first pharyngeal groove.

External carotid artery Main supply of blood to the face, neck, and brain after seven weeks' development.

Extracellular phase Resorption phase in which the mineral is separated from the collagen and is broken into small fragments.

F

Facial sutures A system of articulations developed between each of the major bones of the face to facilitate growth. Categorized as zygomaticomaxillary, frontomaxillary, and zygomaticotemporal.

False denticles Concentric layers of calcified tissue.

Fenestration The area of alveolar bone loss where an apical root penetrates the bone.

Fetal period The embryo from the eighth prenatal week to birth.

Fibroblasts Elongated, ovoid, spindle-shaped, or flattened cells found in connective tissue.

Filiform papillae The most numerous papillae appearing on the dorsum of the tongue. These threadlike elevations point dorsally and toward the throat.

Fluid One of the central components of the body, consisting of blood and lymph.

Foliate papillae Four to eleven vertical grooves or furrows containing taste buds on the lateral posterior sides of the tongue.

Fontanelle One of several membrane-covered spaces found in the incompletely ossified skull of the fetus or newborn.

Foramen cecum Tissue on the surface of the tongue at the junction of the body and base from which cells arise and migrate ventrally in the throat, creating the thyroid gland.

Foramen ovale An opening in the septum between the two atria of the heart.

Fordyce spots A condition characterized by minute yellowish white papules (sebaceous glands) on the oral mucosa commonly observed at the labial commissures and the vermillion border of the lips.

Forebrain, midbrain, and hindbrain The primary brain vesicles formed by closure of the anterior neural tube.

Free gingiva The portion of the gingiva that surrounds the tooth and is not directly attached to the tooth surface; the outer wall of the gingival sulcus.

Frontal process Covering of the brain from which develops the forehead.

Frontal, temporal, and occipital lobes Parts of the forebrain formed by the cerebral hemispheres.

Frontonasal process Frontal area after the fifth week of prenatal development.

Functional eruptive phase Phase in which teeth reach incisal or occlusal contact and then undergo functional eruptive movements, which include compensation for jaw growth and occlusal wear of the enamel.

Fundic bone Bone enclosing the apex of the tooth root.

Fungiform papillae Minute elevations on the dorsum, tip, and sides of the tongue. The papillae are mushroom shaped, with the top being broader than the base.

G

G1 phase The reduplication stage of the interphase after mitosis occurs; the initial resting stage in the cell cycle.

G2 phase The quiescent phase of the post-DNA duplication stage of the cell cycle.

Ganglion A group of nerve cell bodies located outside the central nervous system.

Gap junctions Specialized communicating junction between cells with pores permeable to ions and small molecules up to one kilodalton (KD).

Gastrointestinal tract Tube formed by endodermal cells that eventually becomes pharyngeal pouches, lung buds, liver, gallbladder, pancreas, and urinary bladder.

Gene expression Duplication process in which encoded information for different functions is transferred between molecules.

Genetic mechanisms Processes that help a cell develop and maintain a high degree of order.

Germinal centers Active sites of lymphocyte formation.

Gingiva Soft tissue surrounding the necks of erupted teeth that cover the alveolar process. The gingiva consists of fibrous connective tissue enveloped by mucous membrane. *See also* **attached gingiva, free gingiva, interdental gingiva**.

Gingival fibers One of the principal fiber groups of the periodontal ligament that is located around the necks of the teeth.

Gingival sulcus The shallow, V-shaped trench around each tooth, bound by the tooth on one surface and the epithelium-lined free margin on the other.

Ginglymoarthrodial A type of synovial joint that allows opening and closing, symmetrical protrusion and retrusion, and asymmetrical lateral movement of the mandible, of which the temporomandibular joint is an example.

Gland *See* merocrine gland.

Globular dentin Areas of defective growth with interglobular spaces that underlie the enamel and surface of the root.

Glossopalatine glands The minor salivary glands of the tonsillar folds.

Gnarled enamel The enamel located at the tips of the cusps, in which the rods or groups of rods are twisted, bent, and intertwined. It is seen ultrastructurally.

Golgi apparatus or complex A continuation of the endoplasmic reticulum. A cuplike structure within cells made up of saccules where carbohydrate side chains of glycoproteins form.

Granular layer of Tomes A thin, granular-appearing layer of defective dentin located along the root surface adjacent to the cementum when observed using a microscope.

Granulocyte Any cell containing granules.

Growth factors Chemical substances that induce cells to initiate specific cellular processes, including DNA synthesis in a specific temporal and spatial manner.

Gubernacular cord (gubernaculum dentis) A fibrous tissue band connecting the tooth sac with the alveolar mucosa. This cord may function in tooth eruption.

H

Hard palate Anterior part of the palate consisting of the bony palate bound above by the nasal cavity and below by the mouth. It is covered by keratinized stratified squamous epithelium. In addition, the hard palate contains palatine vessels and nerves, adipose tissue, and mucous glands.

Haversian bone Compact bone containing tubular channels with blood vessels, nerves, and bone cells surrounded by concentrically located lacunae. These structures are termed the *haversian system*.

Haversian canals These nutrient canals are located in cortical bone and extend in the direction of the tooth's long axis.

Hemidesmosome Half of a desmosome that forms a site of attachment between epithelial cells and the basal lamina or between epithelial cells (junctional cells) and the tooth's surface and between other structures throughout the body.

Hemoglobin Complex protein-iron compound in the blood that carries oxygen to the cells from the lungs and carbon dioxide away from the cells to the lungs.

Homeobox gene (genes) A homeobox is a highly conserved DNA sequence found within genes that are responsible for the regulation of patterns of anatomic development in animals and plants (i.e., teeth).

Horizontal fiber group Type of fiber within the dentoalveolar fiber group that extends in a horizontal direction from the midroot cementum to the adjacent alveolar bone proper and resists tipping of the teeth.

Hormone Chemical substance formed in one organ or part of the body and carried by the bloodstream to another part where it stimulates or depresses activity.

Howship's lacunae Absorption lacunae. Tiny cup-shaped depressions on the resorbing front of any hard tissue, the result of resorptive activity by osteoclasts.

Hunter-Schreger bands Alternating dark and light bands in enamel that result from absorption and reflection of light caused by differences in orientation of adjacent groups of enamel rods originating at the dentinoenamel junction and extending toward the outer enamel surface.

Hyaline cartilage A flexible, semitransparent, elastic substance composed of a collagen fibrillar matrix and chondrocytes in lacunae.

Hyalinization Effect of compression that is too great or too rapid on the periodontal ligament; the vascularity is excluded, and the ligament appears colorless.

Hydrodynamics Science of factors determining the flow of liquids. In dentistry, it refers to a theory that pain conduction through dentin results from dentinal fluid movement causing odontoblastic movement and deformation of nerve terminals resulting in an action potential.

Hydroxyapatite An inorganic compound that constitutes bone and teeth.

Hyoid Second arch in the development of the face and neck.

I

Iatrogenic Caused by the actions of a healthcare provider.

IgA A distinct class of immunoglobulins. A protein of animal origin with known antibody activity, synthesized by lymphocytes and plasma cells; found in serum, other body fluids, and tissues.

Imbrication lines Also known as *lines of von Ebner*, incremental lines in dentin that run at right angles to the tubules. These lines, which represent the daily growth pattern, indicate layers of dentin that are less calcified and appear darker than adjacent dentin.

Impaction Position of a tooth in the alveolus that makes it incapable of eruption into the oral cavity.

Implantation The process in which the blastocyst attaches to the wall of the uterus and becomes embedded in its surface.

Incisor liability The succession of larger permanent incisors replacing primary ones. The size ratio of the two incisors of the two dentitions.

Incisor liability factor The replacement of the smaller primary incisors with larger permanent ones.

Increment The amount by which a given quantity is increased. A measurable amount.

Incremental deposition Deposition of material in discrete amounts rather than constant deposition. Rhythmic recurrent deposition of enamel, bone, dentin, or cementum.

Incremental line An evident line produced through a rhythmic, recurrent deposition of successive layers upon present layers.

Incus Cartilage in the first pharyngeal arch that later transforms into bone and functions in the middle ear as hearing bones.

Induction The process in which an undifferentiated cell is instructed by specific organizers to produce a morphogenic effect.

Inferior parathyroids Resulting organ from the third pharyngeal pouch.

Inner enamel epithelium Cells that line the concavity of the enamel organ in the cap and early bell stages of tooth development and differentiate into ameloblasts.

Innervation Presence and distribution of nerves within a part or the supply of nerves stimulating a part.

Intercalated disks Transverse markings that appear on strands of muscle fiber as the heart tube develops.

Intercalated duct Terminal duct that collects secretions from acini.

Intercellular tissue Tissue located between or among cells of any structure.

Interdental gingiva The soft tissue between adjacent contacting teeth in the same arch.

Interdental papilla Gingiva located between the teeth and extending high on the interproximal area of the crowns on the labial and lingual surfaces.

Interdental septa Bony partitions that project into the alveoli between the teeth; interalveolar.

Interdental zone Zone of gingivae between the two adjacent teeth beneath their contact point.

Intermediate cementum A deposition by the epithelial root sheath cells on the root surface formed during root formation. May be termed *enameloid*.

Intermediate junction Type of junctional complex found between adjacent odontoblasts.

Internal carotid Supply of blood to the face, neck, and brain up to seven weeks' development; afterward, it continues to supply the growing brain.

Internasal area The distance between the nostrils.

Interradicular bone Bone that forms between the roots of the multirooted teeth.

Interradicular fibers Group of fibers that are located between the roots of multirooted teeth, extend perpendicular to the tooth's surface and to the adjacent alveolar bone, and resist vertical and lateral forces.

Interstitial growth (endogenous) Growth by expansion of the matrix by cell deposits within the matrix.

Interstitial spaces Spaces between groups or bundles of periodontal fibers.

Intima Inner lining of vessels within the pulp organ.

Intracellular phase Resorption phase in which the osteoclast ingests mineral fragments and continues the dissolution of this mineral.

Intralobular duct system System located inside the lobules that contains intercalated and striated ducts.

Intramembranous Within a membrane. Bone formation occurring within or among connective tissue fibers. It does not replace cartilage, as endochondral bone does.

Intraoral occlusal/incisal movement Fourth event during the prefunctional eruptive phase in which the tooth continues to erupt until clinical contact with the opposing crown occurs.

Intratubular or peritubular dentin The dentinal matrix that immediately surrounds the dentinal tubule.

J

Junctional epithelium Epithelial attachment. That epithelium adhering to the tooth surface at the bottom of the gingival crevice and consisting of one or more layers of nonkeratinizing cells.

K

Keratinized Having developed a horny layer of flattened epithelial cells containing keratin.

Keratinized mucosa Stratified surface of cornified epithelial cells that lack a nucleus and whose cytoplasm is replaced by large amounts of keratohyalin protein.

Keratinocytes Cells of the oral mucosa. These epidermal cells synthesize keratin.

L

Lacunae The very small cavities in bone that are filled with bone cells. *See* **Howship's lacunae.**

Lamella Thin leaf or plate, as of bone. *See also* **enamel lamellae.**

Lamina dura A thin layer of hard, compact bone lining the tooth sockets. Used in radiography to designate a thin, radiopaque line.

Lamina propria Layer of connective tissue underlying the epithelium of skin or a mucous membrane.

Langerhans cells Clear or dendritic cells found in both superficial and deep layers of the epidermis and oral epithelium.

Laryngeal cartilages Cartilage appearing in the fourth arch.

Lateral ligament Ligament that strengthens the fibers of the capsule enclosing the temporomandibular joint to support the joint and limit excursions of the condyles to the normal range.

Lateral nasal process The tissue lateral to the nasal pits.

Lateral palatine processes Processes that develop from the maxillary tissues laterally and grow to the midline to form the palate.

Lateral pterygoid mm Muscle of mastication with two heads that function to protrude the mandible and pull the articular disk forward.

Leeway space The difference in the space in the arch required for the two primary molars and the successional permanent premolars replacing them. The leeway space in the maxilla is 1.3 mm and in the mandible is 3.1 mm.

Leukocytes White blood cells.

Lingual glands Mixed salivary glands at the tip of the tongue.

Lingual tonsils Tonsillar tissue on the floor of the mouth.

Lingula The sharp medial boundary of the mandibular foramen, to which the sphenomandibular ligament is attached.

Lining mucosa Nonkeratinized oral mucosa that covers the surface of the cheeks, lips, soft palate, floor of the mouth, and ventral surface of the tongue.

Lipopolysaccharides (LPS) A type of large molecule found in the outer membrane of gram-negative bacteria which are endotoxins that can cause a strong immune response when bound to the TLR4 receptor.

Lipoteichoic acid (LTA) A major constituent of the cell wall of gram-positive bacteria; is released when the bacteria die and can elicit a strong immune response associated with the TLR2 receptor.

Lobes Groups of salivary gland lobules.

Lobules Groups of salivary acini invested in connective tissue.

Lymphatic system System composed of the lymph nodes, the thymus, and the spleen, as well as the vessels that carry the lymph throughout the body; it is the immunologic defense of the body.

Lymphocytes Type of agranulocyte originating from stem cells and developing in the bone marrow; their numbers increase in response to infection.

Lysosome Small membrane-bound body that contains a variety of acid hydrolases, which function in breaking down substances both inside and outside the cell. It is visible through electron microscopy.

M

Macroglossia Enlargement of the tongue that can be caused by muscular hypertrophy.

Macrognathia Excessive size of the jaw.

Macrophages Any of the large mononuclear phagocytic cells found in various tissues and organs of the body. These cells are a normal constituent of the pulp and function in tissue maintenance.

Macula adherens Discoid desmosomes in the oral mucosa.

Major glands Salivary glands that carry their secretion some distance to the oral cavity by means of a main duct.

Malassez's rests Epithelial cell remnants of Hertwig's sheath in the periodontal ligament. These cell groups appear near the surface of the cementum; they may develop into the epithelial lining of dental cysts.

Malleus Enlarged bulbous structure signaling the termination of Meckel cartilages and, in the adult, is one of the middle ear bones.

Mandible Horseshoe-shaped bone forming the lower jaw and articulating the condyles with the temporal bone on either side; it is derived from the first pharyngeal arch. The mandible is composed of the horizontal body and inclined ramus. The body includes the alveolar process, which contains the teeth.

Mandibular condyle The rounded bony projections of the mandible that articulate with the temporal fossa of the temporal bone in the temporomandibular fossa.

Mantle dentin The initially deposited portions of the dentin formed immediately adjacent to the enamel. It does not contain in the extracellular matrix dentin sialoprotein or dentin phosphoprotein and is mineralized by matrix vesicles.

Masseter mm Muscle of mastication, located at the angle of the mandible.

Masseteric artery One of the large blood vessels stretching from the mandibular notch the deep surface of the masseter muscle.

Masticatory mucosa The mucosa that functions in mastication. It tends to be bound to bone and is therefore immovable. This mucosa covers the hard palate and the gingiva and consists of four layers.

Maturation zone Zone of cartilage characterized by chondrocyte enlargement.

Maxilla Upper jawbone; an irregularly shaped bone articulating with the nasal, lacrimal, zygomatic, palatine, ethmoid, sphenoid, and frontal bones of the face and containing teeth; it is derived from the first pharyngeal arch.

Maxillary processes Processes that are lateral to the oral pit, from which develop the cheeks.

Maxillary sinus Paired sinus cavities occupying the space beneath the floor of the orbit and above the roots of the posterior maxillary molars.

Meckel cartilage The initial skeletal component of the first branchial arch. It is the supporting cartilage of the mandibular arch in the embryo. It articulates with the developing middle ear bones to form the primary temporomandibular joint.

Medial nasal process The area of the nose in the embryo. The tissue medial to the naris.

Medial pterygoid Muscle of mastication that protracts and elevates the mandible.

Median raphe The line denoting union of the palatine bones in the midline of the palate. No submucosa is under the palatal mucosa in this area.

Meiosis Process of reduction division of chromosomes in the daughter cell with half as many as in the parent cell.

Melanocytes Cells responsible for synthesis of melanin that provide pigmentation to the skin and are a derivative of neural crest cells.

Memory cells Another name for lymphocytes because of their ability to retain coding information for antibody production.

Merkel cells Cells located in the basal layer of the gingival epithelium and thought to be epithelial in origin. They function as touch receptors.

Merocrine glands The secreting cells that remain intact during the formation and release of the secretory product. Another name for salivary glands because the basic mode of product excretion is through membrane vesicles passing to the cell's apex.

Mesenchyme Loose, undifferentiated embryonic connective tissue that is a mixture of mesodermal and neural crest cells. The connective tissues of the body form from this tissue.

Mesial drift General movement of a tooth or teeth anteriorly toward the midline of the jaw.

Mesoderm The third primary germ layer of the embryo to differentiate. It is positioned between the ectoderm and the endoderm. From mesoderm are derived connective tissues, bone, cartilage, muscle, blood and blood vessels, lymphatics, notochord, pleura, and peritoneum.

Metaphase The second stage of mitosis in which chromatids become attached centrally at the equatorial plate to a centromere and split into two sets of chromosomes.

Metaphysis The wider part of the diaphysis adjacent to the epiphyseal line.

Microglossia Smallness of the tongue.

Micrognathia Smallness of the jaw, especially the mandible.

Microlamellae The minute spaces between or around enamel rods and through crystal spaces within rods.

Microtubules Small tubular structures found in the cytoplasm and composed of the protein tubulin. They are cylindrical and hollow.

Middle ear Tissue at the end of the external auditory canal, developing from the corresponding first pharyngeal pouch.

Minor salivary glands Salivary glands that empty their products directly into the mouth by means of short ducts.

Mitochondrion Small spherical organelle that is a membrane-bound structure lying free in the cytoplasm and present in all cells. This structure is the principal site of energy generation (ATP) in the cell.

Mixed dentition Simultaneous possession of both primary and permanent teeth.

Mixed glands Salivary glands that contain a combination of serous and mucous secretions.

Monocyte Type of agranulocyte.

Morphogens Chemicals that are present in embryonic tissue that have the ability to directly modify the lineage of the cell and thereby determine the ultimate fate of the cell.

Morula Mass of blastomeres resulting from the early cleavage divisions of the zygote.

MPD Myofascial pain dysfunction.

mRNA An RNA fraction that carries information from deoxyribonucleic acid to the protein-synthesizing ribosomes of cells.

Mucin A glycoprotein that is the primary constituent of mucus.

Mucoceles Retention cysts of the minor salivary gland ducts, which contain mucous secretion. They usually result from rupture of the excretory duct of a minor salivary gland, causing pooling of saliva in the tissues. The resulting vesicular elevation is a mucocele.

Mucogingival junction The separation between attached and free gingiva and alveolar mucosa.

Mucous acinus Minute, saclike, secretory portion of a mucous gland. This is the functional unit of the gland.

Mucous glands Glands that produce viscous proteinaceous secretions, such as the sublingual gland and glands of the hard palate.

Myoblast An embryonic cell that becomes a cell of muscle fiber.

Myoepithelial cells Spindle-shaped, contractile epithelial cells with stellate bodies and processes found in salivary and sweat glands. They are located in the terminal portion of the salivary gland acini and are believed to have contractile ability that facilitates movement of the glandular secretion into the ducts.

Myofibrils Fine longitudinal fibrils (parallel to the long axis) found in a muscle fiber. They are composed of numerous myofilaments.

Myosin A protein that is the most abundant in muscle and is partially responsible for the chemical reaction that allows muscular contraction and movement.

Myotome The intermediate mesoderm.

N

Nasal fin A zone of epithelial contact of the medial nasal and maxillary processes during development.

Nasion A cephalometric landmark located where the intranasal and nasofrontal sutures meet.

Nasolacrimal duct That duct extending from the lacrimal gland of the eye to the internal nasal mucosa.

Neonatal line Accentuated incremental or hesitation line seen in bone, dentin, and enamel, probably caused by changes occurring at or near birth.

Nerve growth factor (NGF) A protein that promotes the growth, organization, and maintenance of sympathetic and some sensory nerve cells.

Nerves Whitish cords composed of fibers arranged in bundles (fascicles) and held together by a connective tissue sheath, the perineurium. The fascicles are surrounded by epineurium. Nerves transmit stimuli from the central nervous system to the periphery by the efferent motor system or from the periphery to the central nervous system by the afferent sensory system.

Neural crest Ganglionic crest, a band of ectodermal cells that appear along either side of the embryonic neural tube at the time of closure.

Neural plate A plate formed by the ectoderm that gives rise to the neural tube.

Neural tube Tube formed by the lateral boundaries of the neural plate, which will eventually become the brain and spinal cord.

Neuroblasts Primitive nerve cells that develop into adult nerve cells, the neurons. They are the functional cells of the brain, spinal cord, and peripheral nerves.

Neurocranium That part of the skull enclosing the brain, as distinguished from the bones of the face.

Neuroglia The supporting structure of the brain and spinal cord, which is composed of specialized cells and their processes.

Neuron A nerve cell, which is any of the conducting cells of the nervous system, consisting of a cell body and containing the nucleus and its surrounding cytoplasm; the dendrite, which carries impulses to the cell body; and the axon that conducts impulses away from the cell body to the area of synapse.

Neutrophils Type of granulocyte.

Nociception The sensory nervous system's response to potential or apparent harm.

Nonkeratinized mucosa Lining mucosa in which the stratified squamous epithelial cells retain their nuclei and cytoplasm. Lining mucosa is found on the inner lips, cheeks, soft palate, vestibular fornix, alveolar mucosa, floor of the mouth, and undersurface of the tongue.

Nonkeratinocytes Cells not producing keratin. Clear or dendritic cells found in oral epithelium, such as pigment cells (melanocytes), Langerhans cells, Merkel cells, and inflammatory cells such as lymphocytes.

Nuclear envelope Membrane bounding the nucleus, composed of two phospholipid layers similar to the plasma membrane of the cell.

Nuclear pores Openings in the nuclear envelope associated with the endoplasmic reticulum that forms at the end of each cell division.

Nucleolus A round, vacuole-like, achromatic body rich in RNA found within the nucleus of a cell.

Nucleus A spheroid body within a cell, containing the genetic matter DNA, organelles, nucleoli, chromatin, linin, and nucleoplasm. It has a thin nuclear membrane vital to protein synthesis.

O

Oblique fiber group Group of fibers that extend in an oblique direction from the area just above the apical zone of the root upward to the alveolar bone and resist vertical or intrusive masticatory forces.

Occlusion Relation of the functional contact of the maxillary and mandibular teeth during activity of the mandible.

Odontoblast One of a layer of columnar cells with long processes extending into the dentinal tubules and lining the peripheral pulp of a tooth. These cells function in dentin formation and vitalize this tissue.

Odontoblastic process A cytoplasmic extension of the cell body of the odontoblasts, some of which extend from the cell as far as the dentinoenamel junction or the cementoenamel junction.

Odontogenic zone This area is peripherally adjacent to the dentin in both the coronal and radicular pulp. It contains the formative cells of dentin known as odontoblasts, the cell-free layer, the cell-rich layer, and it terminates at the parietal plexus of nerves (plexus of Raschkow).

Olfaction The ability to distinguish odors.

Olfactory organ Process that allows the sense of smell by transmitting olfactory impulses to the brain.

Olfactory mucosa Site of most receptors for the sense of smell. It occupies the superior aspect of the nasal cavity between the superior nasal conchae, roof of the nose, and upper part of the nasal septum.

Orbicularis oris The musculature encircling the mouth.

Organelles Living particles located in the cytoplasm of cells. They include mitochondria, Golgi complex, centrosomes, lysosomes, ribosomes, centrioles, endoplasmic reticulum, microtubules, and microfilaments.

Organic matrix Formative portion of a tooth or bone as opposed to mineralized hydroxyapatite.

Organizer The part of an embryo that influences another part to direct histologic and morphologic differentiation.

Oro-naso-optic groove An oblique groove extending from the nostrils to the eyes.

Oropharyngeal membrane Membrane at the deepest extent of the oral pocket that ruptures in the fifth week, opens the oral cavity to the tubular foregut, and soon becomes the oropharynx.

Oropharynx Anatomic division of the pharynx arising from the oropharyngeal membrane.

Osteoblasts Bone-forming cells derived from mesenchyme. They form the osseous matrix, in which they may become enclosed to become osteocytes.

Osteoclasts Multinucleated giant cells larger than osteoblasts and derived from monocytes from the bloodstream. Osteoclasts contain abundant acidophilic cytoplasm formed in bone marrow and function in the absorption and removal of osseous tissue.

Osteocytes Cells of the bone located within lacunae, functioning in maintenance and vitality of bone.

Osteodentin Dentin that appears more like bone than dentin because it contains cells.

Outer enamel epithelial cells Cells that cover the enamel organ.

Oxytalan fibers Type of connective tissue fibers chemically different from collagen fibers and found in the periodontal ligament and gingiva. They appear similar to immature elastic fibers. These fibers are believed to support blood vessels and the principal fibers of the ligament.

P

Pacinian corpuscle Laminated nerve ending that functions in the perception of pressure.

Palatal rugae Transverse ridges located in the mucous membrane of the anterior part of the hard palate. They extend laterally from the incisive papillae and have a core of dense connective tissue.

Palatal shelf elevation Process during the eighth prenatal week by which the posterior shelves push together, forcing the tongue forward and down and causing the palatal shelves to slide over the tongue.

Palate *See* primary palate, secondary palate.

Palatine glands The glands of both the posterior hard palate and soft palate.

Palatine shelf closure or fusion A final growth surge resulting in contact of palatal shelves in the midline.

Palatine tonsils Two large oval masses of lymphoid tissue embedded in the lateral wall of the oropharynx and bilaterally located between the pillars of the fauces.

Papillae Small protuberances on the tongue that are sensitive eminences, possessing a tactile function.

Parasympathetic nervous system The craniosacral portion of the autonomic nervous system; its preganglionic fibers traveling with cranial nerves II, VII, IX, X, and XI and with the second to fourth sacral ventral roots. It innervates the heart, smooth muscle, glands of the head and neck, and thoracic, abdominal, and pelvic viscera.

Parenchyma The functional elements of an organ rather than the supporting framework (stroma) of the organ.

Parietal layer Network composed of both myelinated and nonmyelinated axons (**plexus of Raschkow**).

Parotid Serous-secreting salivary gland anterior to the ear. It is encapsulated and produces 26% of the secretions of the major salivary glands.

Pellicle *See* acquired pellicle.

Penetration Third event during the prefunctional eruptive phase where the tooth's crown tip moves through the fused epithelial layers and allows entrance of the crown enamel into the oral cavity. Only the organic developmental cuticle (primary), secreted earlier by the ameloblasts, covers the enamel.

Perforating fibers (Sharpey's fibers) Penetrating connective tissue fibers by which the tooth is attached to the adjacent alveolar bone. These bundles of collagen fibers penetrate both the cementum and the alveolar bone.

Pericytes Cells found in normal pulp that accompany blood cells.

Perikaryon The cell body of a neuron as distinguished from the nucleus and the processes.

Perikymata Wavelike transverse grooves and ridges that are manifestations of the striae of Retzius on the surface of the enamel. They appear transverse to the long axis of the crown.

Perimysium Connective tissue demarcating a fascicle of skeletal muscle fibers.

Periodontal ligament Connective tissue ligament that is a mode of attachment of the tooth to the alveolus and that consists primarily of type I collagenous fiber bundles. Between the bundles are loose connective tissue, blood vessels, and nerves.

Periodontium Tissue surrounding and supporting the teeth. The tissue has two distinct components: the gingival unit, composed of the free and attached gingivae and the alveolar mucosa, and the component known as the attachment apparatus of the teeth, which includes the cementum, periodontal ligament, and alveolar bone.

Peritubular dentin The zone of dentin forming the wall of the dentinal tubules. This dentin has a 9% higher mineral content than does the remainder of the intertubular dentin.

Phagocyte Any cell capable of ingesting particulate matter.

Phagocytose To engulf and destroy bacteria and other foreign substances; denoting the action of the phagocytic cells.

Pharyngeal arch Tissues that bend around the sides of the pharynx in the shape of bars; each arch is separated by vertical grooves on the lateral sides of the neck at the fifth week.

Pharyngeal pouches Grooves that separate each pharyngeal arch.

Pharyngeal tonsils A collection of more or less closely aggregated lymphoid cells located superficially in the posterior wall of the nasopharynx, the hypertrophy of which results in the glands called adenoids.

Philtrum The vertical groove in the midline of the upper lip.

Plaque See dental plaque.

Plasma cells Cells derived from B lymphocytes, which actively synthesize and secrete immunoglobulins from an extensive rough endoplasmic reticulum. Under appropriate conditions, antigen stimulation induces proliferation and morphologic alteration in B lymphocytes to form plasma cells.

Plasma membrane or plasmalemma (cell membrane) Envelops the entire cell and provides a selective barrier that regulates transport of substances into and out of the cell and contains receptors that bind with various substances that can regulate cell activity.

Pons That part of the central nervous system lying between the medulla oblongata and the mesencephalon, superior to the cerebellum.

Precapillaries Small blood vessels measuring 8 to 12 μm in diameter, present in the peripheral pulp.

Predentin Band of newly formed and as yet unmineralized matrix of dentin, located at the pulpal border of the dentin, consisting mostly of type I collagen.

Preeruptive phase Developmental stage preparatory to eruption of teeth and characterized by movements of the growing teeth within the alveolar process.

Prefunctional eruptive phase Phase of eruption that starts with the initiation of root formation and ends when the teeth reach occlusal contact.

Primary cuticle A thin film on the enamel surface of an unerupted tooth. It is the protein produced by ameloblasts prior to dying and is thought to protect the enamel as it fully matures.

Primary palate That part of the palate formed from the median nasal process. The first palate to form is anterior to the secondary palate.

Prismless enamel Enamel formed without any rods or prism pattern found primarily in the cervical region of the tooth.

Proliferative period Time during which cells grow and increase in number by cell division.

Prophase The first stage in cell reduplication.

Protective stage Stage of plaque formation and attachment.

Pseudostratified epithelium Type of epithelium with all cells in contact with the basal lamina but not with the surface.

Ptyalin Synonymous term for salivary amylase, the enzyme in saliva that catalyzes the hydrolysis of starch into water-soluble carbohydrates.

Pulmonary circulation Blood supplied to the lungs by vessels of the sixth arch.

Pulpal blood vessel Characteristic thin-walled blood vessels of the dental pulp.

Pulp stones or denticles Calcified masses of dentinlike substance located within the pulp or embedded in or attached to the dentinal wall. These stones may appear as a result of aging or trauma. They may be free, embedded, or attached to the dentin.

Pulp bifurcation Zone of branching of the pulp organ resulting in multiple rooted teeth.

Pulp organ Soft tissue within the tooth, consisting of connective tissue, blood vessels, nerves, and lymphatics.

Pulp proliferation zone Zone in the pulp adjacent to the epithelial diaphragm where cellular proliferation occurs and has recently been reported to contain a high proportion of stem cells.

Q

Quiescent stage A period of inactivity.

R

Radiation Transmission of rays, such as light rays, short radio waves, ultraviolet rays, or x-rays.

Radicular pulp The pulp occupying the root canals that extends from the cervical coronal region to the apex of the root.

Ramus General term to designate a smaller structure given off by a larger one or one into which a larger structure divides.

Ramus of mandible Quadrilateral process projecting posteriorly and superiorly from the body of the mandible.

Raphe See median raphe.

Red blood cell (corpuscle, erythrocyte) A nonnucleated biconcave hemoglobin that bears cells and is responsible for transport of oxygen to tissues via the circulatory system.

Reduced enamel epithelium The four layers of the epithelial enamel organ compacted and remaining on the surface of enamel after its formation is complete and that fuses (along with the developmental cuticle) with the oral ectoderm to form the junctional epithelium.

Remodeling Alteration of the structure by reconstruction. The continuous process of turnover of bone carried out by osteoblasts and osteoclasts.

Reparative dentin (tertiary dentin) Deposited after trauma to the tooth by replacement odontoblasts. A defensive reaction whereby hard tissue formation walls off the pulp from the site of injury. Analogous to scar formation in the skin.

Reproduction Duplication or replication; a vital process carried out by the cells in the body.

RER See rough endoplasmic reticulum (RER).

Respiration Process of molecular exchange of oxygen and carbon dioxide within the body's tissues.

Response dentin Deposited after trauma to the tooth by original odontoblasts.

Reticulum A system of membrane-bound cavities in the cytoplasm of a cell. It occurs in two types, granular and agranular surfaces.

Retzius striae Lines reflecting successive incremental deposition of mineralized enamel.

Reversal lines Lines separating layers of bone or cementum deposited in a resorption site, distinguishing it from the scalloped outline of Howship's lacunae.

Ribosomes Particles that translate genetic codes for proteins and activate mechanisms for their production.

RNA (ribonucleic acid) Carries information to sites of actual protein synthesis located in the cell cytoplasm.

Root canal Extension of the pulp from the coronal zone to the root apex. See also **accessory root canal**.

Root formation First event during the prefunctional eruptive phase involving proliferation of the epithelial root sheath, which in time causes initiation of root dentin and formation of the pulp tissues of the forming root. Root formation also causes an increase in the fibrous tissue of the surrounding dental follicle.

Root resorption Dissolution of the root of a tooth by action of osteoclasts. This may occur anywhere along the surface of the tooth root in response to caries or trauma or during the loss of a primary tooth.

Root sheath cells (Hertwig's sheath)   Merged outer and inner epithelial layers of the enamel organ, extending beyond the region of the crown to invest the developing root.

Root trunk   The part of the tooth immediately below the crown neck before division into the roots, covered by cementum and fixed in the alveolus.

Rotation   Type of tooth movement in which the tooth tends to move about a circular axis.

Rough endoplasmic reticulum (RER) (granular)   The ribosomes attached to the endoplasmic reticulum that function in synthesis of secretory protein.

Ruffled border   An area enfolding the plasma membrane of the osteoclast that borders the resorptive zone.

S

Saliva   Clear, slightly alkaline, somewhat viscous mixture of secretions of the salivary glands and gingival fluid exudate. It moistens the mucous membranes and food, facilitating speech and mastication. Consists of water and 0.58% solids.

Salivary calculi   Calcium phosphate concentrations (salivary stones or sialolithiasis) found within a salivary gland or duct, most commonly in the main excretory duct of the submandibular gland (Wharton duct).

Salivary corpuscle   One of the leukocytes or lymphocytes found in saliva.

Salivary glands   Exocrine glands whose secretions flow into the oral cavity.

Schwann cell   Cell forming the myelin sheath of nerves and seen in association with all nerves of the pulp.

Sclerotic (transparent) dentin   Dentin in which the tubules are occluded with mineral. Occurs mostly in elderly people, especially in the roots of the teeth. It is thought that the Ca++ and phosphate supersaturated dentinal fluid, when not maintained by a viable odontoblast, spontaneously crystallizes and occludes the dentinal tubule, preventing further compromise and providing protection from future insults.

Sclerotomes   Part of the somite consisting of mesenchymal tissue that develops into vertebrae and ribs.

Secondary dentin   Circumpulpal dentin deposition formed after tooth eruption.

Secondary palate   The palate proper, formed by fusion of the lateral palatine processes of the maxilla.

Sella turcica   A transverse depression in the midline of the sphenoid bone, containing the hypophysis gland (pituitary gland).

Serous   Relating to, containing, or producing a serum substance with a watery consistency.

Serous demilune   Half-moon or crescent-shaped serous cells associated with the terminal external surface or mucous alveoli.

Serous glands of tongue (von Ebner)   Serous glands opening into the bottom of the trough surrounding the circumvallate papillae and functioning in a cleansing action.

Serumal calculus   Subgingival calculus, so termed because it results in part from exudation of serum.

Sharpey's fibers   *See* perforating fibers (Sharpey's fibers).

Shedding   The loss of the primary dentition caused by the physiologic resorption of the roots and the loss of the bony supporting structure—and therefore the inability of these teeth to withstand the masticatory forces.

Sialography   Diagnostic x-ray technology used to visualize salivary gland ducts by injection of a radiopaque substance into the main excretory duct.

Sjögren syndrome   A chronic autoimmune disease with an unknown etiology in which the white blood cells attack the moisture-producing glands.

Skeletal or voluntary muscle   Type of muscle that allows movement under voluntary control.

Smear layer   The fine particles of cut dentinal debris in dentinal tubules that are produced by cavity preparation.

Smooth muscle   Nonstriated involuntary muscle.

Smooth muscle cells   Cells whose contractility is under control of the autonomic nervous system.

Soft palate   Posterior muscular portion of the palate, forming an incomplete septum between the nasopharynx and the oral cavity.

Somatic nervous system   System that carries impulses to the voluntary muscles, such as the skeletal muscles, which are under conscious control.

Somites   Paired, blocklike masses of mesoderm arranged segmentally along the neural tube in the embryo and forming the dermis, vertebral column, and musculature.

Specialized mucosa   Mucosa found on the dorsum of the tongue. It consists of four types of papillae, which are filiform, fungiform, circumvallate, and foliate.

S-phase (synthesis)   A part of the cell cycle during which DNA is synthesized.

Sphenoid cartilage and bone   Cartilage that is posterior to the ethmoid. It later forms wings of bone that spread out under the brain laterally.

Sphenomandibular ligament   Temporomandibular joint ligament that arises superiorly from the spine of the sphenoid bone and extends downward on the medial side of the ramus to insert on the lingual to limit the inferior movements of the mandible. It is derived from Meckel cartilage.

Spindle fibers   Those fibers not formed between the migrating centrioles during prophase.

Spindles   The termination of dentinal tubules in inner enamel.

Squamous   Relating to flat squama (i.e., the squama of the temporal bone).

Squamous epithelium   Composed of a single layer of flat, scalelike cells, as in the lining of the pulmonary alveoli, or stratified, as in oral epithelium.

Stapes   Third body of cartilage within Meckel cartilages, which later develops into the hearing bones.

Stellate reticulum   A network of star-shaped cells in the center of the enamel organ between the outer and inner enamel epithelia.

Stensen duct   The epithelium-lined duct that drains the parotid gland and exits near the second maxillary molar.

Stomodeum   The embryo's future oral cavity, an invagination lined by surface ectoderm.

Stratified epithelium   A type of epithelium composed of a series of layers. The cells of each may vary in size and shape, as seen in skin and some mucous membranes.

Stratum intermedium   Epithelial cell layer of the enamel organ that lies external and adjacent to the inner enamel epithelium and is attached to it by desmosomes. The stratum intermedium functions as a molecular sieve, allowing specific molecules into or out of ameloblast layer. The stratum intermedium also refers to the intermediate layer of nonkeratinizing epithelia.

Stratum superficiale   Third or superficial layer of the epithelium in the lining mucosa, composed of flattened cells, many of which contain small oval nuclei.

Striae of Retzius   *See* Retzius striae.

Striated duct   An intralobular gland duct that secretes saliva and is involved in ionic transport. The duct is located between the intercalated and interlobular ducts and is named for the basal striations produced by the enfolding of the basal membrane within the cells.

Striated (voluntary) muscles   Groups of muscles with lines across them signifying contraction sites that cause the muscles to function; they supply the dorsal and ventral parts of the limbs and provide both the deep and superficial muscle fibers.

Stroma   Supporting framework of a gland, such as the capsule and trabeculae, rather than the functional parenchyma.

Stylomandibular ligament   Temporomandibular joint ligament that arises from the styloid process and inserts on the posterior border of the ramus.

Sublingual   Refers to the area beneath the anterior lower jaw.

Sublingual gland   The smallest of the three pairs of major salivary glands. A pure mucous gland located in the anterior floor of the mouth.

Submandibular   Refers to the area beneath the angle of the mandible.

Submandibular gland   One of the three paired major salivary glands. The submandibular glands contribute 65% of saliva. These bilateral glands are a mixed seromucous type. These glands demonstrably swell during various types of infections, including mumps, and often after radiation treatment for cancer of surrounding glands and/or tissues.

Submucosa   Layer of tissue that lies beneath the lamina propria underlying the mucous membrane of the lip, cheek, palate, and floor of the mouth.

Successional lamina   That portion of the dental lamina lingual to the developing deciduous teeth that gives rise to the enamel organs of permanent teeth.

Superficial temporal artery   One of the main vessels supplying blood to the temporomandibular joint.

Superior parathyroids   Organs developing from the fourth pharyngeal pouch.

Supporting bone   Bone tissue functionally related to supporting the roots of the teeth. It surrounds, protects, and supports the tooth roots through the alveolar bone proper.

Supporting or sustentacular cells   Cells that lie in the periphery of the taste bud.

Sutures   Articulations between each of the major bones of the face. *See* **facial sutures**.

Sympathetic nervous system   The thoracolumbar part of the autonomic nervous system. Preganglionic fibers arise from cell bodies in the thoracic and first three lumbar segments of the spinal cord. Postganglionic fibers are distributed to the heart, smooth muscle, and glands of the entire body.

Synapse   The region of the junction between two nerve cells where an impulse passes between the axon of one cell and the dendrite of another cell.

Synchondrosis   The union of two bones that have been separated by cartilage.

Syndesmosis   A type of fibrous joint in which opposing surfaces are united in fibrous connective tissue, as in the union between most facial bones.

Synostosis   Fusion of two bones.

Synovial membranes   Membranes that line joint cavities and secrete a small amount of transparent alkaline fluid (synovial fluid) in the articular spaces. Synovial fluid acts as a lubricant and nutrient for the avascular tissue cover (i.e., the condyle and articular tubercle for the temporomandibular joint).

T

T cells   Cells produced by the thymus that destroy invading microbes and are therefore important to the body's immune system.

Taste bud   Receptor of taste on the tongue and in the oropharynx. One of several goblet-shaped cells oriented at right angles to the surface by the epithelium. The taste buds consist of supporting and gustatory cells and are located on the foliate, fungiform, and circumvallate papilla.

Taste   Chemosensory modality translated by the cells of taste buds, including umami, salt, bitter, sweet, and sour.

Telophase   The last of the four stages of mitosis and of the two divisions of meiosis that begins when the chromosomes arrive at the poles of the cell.

Temporal and interoccipital bones   Membrane bones, including frontal, parietal, and squamous portions, forming the protective covering of the brain.

Temporalis mm   Muscle fibers that originate from the floor of the temporal fossa and temporal fascia and work to elevate and retract the mandible and clench the teeth.

Temporomandibular joint (TMJ)   Joint formed between the condyle of the mandible and the mandibular fossa (concavity of the temporal bone).

Temporomandibular ligaments   Four ligaments that include the sphenomandibular on the medial surface, the stylomandibular on the posterior surface, the temporomandibular on the lateral surface, and the capsular surrounding the joint.

Teratogen   Agent or factor that produces physical defects in the developing embryo.

Terminal arterioles   Blood vessels of 10 to 15 μm in diameter present in the pulp organ.

Terminal bar apparatus   Localized condensations of cytoplasmic substance associated with the cell membrane of the apical area of the functional ameloblast.

Terminal sulcus   V-shaped groove separating the surface of the body and base of the tongue.

Tertiary dentin   *See* reparative dentin.

Thymus   A bilaterally symmetric lymphoid organ consisting of two lobes situated in the anterior superior mediastinum.

Thyroglossal duct cyst   A cyst that forms from a persistent thyroglossal duct. Usually, the presenting symptom is a swelling of the thyroglossal duct due to the presence of infection.

Thyroglossal duct   An epithelial cord by which the thyroid gland remains attached to the tongue while descending from the foramen cecum to the front of the trachea; later becomes solid and eventually disappears.

Thyroglossal fistula   A swelling related to the thyroglossal duct that has an opening on the surface of the neck.

Tipping movement   Pressure applied on a specific point on the tooth that causes compression in a limited area between the root and the bone.

TMJ   *See* temporomandibular joint.

Tomes granular layer   This layer of dentin is found only in the tooth root. It is adjacent to the peripheral zone of hyalinized root dentin as a thin, hypomineralized layer, and it is formed by disoriented odontoblasts.

Tomes process   Specialized apical zone of the secretory ameloblasts delineated from the cell body by the desmosomes of the terminal bar apparatus. Tomes process is conical and interdigitates with the forming enamel rods.

Tonofibrils   Systems of fibrils found in the cytoplasm of epithelial cells, which function with the desmosomal plaque to hold adjacent cells together.

Tooth crypt   Space filled by the dental follicle and developing tooth within the alveolar process.

Tooth eruption   Process by which teeth emerge into the oral cavity, a stage coordinated with root growth and maturation of tissues surrounding the tooth, including the alveolar bone.

Traction bands of the palate   Bundles of collagen fibers that firmly attach the oral mucosa to the underlying bone of the hard palate.

Transduction theory   Proposal that odontoblasts are sensory receptors for pain stimuli that are transmitted through the dentin.

Transparent dentin   *See* sclerotic (transparent) dentin.

Transseptal fibers   Fibers that originate in the cervical region of each crown and extend to similar locations on the mesial and distal surfaces of each adjacent tooth. This fiber group functions in resistance to the separation of each tooth.

tRNA   A kind of RNA that carries an anticodon (three nucleotide bases) and a specific amino acid.

Tuberculum impar   Central tissue of the tongue eventually overgrown by the two lateral tissues.

Tuft   *See* enamel tuft.

Tympanic membrane   The membrane at the depth of the external auditory canal.

U

Ultimobranchial body   Tissues resulting from development of the fifth pharyngeal pouch.

Umbilical system   Vascular network connected to the placenta that traverses the umbilical cord and conducts nutrition and oxygen to the embryo while carrying carbon dioxide and wastes to the placenta.

Undifferentiated mesenchymal cells   Cells found in normal pulp that can function and/or differentiate into numerous pulpal cell phenotypes.

V

Vasculature   Refers to the blood vessels and circulating blood system.

Vermilion border   The exposed red portion of the lips. This color is due to a thin epithelium with the presence of eleidin (a clear protein) in the cells and the superficial position of blood vessels.

Vestibular lamina   Lip furrow band located labial and buccal to the dental lamina that forms the oral vestibule between the alveolar portions of the jaws, the lips, and the cheeks.

Visceral mesoderm   Part of the embryonic skeleton formed by dermatome cells that supports the endoderm of the gastrointestinal tract.

Viscerocranial   Refers to those parts of the facial cranial skeleton originating from the branchial arch.

Vitelline vascular system   The blood vascular system of a fertilized egg that overlies the yolk.

Volkmann canals   Perforating canals that enter the bone at right or oblique angles and establish a continuous system that contains the nerves and blood vessels of the bone and connects with the Haversian system.

Vomer flat   Unpaired bone located in the midline of the face, shaped like a trapezoid, and forming the inferior and posterior portions of the nasal septum. It articulates with the sphenoid, ethmoid, two maxillary, and two palatine bones.

von Ebner lines or lines of von Ebner   *See* imbrication lines.

W

Waldeyer ring   A ring of tonsillar tissue surrounding the oropharynx. It is composed of palatine tonsils located laterally, the lingual in the floor of the mouth, and the pharyngeal in the posterior area of the pharynx.

Weil basal layer   *See* cell-free zone.

Wharton duct   The duct that drains the submandibular gland and exits under the tongue after it joins with the duct from the sublingual gland.

Z

Zygoma   The process of the temporal bone that connects with the zygomatic bone.

Zygote   The fertilized cell produced by the union of two gametes.

Zymogen   An inactive precursor that is activated to an enzyme. Granules in serous cells of enzyme-secreting glands, such as the salivary glands and the pancreas.

Note: Page numbers followed by "f" indicate figures, "t" indicate tables, "b" indicate boxes.